Shoulder Arthroplasty: State of the Art and Future Perspectives

Shoulder Arthroplasty: State of the Art and Future Perspectives

Editors

**Markus Scheibel
Alexandre Lädermann
Laurent Audigé**

MDPI • Basel • Beijing • Wuhan • Barcelona • Belgrade • Manchester • Tokyo • Cluj • Tianjin

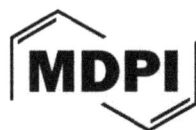

Editors

Markus Scheibel
Shoulder and Elbow Surgery,
Schulthess Clinic
Switzerland

Alexandre Lädermann
Division of Orthopaedics and
Trauma Surgery,
La Tour Hospital
Switzerland

Laurent Audigé
Research and Development
Department,
Schulthess Clinic
Switzerland

Editorial Office
MDPI
St. Alban-Anlage 66
4052 Basel, Switzerland

This is a reprint of articles from the Special Issue published online in the open access journal *Journal of Clinical Medicine* (ISSN 2077-0383) (available at: https://www.mdpi.com/journal/jcm/special_issues/Shoulder_Arthroplasty).

For citation purposes, cite each article independently as indicated on the article page online and as indicated below:

LastName, A.A.; LastName, B.B.; LastName, C.C. Article Title. *Journal Name* **Year**, *Volume Number*, Page Range.

ISBN 978-3-0365-6456-2 (Hbk)
ISBN 978-3-0365-6457-9 (PDF)

© 2023 by the authors. Articles in this book are Open Access and distributed under the Creative Commons Attribution (CC BY) license, which allows users to download, copy and build upon published articles, as long as the author and publisher are properly credited, which ensures maximum dissemination and a wider impact of our publications.

The book as a whole is distributed by MDPI under the terms and conditions of the Creative Commons license CC BY-NC-ND.

Contents

About the Editors . . . . **vii**

Alexandre Lädermann, Laurent Audigé and Markus Scheibel
Innovations in the Realm of Shoulder Arthroplasty
Reprinted from: *J. Clin. Med.* **2023**, *12*, 237, doi:10.3390/jcm12010237 . . . . **1**

Nels Leafblad, Elise Asghar and Robert Z. Tashjian
Innovations in Shoulder Arthroplasty
Reprinted from: *J. Clin. Med.* **2022**, *11*, 2799, doi:10.3390/jcm11102799 . . . . **5**

Alexander Klug, Eva Herrmann, Sebastian Fischer, Reinhard Hoffmann and Yves Gramlich
Projections of Primary and Revision Shoulder Arthroplasty until 2040: Facing a Massive Rise in Fracture-Related Procedures
Reprinted from: *J. Clin. Med.* **2021**, *10*, 5123, doi:10.3390/jcm10215123 . . . . **21**

Alexandre Terrier, Fabio Becce, Frédéric Vauclair, Alain Farron and Patrick Goetti
Association of the Posterior Acromion Extension with Glenoid Retroversion: A CT Study in Normal and Osteoarthritic Shoulders
Reprinted from: *J. Clin. Med.* **2022**, *11*, 351, doi:10.3390/jcm11020351 . . . . **35**

Ismael Coifman, Ulrich H. Brunner and Markus Scheibel
Dislocation Arthropathy of the Shoulder
Reprinted from: *J. Clin. Med.* **2022**, *11*, 2019, doi:10.3390/jcm11072019 . . . . **47**

Jaroslaw Pecold, Mahdi Al-Jeabory, Maciej Krupowies, Ewa Manka, Adam Smereka, Jerzy Robert Ladny and Lukasz Szarpak
Tranexamic Acid for Shoulder Arthroplasty: A Systematic Review and Meta-Analysis
Reprinted from: *J. Clin. Med.* **2022**, *11*, 48, doi:10.3390/jcm11010048 . . . . **65**

Philipp Moroder, Lucca Lacheta, Marvin Minkus, Katrin Karpinski, Frank Uhing, Sheldon De Souza, Michael van der Merwe, et al.
Implant Sizing and Positioning in Anatomical Total Shoulder Arthroplasty Using a Rotator Cuff-Sparing Postero-Inferior Approach
Reprinted from: *J. Clin. Med.* **2022**, *11*, 3324, doi:10.3390/jcm11123324 . . . . **75**

Mariano E. Menendez, Noah Keegan, Brian C. Werner and Patrick J. Denard
COVID-19 as a Catalyst for Same-Day Discharge Total Shoulder Arthroplasty
Reprinted from: *J. Clin. Med.* **2021**, *10*, 5908, doi:10.3390/jcm10245908 . . . . **89**

Joaquin Sanchez-Sotelo
Current Concepts in Humeral Component Design for Anatomic and Reverse Shoulder Arthroplasty
Reprinted from: *J. Clin. Med.* **2021**, *10*, 5151, doi:10.3390/jcm10215151 . . . . **95**

Marko Nabergoj, Shinzo Onishi, Alexandre Lädermann, Houssam Kalache, Rihard Trebše, Hugo Bothorel and Philippe Collin
Can Lateralization of Reverse Shoulder Arthroplasty Improve Active External Rotation in Patients with Preoperative Fatty Infiltration of the Infraspinatus and Teres Minor?
Reprinted from: *J. Clin. Med.* **2021**, *10*, 4130, doi:10.3390/jcm10184130 . . . . **107**

Daniel P. Berthold, Daichi Morikawa, Lukas N. Muench, Joshua B. Baldino, Mark P. Cote, R. Alexander Creighton, Patrick J. Denard, et al.
Negligible Correlation between Radiographic Measurements and Clinical Outcomes in Patients Following Primary Reverse Total Shoulder Arthroplasty
Reprinted from: *J. Clin. Med.* **2021**, *10*, 809, doi:10.3390/jcm10040809 . . . . **115**

Emil Noschajew, Felix Rittenschober, Harald Kindermann and Reinhold Ortmaier
Clinical and Radiologic Outcomes after Anatomical Total Shoulder Replacement Using a Modular Metal-Backed Glenoid after a Mean Follow-Up of 5.7 Years
Reprinted from: *J. Clin. Med.* **2022**, *11*, 6107, doi:10.3390/jcm11206107 . . . . **129**

Anthony Hervé, Mickael Chelli, Pascal Boileau, Gilles Walch, Luc Favard, Christophe Levigne, François Sirveaux, et al.
Clinical and Radiological Results of Hemiarthroplasty and Total Shoulder Arthroplasty for Primary Avascular Necrosis of the Humeral Head in Patients Less than 60 Years Old
Reprinted from: *J. Clin. Med.* **2021**, *10*, 3081, doi:10.3390/jcm10143081 . . . . **143**

Maciej J. K. Simon, Jennifer A. Coghlan and Simon N. Bell
Shoulder Replacement in the Elderly with Anatomic versus Reverse Total Prosthesis? A Prospective 2-Year Follow-Up Study
Reprinted from: *J. Clin. Med.* **2022**, *11*, 540, doi:10.3390/jcm11030540 . . . . **153**

Jan-Philipp Imiolczyk, Ulrich Brunner, Tankred Imiolczyk, Florian Freislederer, David Endell and Markus Scheibel
Reverse Shoulder Arthroplasty for Proximal Humerus Head-Split Fractures—A Retrospective Cohort Study
Reprinted from: *J. Clin. Med.* **2022**, *11*, 2835, doi:10.3390/jcm11102835 . . . . **165**

Marko Nabergoj, Lionel Neyton, Hugo Bothorel, Sean W. L. Ho, Sidi Wang, Xue Ling Chong and Alexandre Lädermann
Reverse Shoulder Arthroplasty with Bony and Metallic versus Standard Bony Reconstruction for Severe Glenoid Bone Loss. A Retrospective Comparative Cohort Study
Reprinted from: *J. Clin. Med.* **2021**, *10*, 5274, doi:10.3390/jcm10225274 . . . . **177**

Alessandro Castagna, Mario Borroni, Luigi Dubini, Stefano Gumina, Giacomo Delle Rose and Riccardo Ranieri
Inverted-Bearing Reverse Shoulder Arthroplasty: Consequences on Scapular Notching and Clinical Results at Mid-Term Follow-Up
Reprinted from: *J. Clin. Med.* **2022**, *11*, 5796, doi:10.3390/jcm11195796 . . . . **191**

Falk Reuther, Ulrich Irlenbusch, Max J. Kääb and Georges Kohut
Conversion of Hemiarthroplasty to Reverse Shoulder Arthroplasty with Humeral Stem Retention
Reprinted from: *J. Clin. Med.* **2022**, *11*, 834, doi:10.3390/jcm11030834 . . . . **201**

Doruk Akgün, Mats Wiethölter, Nina Maziak, Alp Paksoy, Daniel Karczewski, Markus Scheibel and Philipp Moroder
Two-Stage Exchange Arthroplasty for Periprosthetic Shoulder Infection Is Associated with High Rate of Failure to Reimplant and Mortality
Reprinted from: *J. Clin. Med.* **2021**, *11*, 5186, doi:10.3390/jcm10215186 . . . . **211**

Alexandre Lädermann, Rodolphe Eurin, Axelle Alibert, Mehdi Bensouda and Hugo Bothorel
Measuring Patient Value after Total Shoulder Arthroplasty
Reprinted from: *J. Clin. Med.* **2021**, *10*, 5700, doi:10.3390/jcm10235700 . . . . **221**

About the Editors

Markus Scheibel

Prof Markus Scheibel is the chief of the Shoulder and Elbow Department at Schulthess Clinic in Zurich, Switzerland, and Visiting Professor at the Charité-Universitaetsmedizin Berlin. From 2015 to 2021, he served as the president of the German–Austrian–Swiss Association for Shoulder and Elbow Surgery (DVSE), and has recently been appointed as the general secretary of the society. Prof. Scheibel is the chairman of the Berlin International Shoulder Course (BISC) and serves alongside Dr. Philippe Valenti as the chairman of the Paris International Shoulder Course (PISC).

Alexandre Lädermann

Dr. Alexandre Lädermann is Privat Docent at the University of Geneva, founder of BeeMed and Med4Cast, and president of the foundation for Research and Teaching in Orthopedics, Sports Medicine, Trauma, and Imaging (FORE). He is also a member of the Central Committee of the French Arthroscopic Society (SFA), past president of the Swiss Shoulder Society (Expertengruppe Schulter und Ellbogen (Swiss Orthopaedics)), and past president of the Membership Committee and Member of the Central Committee of the European Society for Surgery of the Shoulder and the Elbow (SECEC/ESSSE). Moreover, he is chairman of the 12th Val d'Isère Advanced Shoulder Course and has been president of the congress of the European Society for Shoulder and Elbow Surgery (SECEC/ESSSE) in Geneva and of the International Congress on Adipose Stem cell Treatment (iCAST) in Zurich.

Dr Alexandre Lädermann joined Hôpital de La Tour in 2011, where he oversees shoulder and elbow surgery development in the Division of Orthopaedics and Trauma Surgery. He is particularly responsible for teaching.

He is editor of the journals The Hive, Journal of Shoulder and Elbow Arthroplasty and Journal Clinical Medicine. He is the author of more than 200 publications in journals and books concerning the shoulder and elbow joints.

Laurent Audigé

Laurent Audigé was trained in veterinary medicine in 1986 in France. He gained his PhD in epidemiology in 1996 at Massey University, Palmerston North in New Zealand, and underwent his habilitation at the University of Bern in 2002, after joining the AO Foundation in Davos, Switzerland, in 2000. He then dedicated himself to clinical research in humans, focusing on the treatment of trauma and disorders of the musculoskeletal system. At Schulthess Clinic, he has led the Shoulder and Elbow Surgery department research group since 2012. His own research has been mainly related to the development and validation of fracture classifications, the development of core sets for the documentation and reporting of surgical complications, and the evaluation of outcome and health–economic parameters in surgical patients.

He is active at the University Hospital of Basel as an external scientific collaborator. Laurent Audigé has expertise in multicenter clinical study implementation and is the author of more than 200 peer-reviewed scientific publications.

Clinical research into the evaluation and validation of outcome instruments (e.g., functional scores and quality of life questionnaires) has been a particular strength in clinical research at the Shoulder and Elbow Surgery department in the last 15 years. Selected sets of instruments have been in routine use since 2006 for the long-term follow-up control of patients treated with shoulder prosthesis. Clinical registers were extended to other relevant problems and their treatment, including rotator cuff tears, shoulder instabilities and acromio-clavicular joint instabilities. We seek continuous improvements in the standardization and efficiency of the documentation of surgical interventions in these areas to improve quality control for patients and offer a solid foundation for clinical research.

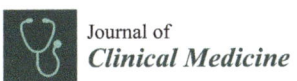

Editorial

Innovations in the Realm of Shoulder Arthroplasty

Alexandre Lädermann [1,2,3,*], Laurent Audigé [4,5,6] and Markus Scheibel [4,7]

1. Division of Orthopaedics and Trauma Surgery, La Tour Hospital, Av. J.-D. Maillard 3, 1217 Meyrin, Switzerland
2. Faculty of Medicine, University of Geneva, 1211 Geneva, Switzerland
3. Division of Orthopaedics and Trauma Surgery, Department of Surgery, Geneva University Hospitals, 1211 Geneva, Switzerland
4. Department of Shoulder and Elbow Surgery, Schulthess Clinic, 8008 Zurich, Switzerland
5. Research and Development Department, Schulthess Clinic, 8008 Zurich, Switzerland
6. Department of Orthopaedic Surgery and Traumatology, University Hospital of Basel, 4031 Basel, Switzerland
7. Center for Musculoskeletal Surgery, Campus Virchow, Charité-Universitaetsmedizin Berlin, 10117 Berlin, Germany
* Correspondence: alexandre.laedermann@gmail.com; Tel.: +41-22-719-75-55; Fax: +41-22-719-60-77

Citation: Lädermann, A.; Audigé, L.; Scheibel, M. Innovations in the Realm of Shoulder Arthroplasty. *J. Clin. Med.* 2023, 12, 237. https://doi.org/10.3390/jcm12010237

Received: 30 November 2022
Accepted: 11 December 2022
Published: 28 December 2022

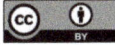

Copyright: © 2022 by the authors. Licensee MDPI, Basel, Switzerland. This article is an open access article distributed under the terms and conditions of the Creative Commons Attribution (CC BY) license (https://creativecommons.org/licenses/by/4.0/).

Introduction

Most of the surgeries regarding the shoulder were established over a century ago. In the 1890s, the understanding of the unstable shoulder was elucidated by Broca and Hartman [1], who introduced the concept of capsulolabral damage following dislocations as a possible cause of recurrent instability [2]. Notably, most of the findings currently considered hallmarks of shoulder instability, including Bankart lesions, bony Bankart lesions, and Kim lesions, as well as anterior and posterior labral periosteal sleeve avulsions and glenoid avulsions of glenohumeral ligaments, were described within research papers decades before their depiction by the eponymous figures to whom these lesions are now commonly assigned [2]. In 1906, Perthes [3] and, a few years later, Bankart [4], emphasized the reattachment of the labrum to stabilize the joint. Current bone grafting techniques are based on the initial descriptions by Noeske in 1921 using the coracoid process [5], Eden [6] in 1918, and Hybinette [7] in 1932, using an autologous iliac crest. Since then, no true paradigm shift has occurred.

Regarding the rotator cuff, a similar observation can be made. Duplay presented the classic description of scapulohumeral periarthritis in 1872, highlighting the potential role of the acromion. Repair of the torn rotator cuff likely dates back to 1898 [8]. Since then, many evolutions regarding these treatments, such as acromioplasty, arthroscopy, or anchors development, have been subsequently observed, but without apparent revolution; 150 years after its first description, the proper place of a procedure such as acromioplasty has yet to be determined [9], and most enhancing technologies (superior capsular reconstruction (SCR) [10], growth factors (PRP) [11], Balloon [12], etc.) for rotator cuff reinforcement or substitution have yet to prove their superiority over simple reattachment of the tendon to the bone.

Interestingly, the former statements are not true within the domain of arthroplasty. Since Themistocles Gluck designed the first shoulder prostheses in 1890, of which Jules Emile Péan implanted the first in 1893 [13], several revolutions have taken place within these last few decades, namely, by Charles Neer and Paul Grammont. Most importantly, the realm of shoulder arthroplasty has undergone significant transformation [14] in recent years, covered in the present Special Issue on shoulder arthroplasty in the *Journal of Clinical Medicine*. It concerns not only surgical indications that have dramatically evolved [15–17], but also planification and navigation with the implementation of artificial intelligence (AI) and augmented reality (AR) [18]. Moreover, the rapid development of surgical techniques [19,20] and new prosthetic designs [21–23], including custom augments with three dimensional (3D) printing, glenoid [24] and humeral [25] reconstruction for various conditions [26], are overviewed. Palpable results of this recent technologic acceleration include improved outcomes [27] and decreased complication rates. Despite the significant progress highlighted in this Special Issue, there is currently a myriad prosthetic designs announcing imminent changes. Indeed, we are only at the dawn of a new era in the history of shoulder arthroplasty, reminding us that a substantial amount of work remains to be carried out in order to see progress.

Author Contributions: A.L.: writing—review and editing, L.A.: writing—review and editing, M.S.: writing—review and editing. All authors have read and agreed to the published version of the manuscript.

Funding: This research was funded by FORE (Foundation for Research and Teaching in Orthopedics, Sports Medicine, Trauma and Imaging in the Musculoskeletal System). Grant number FORE 2022-42.

Acknowledgments: We thank Jeanni Zbinden for her help in editing this editorial.

Conflicts of Interest: A.L. is a paid consultant for Arthrex, Stryker and Medacta. He received royalties from Stryker. He is the founder of FORE, Med4Cast and BeeMed. L.A. declares no conflicts of interest. M.S. is a paid consultant for Arthrex Inc., CONMED Linvatec, DJ Orthopaedics, Exactech, Inc. and Stryker. He received royalties from Stryker, CONMED Linvatec.

References

1. Broca, A.; Hartmann, H. Contribution à l'étude des luxations de l'épaule (luxations anciennes et luxations récidivantes). *Bull. Soc. Anat.* **1890**, *4*, 416–423.
2. Lädermann, A. Anteroinferior Glenohumeral Instability. Available online: https://wiki.beemed.com/view/Anteroinferior_Glenohumeral_Instability#History (accessed on 26 September 2021).
3. Perthes, G. Ueber Operationen beihabitueller Schulterluxation. *Dtsch. Z. Chir.* **1906**, *85*, 199–227. [CrossRef]
4. Bankart, A.S. Recurrent or Habitual Dislocation of the Shoulder-Joint. *Br. Med. J.* **1923**, *2*, 1132–1133. [CrossRef]
5. Lädermann, A.; Bohm, E.; Tay, E.; Scheibel, M. Bone-mediated anteroinferior glenohumeral instability: Current concepts. *Der Orthopade* **2018**, *47*, 129–138. [CrossRef]
6. Eden, R. Zur Operation der habituellen Schulterluxation unter Mitteilung eines neuen Verfahrens bei Abriss am inneren Pfannenrande. *Dsch. Z. Chir.* **1918**, *144*, 269. [CrossRef]
7. Hybinette, S. De la transplantation d'un fragment osseux pour remédier aux luxations récidivantes de l'épaule. *Acta Chir. Scand.* **1932**, *26*, 411–445.
8. Müller, W. *Verletzungen und Krankheiten der oberen Extremität*; Thieme: Leipzig, Germany, 1922.
9. Lädermann, A.; Denard, P.J. Proper Indications for Shoulder Subacromial Decompression Result in Excellent Outcomes. *Arthroscopy* **2021**, *37*, 1705–1707. [CrossRef]
10. Lädermann, A.; Denard, P.J.; Barth, J.; Bonnevialle, N.; Lejeune, E.; Group, S.; Bothorel, H.; Francophone Arthroscopy, S.; Nourrissat, G. Superior capsular reconstruction for irreparable rotator cuff tears: Autografts versus allografts. *Orthop. Traumatol. Surg. Res. OTSR* **2021**, *107*, 103059. [CrossRef]
11. Schwitzguebel, A.J.; Kolo, F.C.; Tirefort, J.; Kourhani, A.; Nowak, A.; Gremeaux, V.; Saffarini, M.; Lädermann, A. Efficacy of Platelet-Rich Plasma for the Treatment of Interstitial Supraspinatus Tears: A Double-Blinded, Randomized Controlled Trial. *Am. J. Sports Med.* **2019**, *47*, 1885–1892. [CrossRef]
12. Metcalfe, A.; Parsons, H.; Parsons, N.; Brown, J.; Fox, J.; Gemperle Mannion, E.; Haque, A.; Hutchinson, C.; Kearney, R.; Khan, I.; et al. Subacromial balloon spacer for irreparable rotator cuff tears of the shoulder (START:REACTS): A group-sequential, double-blind, multicentre randomised controlled trial. *Lancet* **2022**, *399*, 1954–1963. [CrossRef]
13. Bankes, M.J.; Emery, R.J. Pioneers of shoulder replacement: Themistocles Gluck and Jules Emile Pean. *J. Shoulder Elb. Surg.* **1995**, *4*, 259–262. [CrossRef] [PubMed]
14. Leafblad, N.; Asghar, E.; Tashjian, R.Z. Innovations in Shoulder Arthroplasty. *J. Clin. Med.* **2022**, *11*, 2799. [CrossRef] [PubMed]
15. Herve, A.; Chelli, M.; Boileau, P.; Walch, G.; Favard, L.; Levigne, C.; Sirveaux, F.; Clavert, P.; Bonnevialle, N.; Collin, P. Clinical and Radiological Results of Hemiarthroplasty and Total Shoulder Arthroplasty for Primary Avascular Necrosis of the Humeral Head in Patients Less Than 60 Years Old. *J. Clin. Med.* **2021**, *10*, 3081. [CrossRef] [PubMed]
16. Imiolczyk, J.P.; Brunner, U.; Imiolczyk, T.; Freislederer, F.; Endell, D.; Scheibel, M. Reverse Shoulder Arthroplasty for Proximal Humerus Head-Split Fractures-A Retrospective Cohort Study. *J. Clin. Med.* **2022**, *11*, 2835. [CrossRef] [PubMed]
17. Simon, M.J.K.; Coghlan, J.A.; Bell, S.N. Shoulder Replacement in the Elderly with Anatomic versus Reverse Total Prosthesis? A Prospective 2-Year Follow-Up Study. *J. Clin. Med.* **2022**, *11*, 540. [CrossRef]
18. Rojas, J.T.; Lädermann, A.; Ho, S.W.L.; Rashid, M.S.; Zumstein, M.A. Glenoid Component Placement Assisted by Augmented Reality Through a Head-Mounted Display During Reverse Shoulder Arthroplasty. *Arthrosc. Tech.* **2022**, *11*, e863–e874. [CrossRef]

19. Akgun, D.; Wietholter, M.; Maziak, N.; Paksoy, A.; Karczewski, D.; Scheibel, M.; Moroder, P. Two-Stage Exchange Arthroplasty for Periprosthetic Shoulder Infection Is Associated with High Rate of Failure to Reimplant and Mortality. *J. Clin. Med.* **2021**, *10*, 5186. [CrossRef]
20. Moroder, P.; Lacheta, L.; Minkus, M.; Karpinski, K.; Uhing, F.; De Souza, S.; van der Merwe, M.; Akgun, D. Implant Sizing and Positioning in Anatomical Total Shoulder Arthroplasty Using a Rotator Cuff-Sparing Postero-Inferior Approach. *J. Clin. Med.* **2022**, *11*, 3324. [CrossRef]
21. Castagna, A.; Borroni, M.; Dubini, L.; Gumina, S.; Delle Rose, G.; Ranieri, R. Inverted-Bearing Reverse Shoulder Arthroplasty: Consequences on Scapular Notching and Clinical Results at Mid-Term Follow-Up. *J. Clin. Med.* **2022**, *11*, 5796. [CrossRef]
22. Nabergoj, M.; Onishi, S.; Lädermann, A.; Kalache, H.; Trebse, R.; Bothorel, H.; Collin, P. Can Lateralization of Reverse Shoulder Arthroplasty Improve Active External Rotation in Patients with Preoperative Fatty Infiltration of the Infraspinatus and Teres Minor? *J. Clin. Med.* **2021**, *10*, 4130. [CrossRef]
23. Reuther, F.; Irlenbusch, U.; Kaab, M.J.; Kohut, G. Conversion of Hemiarthroplasty to Reverse Shoulder Arthroplasty with Humeral Stem Retention. *J. Clin. Med.* **2022**, *11*, 834. [CrossRef] [PubMed]
24. Nabergoj, M.; Neyton, L.; Bothorel, H.; Ho, S.W.L.; Wang, S.; Chong, X.L.; Lädermann, A. Reverse Shoulder Arthroplasty with Bony and Metallic versus Standard Bony Reconstruction for Severe Glenoid Bone Loss. A Retrospective Comparative Cohort Study. *J. Clin. Med.* **2021**, *10*, 5274. [CrossRef] [PubMed]
25. Sanchez-Sotelo, J. Current Concepts in Humeral Component Design for Anatomic and Reverse Shoulder Arthroplasty. *J. Clin. Med.* **2021**, *10*, 5151. [CrossRef] [PubMed]
26. Coifman, I.; Brunner, U.H.; Scheibel, M. Dislocation Arthropathy of the Shoulder. *J. Clin. Med.* **2022**, *11*, 2019. [CrossRef] [PubMed]
27. Lädermann, A.; Eurin, R.; Alibert, A.; Bensouda, M.; Bothorel, H. Measuring Patient Value after Total Shoulder Arthroplasty. *J. Clin. Med.* **2021**, *10*, 5700. [CrossRef]

Disclaimer/Publisher's Note: The statements, opinions and data contained in all publications are solely those of the individual author(s) and contributor(s) and not of MDPI and/or the editor(s). MDPI and/or the editor(s) disclaim responsibility for any injury to people or property resulting from any ideas, methods, instructions or products referred to in the content.

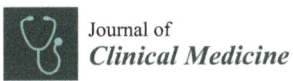

Review

Innovations in Shoulder Arthroplasty

Nels Leafblad, Elise Asghar and Robert Z. Tashjian *

Department of Orthopaedics, School of Medicine, University of Utah, 590 Wakara Way, Salt Lake City, UT 84108, USA; nels.leafblad@hsc.utah.edu (N.L.); elise.asghar@hsc.utah.edu (E.A.)
* Correspondence: robert.tashjian@hsc.utah.edu; Tel.: +1-801-587-5450; Fax: +1-801-587-5411

Abstract: Innovations currently available with anatomic total shoulder arthroplasty include shorter stem designs and augmented/inset/inlay glenoid components. Regarding reverse shoulder arthroplasty (RSA), metal augmentation, including custom augments, on both the glenoid and humeral side have expanded indications in cases of bone loss. In the setting of revision arthroplasty, humeral options include convertible stems and newer tools to improve humeral implant removal. New strategies for treatment and surgical techniques have been developed for recalcitrant shoulder instability, acromial fractures, and infections after RSA. Finally, computer planning, navigation, PSI, and augmented reality are imaging options now available that have redefined preoperative planning and indications as well intraoperative component placement. This review covers many of the innovations in the realm of shoulder arthroplasty.

Keywords: shoulder arthroplasty; stemless; inlay; onlay; augment

Citation: Leafblad, N.; Asghar, E.; Tashjian, R.Z. Innovations in Shoulder Arthroplasty. *J. Clin. Med.* 2022, 11, 2799. https://doi.org/10.3390/jcm11102799

Academic Editors: Markus Scheibel, Alexandre Lädermann and Laurent Audigé

Received: 5 March 2022
Accepted: 12 May 2022
Published: 16 May 2022

Publisher's Note: MDPI stays neutral with regard to jurisdictional claims in published maps and institutional affiliations.

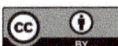

Copyright: © 2022 by the authors. Licensee MDPI, Basel, Switzerland. This article is an open access article distributed under the terms and conditions of the Creative Commons Attribution (CC BY) license (https://creativecommons.org/licenses/by/4.0/).

1. Introduction

The growth in total shoulder arthroplasty over the past 20 years has been exponential. From 1993 to 2007, primary procedures increased 369% [1]. Revision shoulder arthroplasty increased 431% during the same period. During the timing of this explosion, numerous innovations have occurred, most importantly the development of the reverse shoulder arthroplasty (RSA). Currently, RSA accounts for over 70% of the shoulder arthroplasties performed in the U.S. With the expansion of shoulder arthroplasty, and specifically RSA, numerous other innovative designs have been developed in recent years to address more and more complicated pathology to hopefully reduce the increasing revision burden and improve outcomes.

Innovations currently available with anatomic total shoulder arthroplasty include shorter stem designs and augmented inlay glenoid components. Regarding RSA, metal augmentation, including custom augments on both the glenoid and humeral side have expanded indications in cases of bone loss. In the setting of revision arthroplasty, humeral options include convertible stems and newer tools to improve humeral implant removal. New strategies for treatment and surgical techniques have been developed for recalcitrant shoulder instability, acromial fractures, and infections after RSA. Finally, computer planning, navigation, PSI, and augmented reality are imaging options now available that have redefined preoperative planning and indications as well intraoperative component placement.

2. New Perspectives and Innovations in Anatomic Shoulder Arthroplasty

2.1. Humeral Component Innovations

2.1.1. Stemless Implants

There has been a recent trend in the use of stemless humeral components. Rationale for this shift has to do with the reported complications of stemmed implant designs, such as loss of bone stock during revision arthroplasty, malpositioning of the humeral implant, especially in cases of post-traumatic malalignment, intraoperative and postoperative periprosthetic fractures, and an altered center of rotation [2–4]. Several stemless designs are now on the market, all with the aim of providing 3-dimensional reconstruction of the humeral head, recreating the humeral center of rotation independent of the shaft axis [5], avoiding additional greater tuberosity osteotomy in post-traumatic cases, and avoiding the above-listed stem-related complications [4]. Advantages of stemless implants also include decreased surgical time, less blood loss, low stress shielding, and lower risk of diaphyseal stress risers [6,7]. As previously mentioned, particularly in the setting of post-traumatic malalignment or deformities of the glenohumeral joint, stemless designs allow the surgeon to recreate the glenohumeral center of rotation independent of the humeral shaft [5].

Two major stemless designs exist—impaction systems and screw-in systems. Based on work by Habermeyer et al. and Krukenberg et al., there does not appear to be a difference in terms of humeral loosening (n = 0 in both designs), humeral osteophytic exostosis (n = 0 in both designs), or functional outcomes [8,9]. Radiographic medial calcar resorption occurs more often with the impaction design, but there does not appear to be a clinical implication of this, as both designs result in significantly improved Constant and Subjective Shoulder Value (SSV) scores [8,10].

Short- to mid-term (6 months–5 years) results of stemless implants have been favorable with Constant scores ranging from 65–86 and revision rates of 0%–11% [8,9,11–15]. These results seem to translate to the long-term (8–9 years), with constant scores of 62–69 and revision rates of 7%–10% [4,16]. Radiographic evaluation of 49 stemless shoulder arthroplasties at 9 years revealed upward migration of the humeral head in 14.7%, incomplete humeral "radiolucent line" in 2.3%, and no loosening of the humeral implant. There was incomplete glenoid radiolucent line without loosening in 27.3% of the stemless TSA [4]. Hawi et al. also reported a 6.9% revision rate, with secondary cuff insufficiency representing the most common cause (13.9%), and periprosthetic injection (2.3%) and periprosthetic fracture (2.3%) being less common. Interestingly, the humeral implant-related complication rate was 0% [4].

Comparing 20 stemless to 20 stemmed implants with 5-year follow up, Uschock et al. found that both implants provided consistently good functional outcomes. They reported no humeral-related complications in the stemless group, whereas there was one fracture of the greater tuberosity leading to humeral implant loosening in the stemmed group. The stemless group had one case of glenoid loosening. The overall revision rate in both groups was 13.8% [17].

Though there are many potential advantages of stemless implants, several notable limitations remain [7]. These implants lack a convertible platform and therefore require implant removal in the revision to RSA setting. They are dependent on proximal bone quality and there are also concerns regarding lesser tuberosity osteotomies given the dependence of subscapularis fixation strength. Additionally, they may be associated with increased cost. Mixed methodology between various studies of stemless implants makes results somewhat difficult to compare, and yet while further long-term studies are required, stemless implants appear to be a favorable option for TSA. See Figure 1, an X-ray of a stemless humeral implant.

2.1.2. Short Stem Implants

The potential advantages of the short-stemmed prostheses are that they rely less on proximal bone stock than stemless implants and provide a larger surface area with a porous coating for ingrowth into the proximal humerus, are easy to revise given convertible implant options, and have over 10 years of implementation in Europe. Short- to mid-term results with short stem implants are also favorable with Constant scores around 75 and ASES scores around 80, with 0%–9% revision rates [18–21]. Romeo et al. reported on the outcomes of the Apex short stem and concluded that TSA with this anatomic press-fit short-stem results in improved clinical outcomes without component loosening at 2 year follow up [20]. In the anatomic TSA setting, the Aequalis Ascend Flex (Fa. Wright, Memphis, TN, USA) short-stem implant has a relatively high occurrence of radiographic changes around the stem (26%), most commonly cortical thinning and osteopenia at the calcar as well as spot welding laterally. Despite these radiographic findings, no stems were found to be loose and short-term clinical outcomes were favorable and comparable to other short-stem systems [19,22].

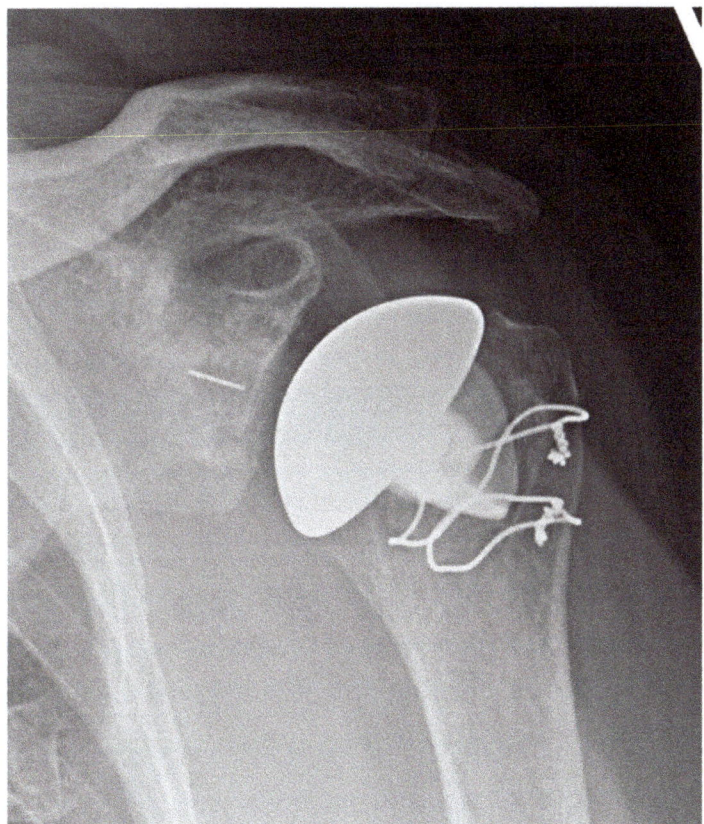

Figure 1. Stemless anatomic TSA. AP X-ray of anatomic TSA with stemless humeral component.

Some have proposed the use of pyrolytic carbon, or pyrocarbon, which has similarities to cortical bone and a low coefficient of friction. There is a theoretical advantage to the less-stiff quality of pyrocarbon, at least in the hemiarthroplasty setting, in that stiff cobalt-chrome humeral heads wear against the less stiff cartilage and subchondral bone of the glenoid. Use of pyrocarbon heads may result in less glenoid bone loss, reducing the complexity of revision surgeries [23–25]. Garrett et al. have reported good short-term outcomes with pyrocarbon head short-stem implants in the hemiarthroplasty setting [21]. Whether these results translate to the anatomic TSA setting is yet to be determined.

The senior author's preference is to use an uncemented short stem (Figure 2) or stemless implant. In poor humeral bone, however, the preference is to cement a short stem.

2.1.3. Convertible Platforms

With the dramatic rise of primary shoulder arthroplasty over the last 15–20 years has come a rise of revision shoulder arthroplasty. Though indications for revision shoulder arthroplasty vary, it remains a technically demanding and challenging procedure regardless of indication. Revision shoulder arthroplasty is associated with increased blood loss and operative times, and frequently requires the use of special implants, augments, and bone grafting [26]. The innovative development of modular platform humeral stems, those that can be converted from an anatomic TSA construct to a reverse TSA, has significantly reduced the complexity of revision shoulder arthroplasty. It theoretically obviates the need to explant the humeral stem that in turn reduces operative time, decreases blood loss, preserves humeral bone stock, and can reduce cost [27]. Crosby et al. found a slightly better postoperative range of motion in those who underwent conversion to RSA with a convertible platform compared to those that required entire humeral implant exchange. The prevalence of intraoperative complications was significantly lower with the convertible-platform group (0% compared to 15%), though rates of reoperation were not different [27].

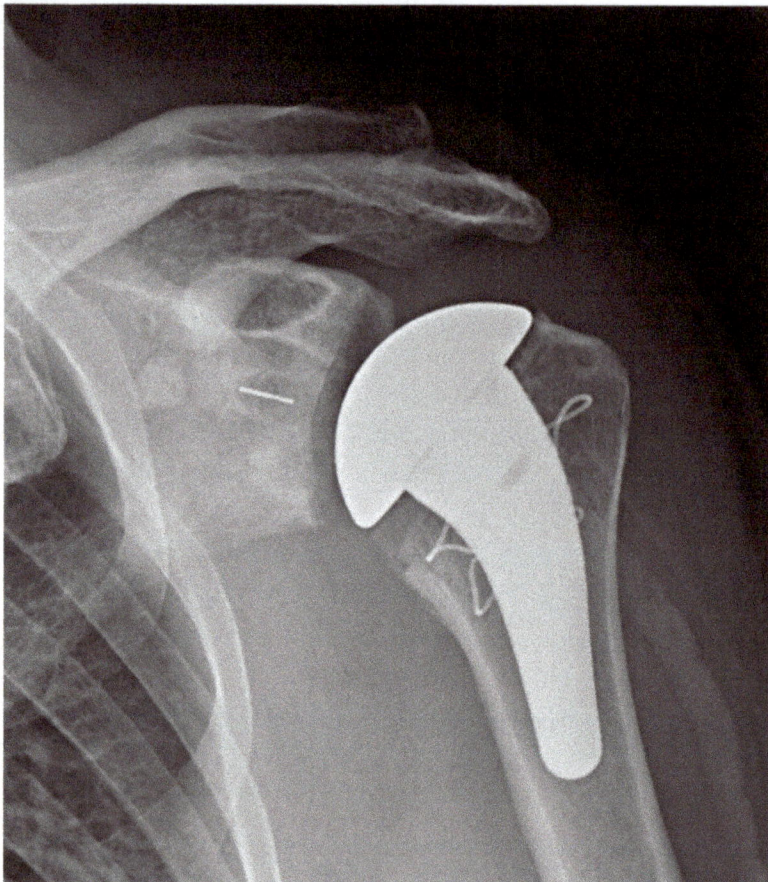

Figure 2. Short stem anatomic TSA. AP X-ray of anatomic TSA with short humeral stem.

It should be noted that not all convertible-platform humeral components can indeed be retained at the revision setting. The convertible platform humeral stem must be well-fixed and well-positioned to be retained. Encouragingly, multiple studies have demonstrated that a vast majority, approximately 80%, can be retained [27–29].

2.2. Glenoid Component Innovations
Augmented Glenoid Components

Excess retroversion and posterior wear of the glenoid present a dilemma for the orthopedic surgeon performing anatomic TSA. Glenoids with posterior wear and formation of a neo-glenoid (Walch B2), and those with >15° retroversion (Walch B3) are at high risk of developing glenoid loosening with standard implants [30]. Glenoid loosening has been the most common cause of anatomic TSA failure and indication for revision. Increased osteolysis has been demonstrated in cases in which the glenoid component is placed in excess retroversion, resulting in decreased implant survival [31].

Glenoid component retroversion beyond 15° leads to decreased contact area and increased contact pressures, placing the glenoid component at high risk of failure [31], and though eccentric reaming can correct small posterior deficits up to 10–15° [32,33], one risks removing excessive native bone when eccentrically reaming for larger deficits. Primary bone grafting has demonstrated variable results and may be associated with clinical and radiographic failure [34–37]. The other remaining option to deal with excessive posterior wear and retroversion even in the setting of an intact rotator cuff is to perform RSA, and some authors prefer this method [30].

For these reasons, there has been the introduction of augmented glenoid components that theoretically reduce bone removal and shear stresses, while retaining the benefits of anatomic TSA over RSA. Full wedge and partial wedge augments of varying degrees exist. Older designs included a keel that was angled in line with the neo-glenoid face, thus directing fixation toward the anterior neck of the glenoid. Newer implants have placed vault fixation angled with the paleo-glenoid to improve fixation [38]. Strong long-term data is lacking for augmented glenoid components. However, the short-term results are encouraging with multiple studies citing revision rates of 0%–5% at 2–3-year follow-up [38–43]. Larger-degree augments may be at higher risk of failure, as demonstrated by Priddy et al. in their retrospective study of full-wedge glenoid augmented TSA compared to non-augmented TSA, in which all failures of the augmented glenoids requiring revision came with the 16° augment, with no failures of the 8° or 12° augments. There were no differences in radiographic lucencies around the pegs, postop ROM or patient reported outcome measures [38].

The senior author's preference for managing glenoid retroversion includes high-side reaming a B2 or B3 glenoid for retroversion <25°. When retroversion is 25° to 35°, the preference is to use an augmented glenoid component (Figure 3). For retroversion >35°, the senior author will perform an RSA with bone grafting of the glenoid.

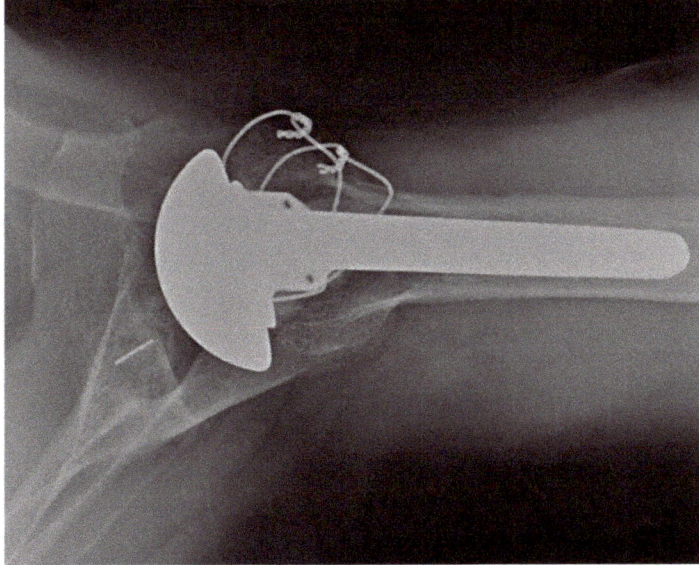

Figure 3. Anatomic TSA with posteriorly augmented glenoid polyethylene. Axillary X-ray of posteriorly augmented glenoid polyethylene.

2.3. Inlay versus Onlay Glenoid Components

Traditional onlay glenoid prostheses exhibit signs of loosening at relatively high rates, even when optimally placed [44–46]. Metal-backed glenoids have fallen out of favor due to the unacceptably high failure rates [47], so all-polyethylene designs are the gold standard. Though somewhat controversial, pegged onlay glenoids appear to have superior survivorship to keeled glenoids [45,48]. The "rocking-horse" phenomenon at the glenoid-bone interface can result in edge loading, liftoff, and subsequent component loosening. With radiolucent lines occurring in approximately 30%–75% of TSAs with onlay glenoids by 10-year follow up, and loosening resulting in clinical failure requiring revision TSA 2%–10% of the time [49–51], there indeed is need for improvement in implant design. This has led to the development of the inlay glenoid design, in which the polyethylene component is implanted flush with the glenoid bone surface. Its theoretical advantages are those of less glenoid bone removal and improved mechanical characteristics due to less implant edge loading and lift off.

In a cadaveric study by Gagliono et al., onlay glenoid components exhibited gross loosening during fatigue testing, whereas the inlay glenoid components did not, and the onlay glenoids experienced significantly higher forces acting on them than did the native or inlay glenoids [52]. Short term results are promising, with good improvement in PROs, function, and ROM, without increased complication rates, and low reoperation rates [53]. This has been true even in the setting of posterior glenoid erosion, with no differences in short term clinical and radiographic outcomes evaluating non-spherical humeral head and inlay glenoid components in concentric (Walch A) glenoids compared to non-concentric (Walch B1 and B2) glenoids, according to the work of Egger et al. [54]. Inlay components may be of particular benefit in the younger, athletic, weight-lifting population given the theoretical decrease in mechanical loosening and resultant lack of restrictions afforded to them. Early clinical results have been excellent, and most of these patients are able to return to sports and lifting at the same or higher level [53,55].

Longer term data is required to definitively say whether inlay glenoid components are superior to onlay components, but early evidence suggests that this may turn out to be the case.

The senior author typically uses an onlay glenoid component, except when glenoid dysplasia exists, in which case the preference is to use an inlay glenoid component. See Figure 4, which depicts an X-ray appearance of an inlay glenoid component.

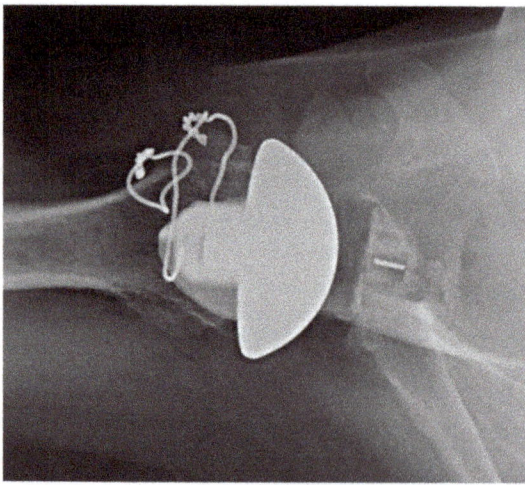

Figure 4. Inlay glenoid polyethylene in setting of glenoid dysplasia. Axillary X-ray of inlay glenoid polyethylene in setting of glenoid dysplasia.

2.4. Convertible Glenoid Components in Anatomic TSA

Cemented all-polyethylene glenoid components have represented the gold standard in anatomic TSA, given the historically unreliable results of cementless glenoid components. However, given the challenges and risks of revising a cemented glenoid component, there has been a resurgence of interest in convertible metal-backed glenoid components for anatomic TSA. The new generation of convertible metal-backed trays feature improved designs including a highly stable anchorage mechanism of the metal carrier in the glenoid vault, with larger bone-implant contact area and improved stability against shear forces [56]. Short and midterm follow-up results of the latest generation of convertible glenoid systems are encouraging, with revision rates ranging from 0%–11% [56–58]. Magosch et al. reported no glenoid loosening, an implant related revision rate of 4.2%, polyethylene dissociated in 4.2%, and no complications in cases requiring revision to RSA, in their prospective study of 48 patients at a mean follow up of 49 months [56]. In the setting of failed anatomic TSA, conversion to RSA may be facilitated by convertible glenoid systems, while maintaining improvements in pain and shoulder function [59]. Long-term follow-up data is needed, but there may indeed be a role for these convertible glenoid components moving forward.

3. New Perspectives and Innovations in Reverse Shoulder Arthroplasty

Reverse shoulder arthroplasty was approved by the FDA in the US in 2003. Since then, the prevalence has increased significantly by more than 2.5 times from 7.3 cases per 100,000 persons to 19.3 cases per 100,000 persons between 2012 to 2017 [60]. Its original indication was rotator cuff arthropathy in older patients [61], but this has since been expanded as prostheses have improved and surgeon experience has become more ubiquitous. Indications now include fracture, revision shoulder surgery, rotator cuff arthropathy in relatively younger patients, tumor, and glenoid bone loss. As these indications expand, more options have developed to assist in decreasing complications and improving complex or revision surgeries.

3.1. Combined Humeral and Glenoid Component Innovations
Lateralization

Reverse shoulder arthroplasty designs have evolved over the last 15 years. One major evolution has been increased lateralization of the glenoid component. Typically, in RSA, the glenoid center of rotation (COR) is still medialized relative to the native shoulder COR. The increased lateralization is in reference to the preoperative humeral position rather than the COR. The current trend is to increase lateralization to increase soft tissue tension, particularly the rotator cuff. This lateralization can be achieved by one of three methods: lateralized glenoid baseplate, lateralized glenosphere or glenoid bone grafts (e.g., BIORSA).

Lateralization can have negative and positive effects on both the glenoid and humerus. Glenoid lateralization decreases adduction impingement thereby decreasing scapular notching and improving adduction, ER and extension motion [62–66]. It also improves rotator cuff tension and prosthetic stability [67,68]. Glenoid lateralization does, however, decrease the mechanical advantage of the deltoid, increase the shear forces across the implant interface and increase acromial strain, potentially increasing the risk of stress fracture [69–74]. Humeral lateralization on the other hand improves the deltoid mechanical advantage as well as improves the posterior cuff tension and the deltoid wrap by providing a more anatomic vector of muscle pull [67,70,75,76]. The negative effects of humeral lateralization are potentially too much soft tissue tension when combined with glenoid lateralization.

3.2. Humeral Component Innovations
3.2.1. Stemless Implants

Stemless RSA implants are not currently FDA approved in the United States, however they have been approved and studied in Europe and Canada. The appeal of a stemless RSA implant is similar to their appeal in anatomic TSA, namely preserving proximal bone stock and easier implantation in the setting of altered distal anatomy, as well as potentially decreasing implant malposition and periprosthetic fractures [77,78]. International literature has found no significant difference in ROM and clinical outcomes scores between stemmed and stemless RSA in early to mid-term results [79,80]. Osteopenia was noted to be a relative contraindication for stemless implantation due to an association with early humeral component loosening [81,82]. Long-term survivorship of these implants is still under investigation.

3.2.2. Inlay vs. Onlay Implants

The original Grammont style implant was designed as a 155° inlay prosthesis. With the inlay component, the metaphyseal portion of the stem is inset into the humeral metaphysis. The thought behind this original design was to increase the surface area contact and medialize the humerus. The humeral stem onlay prosthesis was then developed with the metaphyseal tray sitting on top of the humeral cut surface. This allows for more lateralized and distalized humeral designs, preserved proximal bone stock, and the potential for stem conversion between RSA, TSA, and hemiarthroplasty [83–85].

In a biomechanical study by Walch, when compared to 155° inlay and 135°/155° onlay stems, only the 145° onlay humeral stem restored >50% of the native ROM and maximally lengthened the cuff [83]. Clinical studies have demonstrated improved adduction, extension, and ER with onlay humerus compared to the traditional inlay component [86,87]. In one of these studies, there was no difference in complications, however increased scapular fractures have been noted in other studies of the onlay stems, particularly with distalizing designs [84,87,88]. Ultimately, further clinical trials are needed to fully delineate the outcomes of inlay versus onlay, but the data so far suggests that onlay stems, particularly with lower neck shaft angle, offer improved outcomes and more revision versatility, but with the increased risk of scapular fracture.

The senior author's preference is to use an inlay short stem humeral component with a lateralized glenoid baseplate (Figure 5). If, however, there is significant proximal humeral bone loss, the senior author's preference is to use a standard length or long stem with proximal humeral allograft when necessary.

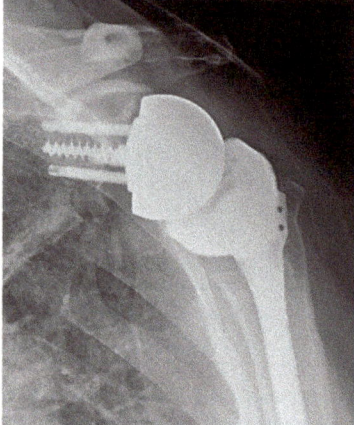

Figure 5. Lateralized RSA. AP X-ray of lateralized glenoid baseplate.

3.2.3. Vitamin E Polyethylene Implants

Vitamin E has become the most common antioxidant used in polyethylene components for all joint replacements including reverse shoulder arthroplasty [89]. It is added as an antioxidant stabilizer to inhibit oxidative degradation in ultra-high molecular weight polyethylene (UHMWPE). Vitamin E enhanced UHMWPE demonstrates more stability than gamma sterilized or high-dose irradiated UHMWPE implants under accelerated aging conditions [90–92] and more mechanical and fatigue strength [93]. Vitamin E implants that were evaluated in a wear stimulator for shoulder implants demonstrated a significant reduction in wear compared to non-vitamin E enhanced implants [94].

3.2.4. Ceramic Implants

Ceramic RSA components do not yet have FDA approval in the United States, however they are approved internationally. Internationally, ceramic humeral heads have been evaluated in anatomic TSA and shown to have reduced wear and osteolysis [95,96].

3.3. Glenoid Component Innovations

Augmented Glenoid Components

As discussed in the section on glenoid augmentation for the anatomic shoulder arthroplasty, glenoid bone loss presents a difficult problem for anatomic and reverse shoulder arthroplasty. With existing bone loss, many prefer to perform an RSA. This is thought to be a better option due to the decreased humeral migration and ultimately asymmetric poly wear with the more constrained RSA component as compared to the TSA. Even with the advantage of RSA glenoid implants, there are still minimum requirements for baseplate placement. The implant goals are typically cited as version within 5–10 degrees of neutral, neutral to mildly inferior inclination, a minimum of 50% baseplate contact with possibly more with augmented baseplates [97,98].

Glenoid augments assist in achieving these goals by increasing the baseplate support with less glenoid reaming. This also has the added benefit of preserving more native bone stock and increasing glenoid lateralization. When evaluating glenoid bone loss, cases are typically broken down into primary cases with bone loss or erosion and revision cases.

For primary cases, the bone loss is usually angular deformities—either version or inclination. Version abnormalities are associated with primary osteoarthritis, post-traumatic arthritis and post-capsulorrhaphy arthritis. Version change of >20 degrees requires either an augment or bone graft to avoid excessive reaming and to achieve the ideal baseplate position. Inclination deformities are associated with cuff tear arthropathy. Hamada 4 and 5 changes are usually associated with superior erosion but can occasionally be central erosion. Again, an augmented baseplate can improve the seating with less glenoid reaming, and inclination of >10–15° requires augment or bone graft rather than asymmetric reaming.

For revision cases, augments are more frequently used as opposed to autograft due to the lack of excess bone graft (e.g., humeral head) available. Bone loss in revision cases can be complex and variable including peripheral bone loss, cavitary ventral bone loss, angular erosive deformities and, most complex, combined defects.

Several augment options exist to address these bone loss patterns. First, there are non-custom implants. These require some glenoid reaming and are angled metallic augments that can be either a full or half wedge ranging from 10–30 degrees. These augments increase the baseplate thickness, so lateralized glenospheres may not be required. Second, there are custom implants. These are designed pre-operatively off a CT scan platform and are based on an individual patient's deformity. They typically do not require glenoid reaming. Custom implants are best used in the setting of complex, combined glenoid bone loss patterns (e.g., peripheral and cavitary), severe peripheral defects severely compromising the glenoid vault walls and severe angular deformity with central bone loss. This is more often indicated in the revision setting.

The senior author's preference in cases without glenoid bone loss is to use a standard lateralized baseplate. In cases of glenoid bone loss, he will use an off-the-shelf augment for <5 mm bone loss (Figure 6), BIORSA for 5–10 mm of bone loss, structural allograft or autograft on the glenoid for 10–20 mm of bone loss, and a custom baseplate (Figure 7) or 2-stage iliac crest bone graft (ICBG) reconstruction for >20 mm of bone loss.

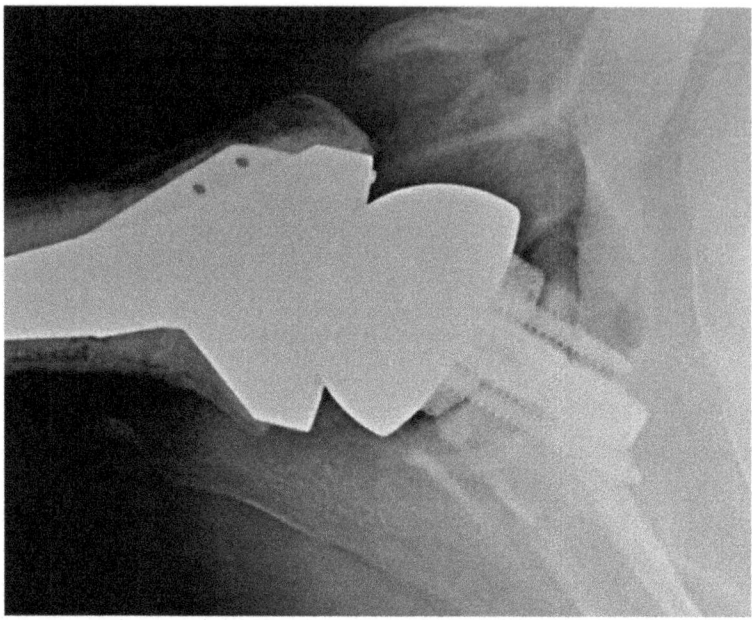

Figure 6. RSA with augmented baseplate. Axillary X-ray of augmented glenoid baseplate.

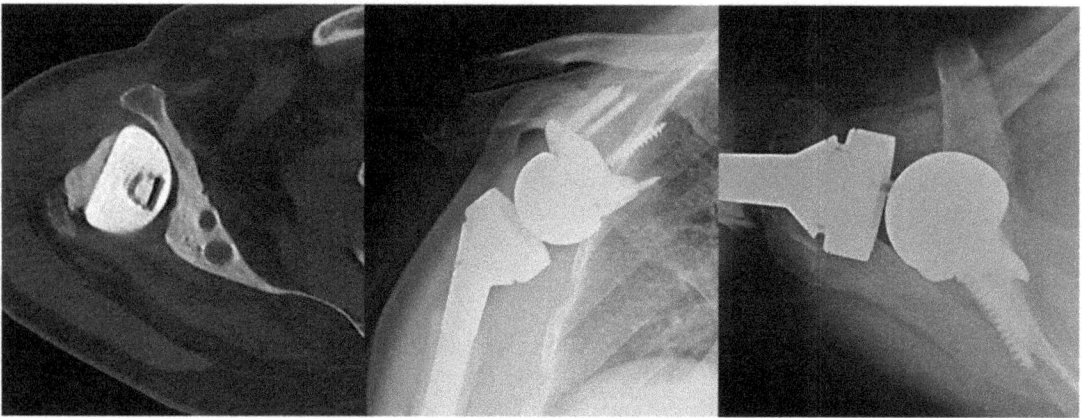

Figure 7. Case of severe glenoid bone loss treated with RSA with custom glenoid component. (**Left**) Axial CT scan of right shoulder status post antibiotic hemiarthroplasty spacer for prior prosthetic joint infection. (**Middle**) AP X-ray of RSA with custom glenoid component. (**Right**) Axillary X-ray of RSA with custom glenoid component.

4. New Perspectives and Innovations in Revision Shoulder Arthroplasty and Complications

4.1. Convertible Implants

Humeral revision can be as complicated as glenoid revision in revision shoulder arthroplasty. Humeral revision is complicated by humeral stems that are challenging to remove and at the same time complicated by bone loss leading to the inability to place new implants with adequate fixation. Solutions on the humeral side include stemmed implants that are convertible, so removal does not need to be performed. Convertible systems have the benefits of an easier revision but can be complicated by improper positioning of the original stem or failure of ability to reduce the implant at the time of revision. Component removal, if required, can be challenging depending on fixation methods and adequacy of fixation. Options include breaking up the fixation from above, osteotomy or windows. In the setting of cement, removal systems can significantly improve the ease of revision as well as eliminate the need for windows to remove cement and plugs. This is especially true in the setting of infection. In the setting of bone loss proximally, options for humeral revision include long-stem cemented or uncemented stems with or without proximal replacement using bone or metal. Various options have their own advantages and disadvantages.

4.2. Humeral Bone Loss

Humeral bone loss is usually seen in the revision setting after failed ORIF, hemiarthroplasty for fracture and failed anatomic TSA, as well as sequalae from a fracture malunion or nonunion or oncologic resection. Like glenoid bone loss, humeral bone loss is a difficult problem associated with several complications post-operatively after an RSA. One commonly cited complication is the loss of rotator cuff function, particularly ER, due to the loss of tuberosities. Loss of the tuberosity is also associated with decreased contour that decreases the deltoid wrap and subsequently alters the deltoid vector. Lastly, aseptic humeral loosening is seen due to the lack of metaphyseal osseous support which increases the torsional forces in the diaphysis.

Treatment options for this include humeral allograft prosthetic composite implants or proximal humeral replacement systems. For the replacement systems, metallic augmentation is used to restore the absent proximal humerus bone to restore the deltoid wrap. These systems also have built in modularity to allow for adjusted length and offset as needed. They rely on diaphyseal fixation and can be either cemented or cementless depending on the quantity and quality of bone available distally. These require bilateral full length humerus films to quantify the amount of bone loss requiring restoration.

5. Innovations in Arthroplasty Technologies

5.1. Patient-Specific Instrumentation and Pre-Operative Planning

Patient-Specific Instrumentation (PSI) systems have been developed to help surgeons more accurately implant the glenoid prosthesis. A patient's preoperative 3D CT scan is used to create a 3D virtual surgery tool that enhances the surgeon's ability to prepare the glenoid surface as well as fix the implant and screws. A meta-analysis of 12 studies comprising 227 participants found that PSI, compared to standard instrumentation methods, significantly improved glenoid positioning and decreased the number of malpositioned components from 68.6% to 15.3% [99]. These systems can be particularly helpful in cases of altered glenoid morphology. Hendel et al. found that in patients with preoperative retroversion >16°, surgeons utilizing PSI were able to place the glenoid component within 1.2° of the ideal position [100]. Though implantation accuracy may be improved with PSI, the long-term clinical outcomes remain to be seen. In knee arthroplasty, for instance, PSI and robotic-assisted surgery have failed to demonstrate improvements in long-term clinical outcomes [101,102]. Robotic-assisted total shoulder arthroplasty is on the horizon, but prior to its widespread implementation, there must be careful consideration of its costs, benefits, and long-term outcomes.

Patient-specific computer modeling and surgeon-controlled 3D planning software have emerged as valuable tools for preoperative planning in shoulder arthroplasty. Statistical shape modeling technology can help quantify glenoid bone defects and virtually reconstruct the glenoid, thus assisting the surgeon to choose a suitable glenoid implant. 3D technologies can predict impingement-free ROM, which could help prevent notching or possible instability secondary to impingement. They also allow the surgeon to virtually plan implant size, implant seating and positioning, appropriate reaming depth, and compare different implant designs before even entering the OR. Patient specific guides can also be created based on these virtual models for use in the OR. The senior author's current preference is to use Blueprint ™ (Stryker, Kalamazoo, MI, USA) 3D planning software for a vast majority of cases.

5.2. Augmented and Mixed Reality Applications in Total Shoulder Arthroplasty

Augmented reality (AR) that is a "digital display overlay on real-world surfaces, allowing for depth perception" can be used in preoperative planning and intraoperative guidance during shoulder arthroplasty [103]. AR has been used in multiple orthopedic procedures and its applications are broadening. Ponce et al. utilized an AR device to enable a surgeon to interact remotely with another surgeon during a TSA via livestreamed video, allowing remote mentoring and guidance [104].

Mixed reality (MR), which consists of a "digital display overlay combined with interactive projected holograms", allows the surgeon to view the real world while manipulating the digital content generated by the device [103]. Gregory et al., in their proof-of-concept study, successfully utilized the HoloLens MR system (Microsoft) to perform a standard RSA, with an operative time of 90 min and a post-op CT confirming proper prosthetic positioning [105].

The ability to visualize data in real time and improve the accuracy of surgical intervention make these reality technologies promising tools for the shoulder arthroplasty surgeon. However, the prohibitive costs of these tools, for now at least, limit their widespread application.

6. Conclusions

As our understanding of the biomechanics of shoulder arthroplasty has expanded over the past decades, as has surgical innovation and the state of the art. Shorter stem or stemless anatomic TSA decreases humeral bone loss and can be beneficial in situations of proximal humerus deformity. Augmented glenoid components reduce bone removal and shear stresses in cases of excess glenoid retroversion, while retaining the benefits of anatomic TSA over RSA. Regarding RSA, metal augmentation, including custom augments, on both the glenoid and humeral side have expanded indications in cases of bone loss. In the setting of revision shoulder arthroplasty, convertible stems and newer tools to improve humeral implant removal can help simplify an already complex surgery. We have now entered an era of computer planning, navigation, PSI, and augmented reality that has redefined preoperative planning and indications, while aiding the surgeon in their operative execution.

Funding: This research received no external funding.

Institutional Review Board Statement: Not applicable.

Informed Consent Statement: Not applicable.

Data Availability Statement: Not applicable.

Conflicts of Interest: The authors declare no conflict of interest.

References

1. Day, J.S.; Lau, E.; Ong, K.L.; Williams, G.R.; Ramsey, M.L.; Kurtz, S.M. Prevalence and projections of total shoulder and elbow arthroplasty in the United States to 2015. *J. Shoulder Elb. Surg.* **2010**, *19*, 1115–1120. [CrossRef] [PubMed]
2. Boileau, P.; Walch, G. The Three-Dimensional Geometry of the Proximal Humerus. *J. Bone Jt. Surg. Br. Vol.* **1997**, *79-B*, 857–865. [CrossRef]
3. Heers, G.; Grifka, J.; An, K.N. Biomechanical considerations on shoulder joint prosthesis implantation. *Der Orthop.* **2001**, *30*, 346–353. [CrossRef] [PubMed]
4. Hawi, N.; Magosch, P.; Tauber, M.; Lichtenberg, S.; Habermeyer, P. Nine-year outcome after anatomic stemless shoulder prosthesis: Clinical and radiologic results. *J. Shoulder Elb. Surg.* **2017**, *26*, 1609–1615. [CrossRef]
5. Kadum, B.; Hassany, H.; Wadsten, M.; Sayed-Noor, A.; Sjödén, G. Geometrical analysis of stemless shoulder arthroplasty: A radiological study of seventy TESS total shoulder prostheses. *Int. Orthop.* **2016**, *40*, 751–758. [CrossRef]
6. Athwal, G.S. Spare the Canal: Stemless Shoulder Arthroplasty Is Finally Here. *J. Bone Jt. Surg.* **2016**, *98*, e28. [CrossRef]

7. Brabston, E.W.; Fehringer, E.V.; Owen, M.T.; Ponce, B.A. Stemless Humeral Implants in Total Shoulder Arthroplasty. *J. Am. Acad. Orthop. Surg.* **2020**, *28*, e277–e287. [CrossRef]
8. Krukenberg, A.; McBirnie, J.; Bartsch, S.; Böhler, N.; Wiedemann, E.; Jost, B.; Mansat, P.; Bellon-Champel, P.; Angeloni, R.; Scheibel, M. Sidus Stem-Free Shoulder System for primary osteoarthritis: Short-term results of a multicenter study. *J. Shoulder Elb. Surg.* **2018**, *27*, 1483–1490. [CrossRef]
9. Habermeyer, P.; Lichtenberg, S.; Tauber, M.; Magosch, P. Midterm results of stemless shoulder arthroplasty: A prospective study. *J. Shoulder Elb. Surg.* **2015**, *24*, 1463–1472. [CrossRef]
10. Alikhah, A.; Imiolczyk, J.P.; Krukenberg, A.; Scheibel, M. Screw fixation in stemless shoulder arthroplasty for the treatment of primary osteoarthritis leads to less osteolysis when compared to impaction fixation. *BMC Musculoskelet. Disord.* **2020**, *21*, 295. [CrossRef]
11. Huguet, D.; DeClercq, G.; Rio, B.; Teissier, J.; Zipoli, B. Results of a new stemless shoulder prosthesis: Radiologic proof of maintained fixation and stability after a minimum of three years' follow-up. *J. Shoulder Elb. Surg.* **2010**, *19*, 847–852. [CrossRef] [PubMed]
12. Berth, A.; Pap, G. Stemless shoulder prosthesis versus conventional anatomic shoulder prosthesis in patients with osteoarthritis. *J. Orthop. Traumatol.* **2013**, *14*, 31–37. [CrossRef] [PubMed]
13. Bell, S.N.; Coghlan, J.A. Short stem shoulder replacement. *Int. J. Shoulder Surg.* **2014**, *8*, 72–75. [CrossRef] [PubMed]
14. Churchill, R.S.; Chuinard, C.; Wiater, J.M.; Friedman, R.; Freehill, M.; Jacobson, S.; Spencer, E.; Holloway, G.B.; Wittstein, J.; Lassiter, T.; et al. Clinical and Radiographic Outcomes of the Simpliciti Canal-Sparing Shoulder Arthroplasty System. *J. Bone Jt. Surg.* **2016**, *98*, 552–560. [CrossRef] [PubMed]
15. Collin, P.; Matsukawa, T.; Boileau, P.; Brunner, U.; Walch, G. Is the humeral stem useful in anatomic total shoulder arthroplasty? *Int. Orthop.* **2017**, *41*, 1035–1039. [CrossRef]
16. Beck, S.; Beck, V.; Wegner, A.; Dudda, M.; Patsalis, T.; Jäger, M. Long-term survivorship of stemless anatomical shoulder replacement. *Int. Orthop.* **2018**, *42*, 1327–1330. [CrossRef]
17. Uschok, S.; Magosch, P.; Moe, M.; Lichtenberg, S.; Habermeyer, P. Is the stemless humeral head replacement clinically and radiographically a secure equivalent to standard stem humeral head replacement in the long-term follow-up? A prospective randomized trial. *J. Shoulder Elb. Surg.* **2017**, *26*, 225–232. [CrossRef]
18. Aibinder, W.R.; Bartels, D.W.; Sperling, J.W.; Sanchez-Sotelo, J. Mid-term radiological results of a cementless short humeral component in anatomical and reverse shoulder arthroplasty. *Bone Jt. J.* **2019**, *101-B*, 610–614. [CrossRef]
19. Schnetzke, M.; Preis, A.; Coda, S.; Raiss, P.; Loew, M. Anatomical and reverse shoulder replacement with a convertible, uncemented short-stem shoulder prosthesis: First clinical and radiological results. *Arch. Orthop. Trauma Surg.* **2017**, *137*, 679–684. [CrossRef]
20. Romeo, A.A.; Thorsness, R.J.; Sumner, S.A.; Gobezie, R.; Lederman, E.S.; Denard, P.J. Short-term clinical outcome of an anatomic short-stem humeral component in total shoulder arthroplasty. *J. Shoulder Elb. Surg.* **2018**, *27*, 70–74. [CrossRef]
21. Garret, J.; Harly, E.; le Huec, J.C.; Brunner, U.; Rotini, R.; Godenèche, A. Pyrolytic carbon humeral head in hemi-shoulder arthroplasty: Preliminary results at 2-year follow-up. *JSES Open Access* **2019**, *3*, 37–42. [CrossRef]
22. Schnetzke, M.; Wittmann, T.; Raiss, P.; Walch, G. Short-term results of a second generation anatomic short-stem shoulder prosthesis in primary osteoarthritis. *Arch. Orthop. Trauma Surg.* **2019**, *139*, 149–154. [CrossRef] [PubMed]
23. Rasmussen, J.V.; Olsen, B.S.; Al-Hamdani, A.; Brorson, S. Outcome of Revision Shoulder Arthroplasty After Resurfacing Hemiarthroplasty in Patients with Glenohumeral Osteoarthritis. *J. Bone Jt. Surg.* **2016**, *98*, 1631–1637. [CrossRef] [PubMed]
24. Hannoun, A.; Ouenzerfi, G.; Brizuela, L.; Mebarek, S.; Bougault, C.; Hassler, M.; Berthier, Y.; Trunfio-Sfarghiu, A.-M. Pyrocarbon versus cobalt-chromium in the context of spherical interposition implants: An in vitro study on cultured chondrocytes. *Eur. Cells Mater.* **2019**, *37*, 1–15. [CrossRef] [PubMed]
25. Klawitter, J.J.; Patton, J.; More, R.; Peter, N.; Podnos, E.; Ross, M. In vitro comparison of wear characteristics of PyroCarbon and metal on bone: Shoulder hemiarthroplasty. *Shoulder Elb.* **2020**, *12*, 11–22. [CrossRef]
26. Hsu, S.H.; Byram, I.R.; Bigliani, L.U. Implant Removal in Revision Arthroplasty: A Tour de Force. *Semin. Arthroplast.* **2012**, *23*, 118–124. [CrossRef]
27. Crosby, L.A.; Wright, T.W.; Yu, S.; Zuckerman, J.D. Conversion to Reverse Total Shoulder Arthroplasty with and without Humeral Stem Retention: The Role of a Convertible-Platform Stem. *J. Bone Jt. Surg.* **2017**, *99*, 736–742. [CrossRef]
28. Wieser, K.; Borbas, P.; Ek, E.T.; Meyer, D.C.; Gerber, C. Conversion of Stemmed Hemi- or Total to Reverse Total Shoulder Arthroplasty: Advantages of a Modular Stem Design. *Clin. Orthop. Relat. Res.* **2015**, *473*, 651–660. [CrossRef]
29. Dilisio, M.F.; Miller, L.R.; Siegel, E.J.; Higgins, L.D. Conversion to Reverse Shoulder Arthroplasty: Humeral Stem Retention Versus Revision. *Orthopedics* **2015**, *38*, e773–e779. [CrossRef]
30. Bercik, M.J.; Kruse, K.; Yalizis, M.; Gauci, M.O.; Chaoui, J.; Walch, G. A modification to the Walch classification of the glenoid in primary glenohumeral osteoarthritis using three-dimensional imaging. *J. Shoulder Elb. Surg.* **2016**, *25*, 1601–1606. [CrossRef]
31. Shapiro, T.A.; McGarry, M.H.; Gupta, R.; Lee, Y.S.; Lee, T.Q. Biomechanical effects of glenoid retroversion in total shoulder arthroplasty. *J. Shoulder Elb. Surg.* **2007**, *16*, S90–S95. [CrossRef] [PubMed]
32. Iannotti, J.P.; Greeson, C.; Downing, D.; Sabesan, V.; Bryan, J.A. Effect of glenoid deformity on glenoid component placement in primary shoulder arthroplasty. *J. Shoulder Elb. Surg.* **2012**, *21*, 48–55. [CrossRef] [PubMed]

33. Sabesan, V.; Callanan, M.; Sharma, V.; Iannotti, J.P. Correction of acquired glenoid bone loss in osteoarthritis with a standard versus an augmented glenoid component. *J. Shoulder Elb. Surg.* **2014**, *23*, 964–973. [CrossRef] [PubMed]
34. Hill, J.M.; Norris, T.R. Long-term results of total shoulder arthroplasty following bone-grafting of the glenoid. *J. Bone Jt. Surg. Am. Vol.* **2001**, *83*, 877–883. [CrossRef]
35. Iannotti, J.P.; Frangiamore, S.J. Fate of large structural allograft for treatment of severe uncontained glenoid bone deficiency. *J. Shoulder Elb. Surg.* **2012**, *21*, 765–771. [CrossRef]
36. Klika, B.J.; Wooten, C.W.; Sperling, J.W.; Steinmann, S.P.; Schleck, C.D.; Harmsen, W.S.; Cofield, R.H. Structural bone grafting for glenoid deficiency in primary total shoulder arthroplasty. *J. Shoulder Elb. Surg.* **2014**, *23*, 1066–1072. [CrossRef]
37. Walch, G.; Moraga, C.; Young, A.; Castellanos-Rosas, J. Results of anatomic nonconstrained prosthesis in primary osteoarthritis with biconcave glenoid. *J. Shoulder Elb. Surg.* **2012**, *21*, 1526–1533. [CrossRef]
38. Priddy, M.; Zarezadeh, A.; Farmer, K.W.; Struk, A.M.; King, J.J.; Wright, T.W.; Schoch, B.S. Early results of augmented anatomic glenoid components. *J. Shoulder Elb. Surg.* **2019**, *28*, S138–S145. [CrossRef]
39. Mizuno, N.; Denard, P.J.; Raiss, P.; Walch, G. Reverse total shoulder arthroplasty for primary glenohumeral osteoarthritis in patients with a biconcave glenoid. *J. Bone Jt. Surg. Am. Vol.* **2013**, *95*, 1297–1304. [CrossRef]
40. Favorito, P.J.; Freed, R.J.; Passanise, A.M.; Brown, M.J. Total shoulder arthroplasty for glenohumeral arthritis associated with posterior glenoid bone loss: Results of an all-polyethylene, posteriorly augmented glenoid component. *J. Shoulder Elb. Surg.* **2016**, *25*, 1681–1689. [CrossRef]
41. Stephens, S.P.; Spencer, E.E.; Wirth, M.A. Radiographic results of augmented all-polyethylene glenoids in the presence of posterior glenoid bone loss during total shoulder arthroplasty. *J. Shoulder Elb. Surg.* **2017**, *26*, 798–803. [CrossRef] [PubMed]
42. Lenart, B.A.; Namdari, S.; Williams, G.R. Total shoulder arthroplasty with an augmented component for anterior glenoid bone deficiency. *J. Shoulder Elb. Surg.* **2016**, *25*, 398–405. [CrossRef] [PubMed]
43. Sandow, M.; Schutz, C. Total shoulder arthroplasty using trabecular metal augments to address glenoid retroversion: The preliminary result of 10 patients with minimum 2-year follow-up. *J. Shoulder Elb. Surg.* **2016**, *25*, 598–607. [CrossRef] [PubMed]
44. Norris, T.R.; Iannotti, J.P. Functional outcome after shoulder arthroplasty for primary osteoarthritis: A multicenter study. *J. Shoulder Elb. Surg.* **2002**, *11*, 130–135. [CrossRef] [PubMed]
45. Papadonikolakis, A.; Neradilek, M.B.; Matsen, F.A. Failure of the glenoid component in anatomic total shoulder arthroplasty: A systematic review of the English-language literature between 2006 and 2012. *J. Bone Jt. Surg. Am. Vol.* **2013**, *95*, 2205–2212. [CrossRef]
46. Strauss, E.J.; Roche, C.; Flurin, P.H.; Wright, T.; Zuckerman, J.D. The glenoid in shoulder arthroplasty. *J. Shoulder Elb. Surg.* **2009**, *18*, 819–833. [CrossRef]
47. Taunton, M.J.; McIntosh, A.L.; Sperling, J.W.; Cofield, R.H. Total shoulder arthroplasty with a metal-backed, bone-ingrowth glenoid component. Medium to long-term results. *J. Bone Jt. Surg. Am. Vol.* **2008**, *90*, 2180–2188. [CrossRef]
48. Vavken, P.; Sadoghi, P.; von Keudell, A.; Rosso, C.; Valderrabano, V.; Müller, A.M. Rates of radiolucency and loosening after total shoulder arthroplasty with pegged or keeled glenoid components. *J. Bone Jt. Surg. Am. Vol.* **2013**, *95*, 215–221. [CrossRef]
49. Clitherow, H.D.S.; Frampton, C.M.A.; Astley, T.M. Effect of glenoid cementation on total shoulder arthroplasty for degenerative arthritis of the shoulder: A review of the New Zealand National Joint Registry. *J. Shoulder Elb. Surg.* **2014**, *23*, 775–781. [CrossRef]
50. Fox, T.J.; Foruria, A.M.; Klika, B.J.; Sperling, J.W.; Schleck, C.D.; Cofield, R.H. Radiographic survival in total shoulder arthroplasty. *J. Shoulder Elb. Surg.* **2013**, *22*, 1221–1227. [CrossRef]
51. Wirth, M.A.; Loredo, R.; Garcia, G.; Rockwood, C.A.; Southworth, C.; Iannotti, J.P. Total shoulder arthroplasty with an all-polyethylene pegged bone-ingrowth glenoid component: A clinical and radiographic outcome study. *J. Bone Jt. Surg. Am. Vol.* **2012**, *94*, 260–267. [CrossRef] [PubMed]
52. Gagliano, J.R.; Helms, S.M.; Colbath, G.P.; Przestrzelski, B.T.; Hawkins, R.J.; DesJardins, J.D. A comparison of onlay versus inlay glenoid component loosening in total shoulder arthroplasty. *J. Shoulder Elb. Surg.* **2017**, *26*, 1113–1120. [CrossRef] [PubMed]
53. Cvetanovich, G.L.; Naylor, A.J.; O'Brien, M.C.; Waterman, B.R.; Garcia, G.H.; Nicholson, G.P. Anatomic total shoulder arthroplasty with an inlay glenoid component: Clinical outcomes and return to activity. *J. Shoulder Elb. Surg.* **2020**, *29*, 1188–1196. [CrossRef] [PubMed]
54. Egger, A.C.; Peterson, J.; Jones, M.H.; Miniaci, A. Total shoulder arthroplasty with nonspherical humeral head and inlay glenoid replacement: Clinical results comparing concentric and nonconcentric glenoid stages in primary shoulder arthritis. *JSES Open Access* **2019**, *3*, 145–153. [CrossRef]
55. Uribe, J.; Luis Vargas John, Z. Minimum 2 Years Outcomes of Powerlifters and Bodybuilders with advanced Glenohumeral arthritis, managed with Stemless aspherical humeral head resurfacing and inlay glenoid. *Orthop. J. Sports Med.* **2020**, *8*. [CrossRef]
56. Magosch, P.; Lichtenberg, S.; Tauber, M.; Martetschläger, F.; Habermeyer, P. Prospective midterm results of a new convertible glenoid component in anatomic shoulder arthroplasty: A cohort study. *Arch. Orthop. Trauma Surg.* **2021**, *141*, 717–724. [CrossRef]
57. Merolla, G.; Chin, P.; Sasyniuk, T.M.; Paladini, P.; Porcellini, G. Total shoulder arthroplasty with a second-generation tantalum trabecular metal-backed glenoid component: Clinical and radiographic outcomes at a mean follow-up of 38 months. *Bone Jt. J.* **2016**, *98-B*, 75–80. [CrossRef]
58. Watson, S.T.; Gudger, G.K.; Long, C.D.; Tokish, J.M.; Tolan, S.J. Outcomes of Trabecular Metal-backed glenoid components in anatomic total shoulder arthroplasty. *J. Shoulder Elb. Surg.* **2018**, *27*, 493–498. [CrossRef]

59. Valenti, P.; Katz, D.; Kany, J.; Werthel, J.D. Convertible Glenoid Components Facilitate Revisions to Reverse Shoulder Arthroplasty Easier: Retrospective Review of 13 Cases. *Am. J. Orthop.* **2018**, *47*. [CrossRef]
60. Best, M.J.; Aziz, K.T.; Wilckens, J.H.; McFarland, E.G.; Srikumaran, U. Increasing incidence of primary reverse and anatomic total shoulder arthroplasty in the United States. *J. Shoulder Elb. Surg.* **2021**, *30*, 1159–1166. [CrossRef]
61. Grammont, P.M.; Baulot, E. Delta shoulder prosthesis for rotator cuff rupture. *Orthopedics* **1993**, *16*, 65–68. [CrossRef] [PubMed]
62. Gutiérrez, S.; Comiskey, C.A.; Luo, Z.P.; Pupello, D.R.; Frankle, M.A. Range of impingement-free abduction and adduction deficit after reverse shoulder arthroplasty. Hierarchy of surgical and implant-design-related factors. *J. Bone Jt. Surg. Am. Vol.* **2008**, *90*, 2606–2615. [CrossRef] [PubMed]
63. Gutiérrez, S.; Levy, J.C.; Frankle, M.A.; Cuff, D.; Keller, T.S.; Pupello, D.R.; Lee, W.E. Evaluation of abduction range of motion and avoidance of inferior scapular impingement in a reverse shoulder model. *J. Shoulder Elb. Surg.* **2008**, *17*, 608–615. [CrossRef] [PubMed]
64. Keener, J.D.; Patterson, B.M.; Orvets, N.; Aleem, A.W.; Chamberlain, A.M. Optimizing reverse shoulder arthroplasty component position in the setting of advanced arthritis with posterior glenoid erosion: A computer-enhanced range of motion analysis. *J. Shoulder Elb. Surg.* **2018**, *27*, 339–349. [CrossRef]
65. Tashjian, R.Z.; Burks, R.T.; Zhang, Y.; Henninger, H.B. Reverse total shoulder arthroplasty: A biomechanical evaluation of humeral and glenosphere hardware configuration. *J. Shoulder Elb. Surg.* **2015**, *24*, e68–e77. [CrossRef]
66. Werner, B.S.; Chaoui, J.; Walch, G. The influence of humeral neck shaft angle and glenoid lateralization on range of motion in reverse shoulder arthroplasty. *J. Shoulder Elb. Surg.* **2017**, *26*, 1726–1731. [CrossRef]
67. Roche, C.P.; Diep, P.; Hamilton, M.; Crosby, L.A.; Flurin, P.-H.; Wright, T.W.; Zuckerman, J.D.; Routman, H.D. Impact of inferior glenoid tilt, humeral retroversion, bone grafting, and design parameters on muscle length and deltoid wrapping in reverse shoulder arthroplasty. *Bull. Hosp. Jt. Dis.* **2013**, *71*, 284–293.
68. Chan, K.; Langohr, G.D.G.; Mahaffy, M.; Johnson, J.A.; Athwal, G.S. Does Humeral Component Lateralization in Reverse Shoulder Arthroplasty Affect Rotator Cuff Torque? Evaluation in a Cadaver Model. *Clin. Orthop. Relat. Res.* **2017**, *475*, 2564–2571. [CrossRef]
69. Henninger, H.B.; Barg, A.; Anderson, A.E.; Bachus, K.N.; Burks, R.T.; Tashjian, R.Z. Effect of lateral offset center of rotation in reverse total shoulder arthroplasty: A biomechanical study. *J. Shoulder Elb. Surg.* **2012**, *21*, 1128–1135. [CrossRef]
70. Giles, J.W.; Langohr, G.D.G.; Johnson, J.A.; Athwal, G.S. Implant Design Variations in Reverse Total Shoulder Arthroplasty Influence the Required Deltoid Force and Resultant Joint Load. *Clin. Orthop. Relat. Res.* **2015**, *473*, 3615–3626. [CrossRef]
71. Wong, M.T.; Langohr, G.D.G.; Athwal, G.S.; Johnson, J.A. Implant positioning in reverse shoulder arthroplasty has an impact on acromial stresses. *J. Shoulder Elb. Surg.* **2016**, *25*, 1889–1895. [CrossRef] [PubMed]
72. Costantini, O.; Choi, D.S.; Kontaxis, A.; Gulotta, L.V. The effects of progressive lateralization of the joint center of rotation of reverse total shoulder implants. *J. Shoulder Elb. Surg.* **2015**, *24*, 1120–1128. [CrossRef] [PubMed]
73. Yang, C.-C.; Lu, C.-L.; Wu, C.-H.; Wu, J.-J.; Huang, T.-L.; Chen, R.; Yeh, M.-K. Stress analysis of glenoid component in design of reverse shoulder prosthesis using finite element method. *J. Shoulder Elb. Surg.* **2013**, *22*, 932–939. [CrossRef] [PubMed]
74. Virani, N.A.; Harman, M.; Li, K.; Levy, J.; Pupello, D.R.; Frankle, M.A. In vitro and finite element analysis of glenoid bone/baseplate interaction in the reverse shoulder design. *J. Shoulder Elb. Surg.* **2008**, *17*, 509–521. [CrossRef] [PubMed]
75. Hamilton, M.A.; Diep, P.; Roche, C.; Flurin, P.H.; Wright, T.W.; Zuckerman, J.D.; Routman, H. Effect of reverse shoulder design philosophy on muscle moment arms. *J. Orthop. Res. Off. Publ. Orthop. Res. Soc.* **2015**, *33*, 605–613. [CrossRef]
76. Liou, W.; Yang, Y.; Petersen-Fitts, G.R.; Lombardo, D.J.; Stine, S.; Sabesan, V.J. Effect of lateralized design on muscle and joint reaction forces for reverse shoulder arthroplasty. *J. Shoulder Elb. Surg.* **2017**, *26*, 564–572. [CrossRef]
77. Upfill-Brown, A.; Satariano, N.; Feeley, B. Stemless shoulder arthroplasty: Review of short and medium-term results. *JSES Open Access* **2019**, *3*, 154–161. [CrossRef]
78. Levy, O.; Panagopoulos, G.N.; Leonidou, A.; Atoun, E. Stemless reverse shoulder arthroplasty: Indications, technique and European experience. *Ann. Jt.* **2018**, *3*, 108. [CrossRef]
79. Liu, E.Y.; Kord, D.; Yee, N.J.; Horner, N.S.; Al Mana, L.; Leroux, T.; Alolabi, B.; Khan, M. Stemless reverse total shoulder arthroplasty: A systematic review of short- and mid-term results. *Shoulder Elb.* **2021**, *13*, 482–491. [CrossRef]
80. Leonidou, A.; Virani, S.; Buckle, C.; Yeoh, C.; Relwani, J. Reverse shoulder arthroplasty with a cementless short metaphyseal humeral prosthesis without a stem: Survivorship, early to mid-term clinical and radiological outcomes in a prospective study from an independent centre. *Eur. J. Orthop. Surg. Traumatol. Orthop. Traumatol.* **2020**, *30*, 89–96. [CrossRef]
81. Ballas, R.; Béguin, L. Results of a stemless reverse shoulder prosthesis at more than 58 months mean without loosening. *J. Shoulder Elb. Surg.* **2013**, *22*, e1–e6. [CrossRef] [PubMed]
82. Kadum, B.; Mukka, S.; Englund, E.; Sayed-Noor, A.; Sjödén, G. Clinical and radiological outcome of the Total Evolutive Shoulder System (TESS®) reverse shoulder arthroplasty: A prospective comparative non-randomised study. *Int. Orthop.* **2014**, *38*, 1001–1006. [CrossRef] [PubMed]
83. Lädermann, A.; Denard, P.J.; Collin, P.; Zbinden, O.; Chiu, J.C.-H.; Boileau, P.; Olivier, F.; Walch, G. Effect of humeral stem and glenosphere designs on range of motion and muscle length in reverse shoulder arthroplasty. *Int. Orthop.* **2020**, *44*, 519–530. [CrossRef]

84. Haidamous, G.; Lädermann, A.; Frankle, M.A.; Gorman, R.A.; Denard, P.J. The risk of postoperative scapular spine fracture following reverse shoulder arthroplasty is increased with an onlay humeral stem. *J. Shoulder Elb. Surg.* **2020**, *29*, 2556–2563. [CrossRef] [PubMed]
85. Cho, N.S.; Nam, J.H.; Hong, S.J.; Kim, T.W.; Lee, M.G.; Ahn, J.T.; Rhee, Y.G. Radiologic Comparison of Humeral Position according to the Implant Designs Following Reverse Shoulder Arthroplasty: Analysis between Medial Glenoid/Medial Humerus, Lateral Glenoid/Medial Humerus, and Medial Glenoid/Lateral Humerus Designs. *Clin. Shoulder Elb.* **2018**, *21*, 192–199. [CrossRef] [PubMed]
86. Beltrame, A.; di Benedetto, P.; Cicuto, C.; Cainero, V.; Chisoni, R.; Causero, A. Onlay versus Inlay humeral steam in Reverse Shoulder Arthroplasty (RSA): Clinical and biomechanical study. *Acta Bio-Med. Atenei Parm.* **2019**, *90*, 54–63. [CrossRef]
87. Merolla, G.; Walch, G.; Ascione, F.; Paladini, P.; Fabbri, E.; Padolino, A.; Porcellini, G. Grammont humeral design versus onlay curved-stem reverse shoulder arthroplasty: Comparison of clinical and radiographic outcomes with minimum 2-year follow-up. *J. Shoulder Elb. Surg.* **2018**, *27*, 701–710. [CrossRef] [PubMed]
88. Ascione, F.; Kilian, C.M.; Laughlin, M.S.; Bugelli, G.; Domos, P.; Neyton, L.; Godeneche, A.; Edwards, T.B.; Walch, G. Increased scapular spine fractures after reverse shoulder arthroplasty with a humeral onlay short stem: An analysis of 485 consecutive cases. *J. Shoulder Elb. Surg.* **2018**, *27*, 2183–2190. [CrossRef]
89. Mehta, N.; Hall, D.J.; Pourzal, R.; Garrigues, G.E. The Biomaterials of Total Shoulder Arthroplasty. *JBJS Rev.* **2020**, *8*, e19.00212. [CrossRef]
90. Bracco, P.; Brunella, V.; Zanetti, M.; Luda, M.P.; Costa, L. Stabilisation of ultra-high molecular weight polyethylene with Vitamin E. *Polym. Degrad. Stab.* **2007**, *92*, 2155–2162. [CrossRef]
91. Wolf, C.; Macho, C.; Lederer, K. Accelerated ageing experiments with crosslinked and conventional ultra-high molecular weight polyethylene (UHMW-PE) stabilised with alpha-tocopherol for total joint arthroplasty. *J. Mater. Sci. Mater. Med.* **2006**, *17*, 1333–1340. [CrossRef] [PubMed]
92. Oral, E.; Christensen, S.D.; Malhi, A.S.; Wannomae, K.K.; Muratoglu, O.K. Wear resistance and mechanical properties of highly cross-linked, ultrahigh-molecular weight polyethylene doped with vitamin E. *J. Arthroplast.* **2006**, *21*, 580–591. [CrossRef] [PubMed]
93. Oral, E.; Wannomae, K.K.; Hawkins, N.; Harris, W.H.W.H.; Muratoglu, O.K.O.K. Alpha-tocopherol-doped irradiated UHMWPE for high fatigue resistance and low wear. *Biomaterials* **2004**, *25*, 5515–5522. [CrossRef] [PubMed]
94. Alexander, J.J.; Bell, S.N.; Coghlan, J.; Lerf, R.; Dallmann, F. The effect of vitamin E-enhanced cross-linked polyethylene on wear in shoulder arthroplasty-a wear simulator study. *J. Shoulder Elb. Surg.* **2019**, *28*, 1771–1778. [CrossRef] [PubMed]
95. Mueller, U.; Braun, S.; Schroeder, S.; Schroeder, M.; Sonntag, R.; Jaeger, S.; Kretzer, J.P. Influence of humeral head material on wear performance in anatomic shoulder joint arthroplasty. *J. Shoulder Elb. Surg.* **2017**, *26*, 1756–1764. [CrossRef]
96. Bell, S.N.; Christmas, M.U.S.I.; Coghlan, J.A. Proximal humeral osteolysis and glenoid radiolucent lines in an anatomic shoulder arthroplasty: A comparison of a ceramic and a metal humeral head component. *J. Shoulder Elb. Surg.* **2020**, *29*, 913–923. [CrossRef]
97. Formaini, N.T.; Everding, N.G.; Levy, J.C.; Santoni, B.G.; Nayak, A.N.; Wilson, C.; Cabezas, A.F. The effect of glenoid bone loss on reverse shoulder arthroplasty baseplate fixation. *J. Shoulder Elb. Surg.* **2015**, *24*, e312–e319. [CrossRef]
98. Martin, E.J.; Duquin, T.R.; Ehrensberger, M.T. Reverse total shoulder glenoid baseplate stability with superior glenoid bone loss. *J. Shoulder Elb. Surg.* **2017**, *26*, 1748–1755. [CrossRef]
99. Villatte, G.; Muller, A.S.; Pereira, B.; Mulliez, A.; Reilly, P.; Emery, R. Use of Patient-Specific Instrumentation (PSI) for glenoid component positioning in shoulder arthroplasty. A systematic review and meta-analysis. *PLoS ONE* **2018**, *13*, e0201759. [CrossRef]
100. Hendel, M.D.; Bryan, J.A.; Barsoum, W.K.; Rodriguez, E.J.; Brems, J.J.; Evans, P.J.; Iannotti, J.P. Comparison of patient-specific instruments with standard surgical instruments in determining glenoid component position: A randomized prospective clinical trial. *J. Bone Jt. Surg. Am. Vol.* **2012**, *94*, 2167–2175. [CrossRef]
101. Turgeon, T.R.; Cameron, B.; Burnell, C.D.; Hedden, D.R.; Bohm, E.R. A double-blind randomized controlled trial of total knee replacement using patient-specific cutting block instrumentation versus standard instrumentation. *Can. J. Surg. J. Can. Chir.* **2019**, *62*, 460–467. [CrossRef] [PubMed]
102. Trivedi, N.N.; Shimberg, J.L.; Sivasundaram, L.; Mengers, S.; Salata, M.J.; Voos, J.E.; Gillespie, R.J. Advances in Glenoid Design in Anatomic Total Shoulder Arthroplasty. *J. Bone Jt. Surg. Am. Vol.* **2020**, *102*, 1825–1835. [CrossRef] [PubMed]
103. Verhey, J.T.; Haglin, J.M.; Verhey, E.M.; Hartigan, D.E. Virtual, augmented, and mixed reality applications in orthopedic surgery. *Int. J. Med. Robot. Comput. Assist. Surg. MRCAS* **2020**, *16*, e2067. [CrossRef] [PubMed]
104. Ponce, B.A.; Brabston, E.W.; Zu, S.; Watson, S.L.; Baker, D.; Winn, D.; Guthrie, B.L.; Shenai, M.B. Telemedicine with mobile devices and augmented reality for early postoperative care. In Proceedings of the Annual International Conference of the IEEE Engineering in Medicine and Biology Society, Orlando, FL, USA, 16–20 August 2016; pp. 4411–4414. [CrossRef]
105. Gregory, T.M.; Gregory, J.; Sledge, J.; Allard, R.; Mir, O. Surgery guided by mixed reality: Presentation of a proof of concept. *Acta Orthop.* **2018**, *89*, 480–483. [CrossRef]

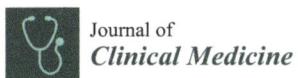

Article

Projections of Primary and Revision Shoulder Arthroplasty until 2040: Facing a Massive Rise in Fracture-Related Procedures

Alexander Klug [1,*], Eva Herrmann [2], Sebastian Fischer [1], Reinhard Hoffmann [1] and Yves Gramlich [1]

[1] Abteilung für Unfallchirurgie und Orthopädische Chirurgie, BG Unfallklinik Frankfurt am Main gGmbH, Friedberger Landstrasse 430, 60389 Frankfurt am Main, Germany; sebastian.fischer@bgu-frankfurt.de (S.F.); reinhard.hoffmann@bgu-frankfurt.de (R.H.); yves.gramlich@bgu-frankfurt.de (Y.G.)

[2] Institut für Biostatistik und Mathematische Modellierung, Goethe-Universität Frankfurt am Main, Theodor-Stern-Kai 7, 60596 Frankfurt am Main, Germany; herrmann@med.uni-frankfurt.de

* Correspondence: alexander.klug@bgu-frankfurt.de; Tel.: +49-69-475-1594

Abstract: Although the demand for shoulder arthroplasties has reached its highest number worldwide, there remains a lack of epidemiologic data regarding recent and future trends. In this study, data for all shoulder arthroplasties (hemiarthroplasty, reverse/anatomic shoulder arthroplasty) from the nationwide inpatient statistics of Germany (2010–2019) and population forecasts until 2040 were gathered. A Poisson and a negative binomial approach using monotone B-splines were modeled for all types of prostheses to project the annual number and incidence of primary and revision arthroplasty. Additionally, trends in main indicators were also gathered and expected changes were calculated. Overall, the number of primary shoulder replacements is set to increase significantly by 2040, reaching at least 37,000 (95% CI 32,000–44,000) procedures per year. This trend is mainly attributable to an about 10-fold increased use of fracture-related reverse shoulder arthroplasty in patients over 80 years of age, although the number of procedures in younger patients will also rise substantially. In contrast, hemiarthroplasties will significantly decrease. The number of revision procedures is projected to increase subsequently, although the revision burden is forecast to decline. Using these country-specific projection approaches, a massive increase of primary and revision shoulder arthroplasties is expected by 2040, mainly due to a rising number of fracture-related procedures. These growth rates are substantially higher than those from hip or knee arthroplasty. As these trends are similar in most Western countries, this draws attention to the international issue, of: if healthcare systems will be able to allocate human and financial resources adequately, and if future research and fracture-prevention programs may help to temper this rising burden in the upcoming decades.

Keywords: shoulder arthroplasty; reverse shoulder arthroplasty; proximal humerus fracture; hemiarthroplasty; projections; revision

1. Introduction

With the baby boomer generation reaching 65 years of age, the socioeconomic issues of an aging population, with higher incidences of degenerative joint diseases [1] and fractures, will certainly affect inpatient care. While the increase in the number of hip and knee arthroplasties is predicted to slow down over the next decades [2–7], only a few studies have examined national trends for upper extremity arthroplasties [8,9]. However, in contrast to hip and knee arthroplasty, the demand and impact of shoulder arthroplasty have been underestimated in the past, probably due to a smaller number of arthroplasties performed per year. In the United States, which is commonly used as a reference in other orthopedic studies, current growth rates for shoulder arthroplasties are reported to be comparable with, or even higher than the growth rates for total hip and knee procedures [8,10]. Furthermore, the projected demand for shoulder arthroplasty is

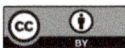

anticipated to increase more rapidly over the next decade based on the future demographic development of the U.S. [9]. However, in contrast to the United States, Germany and many other Western (European) countries face population declines in the near future due to lower birth and immigration rates, which are unable to make up for the aging of the population. Based on current projections, many other countries will likely be heading in the same direction within the next few decades [11,12]. As the incidence of shoulder arthroplasty is higher for older patients, an increased burden in the future has to be expected, as age-related diseases, like osteoarthritis, osteoporosis, frailty-syndrome or injuries are becoming increasingly important. In Germany, the incidence of shoulder arthroplasty is amongst the highest around the world [13], due to a relatively old population and a social healthcare system, which provides almost unlimited access to all parts of orthopedic treatment. However, as the working population is shrinking and increasingly aging, the healthcare system faces the challenge of higher demand and costs.

Furthermore, newer implant designs and expanded indications, such as the use of reverse total shoulder arthroplasty (rTSA) for proximal humerus fractures [14,15], have also led to the rising surgical volume of shoulder arthroplasties in recent years. A shift towards total shoulder arthroplasty (TSA) and away from hemiarthroplasty (HA) procedures have also been reported, presumably because of better outcomes both in degenerative and traumatic conditions [16,17]. However, the contribution of rTSA to future projections of shoulder arthroplasties has not been evaluated yet. Furthermore, the revision burden of these procedures appears to be rising as well [8], which is of particular concern because revision surgery tends to be more complex and cost-intensive than primary arthroplasty [18].

Therefore, the aim of this study was to provide a reliable projection of the future need for primary and revision shoulder arthroplasty to assist orthopedic surgeons, politicians, healthcare providers and other stakeholders (insurances, industry) in providing enough human and financial resources to maintain the current standard of care.

2. Materials and Methods

2.1. Data Collection

An analysis of the data from the national inpatient statistics of Germany (DeStatis) was conducted. This database includes all annual inpatient treatment reports from all German hospitals and medical institutions, making this study a nationwide survey (except military and psychiatric facilities). The data are based on the International Statistical Classification of Diseases and Related Health Problems, Tenth Edition (ICD-10) and the German procedure classification system (OPS), which is the official classification system for encoding surgical procedures in Germany. These statistics contain anonymized data sustaining plausibility checks and data validation on a medical and economic level. All cases reported between 2010 and 2019 were analyzed based on the corresponding OPS codes in its most recent version [19], as well as their associated ICD diagnosis. Data after 2019 was intentionally excluded because of the interference due to the COVID-19 pandemic, which led to a massive reorganization of the medical system in 2020 and early 2021. All patients with shoulder arthroplasty, including either anatomic or reverse arthroplasty and all hemiarthroplasties, as well as all revision shoulder arthroplasties and explanations, were identified. During the study period, no coding changes were performed. Age was categorized in the following groups: <55, 55–59, 60–64, 65–69, 70–74, 75–79, 80–84, 85–89, and older than 90 years.

Population data was available from official population projection statistics until 2040 [20]. These population projections consider the future mortality and increased life expectancy for the oldest population groups, and the immigration rate.

2.2. Data Analysis

Data from 2010 to 2019 (baseline years) and population forecasts up to the year 2040 were used to project the annual incidence of shoulder arthroplasty in Germany. A linear

(Poisson, "classic approach") regression analysis was performed to estimate the expected incidence with the calendar year, sex, and patient age as covariates. The incidence was calculated by dividing the estimated number of arthroplasties for the national total and for each age subgroup by the corresponding official population forecast. An offset variable for the size of the population was chosen to ensure that the procedural number did not exceed the total population number. To overcome overdispersion problems that could result in an underestimation of the variance, we used a robust sandwich covariance matrix estimator for variance calculation. To minimize the error of variance underestimation of the estimated parameter because of overdispersion, we applied a quasi-Poisson regression to our data in accordance with the theory of quasi-likelihood.

As regressions based on logarithm, or an exponent, like Poisson, will only fit optimally when that is the exact nature of the true relationship, they might not be economically plausible, as in principle the projected counts can rise to infinity. In contrast, it seems quite reasonable to imagine that there might rather be an asymptotic or curvilinear relationship. To overcome this issue, an alternative estimate of the TSA projections was also determined by fitting the incidence rates (counts per 100,000 persons and year) with a negative binomial regression model using a monotone B-spline approach ("new approach") for modeling time effects and accounting for respective gender and age groups. Splines are used in statistics in order to mathematically reproduce flexible shapes. Knots are placed at several places within the data range, to identify the points where adjacent functional pieces join each other. The advantage of using splines for yearly data compared to the traditional approach is the more accurate curve estimation for the nonlinear trend changes and the simple way of modeling interactions between the time variables.

To compare the prediction accuracy of each model, the dataset was then split into training (years 2010–2017) and testing subsets (years 2018–2019). Both models were analyzed regarding common forecast accuracy measurement instruments (mean squared error (MSE), root mean squared error (RMSE), the mean absolute percentage error (MAPE) and Theil's U inequality coefficients, of which the first (U1) is a measure of forecast accuracy and the second (U2) is a measure of forecast quality [21]), which showed lower and thus more accurate values for the negative binomial approach using monotone B-splines (Table 1).

Table 1. Two-year forecast accuracy using an out-of-sample training-test validation set (minor numbers indicating greater forecast quality).

Model	MSE	RMSE	MAPE	U1	U2
Poisson	48,816.735	220.945	6.595	0.018	0.009
B-spline	19,724.682	140.445	3.108	0.012	0.006

MSE: mean squared error; RMSE: root mean squared error; MAPE: mean absolute percentage error; U1/2: Thiel's U inequality coefficients.

Because of the anonymization of the diagnosis-related group DRG data, arthroplasty patients who underwent a revision (replacement or explanation) could not be individually followed and therefore, actual revision rates could not be calculated. Instead, we estimated the revision burden (RB) by dividing the number of revisions in the form of replacements or explanations by the number of all primary and revision shoulder arthroplasties (HA and TSA), as described previously [22]. Future projections for revision arthroplasty were also calculated, as mentioned above. For better comparison, a "constant rate" approach was used, based on the average revision burden during the baseline years and the projections of shoulder replacements in 2040.

All statistical analyses were performed using R Version 3.4.0 (R Development Core Team, The R Foundation for Statistical Computing, Vienna, Austria).

3. Results

3.1. Historical Data: Baseline Years 2010–2019

The procedural volume of primary shoulder arthroplasties increased by approximately 14% each year from 13,678 to 25,294 patients, amounting to an incidence rate of 30.4 per 100,000 in 2019 (Figure 1). This development has mainly been attributed to increased utilization of rTSA, for which the number of procedures has almost quadrupled since 2010. In addition, the use of HA decreased by over 70%, while the number and incidence of anatomic total shoulder arthroplasty procedures (aTSA) showed almost steady progress over time. Regarding the demand in different age groups, in 2010, 5.2% of all primary shoulder arthroplasties and only 1.8% of all rTSA procedures were performed in younger patients (55 years or younger). By the end of 2019, the relative size of this population had decreased to 4.1% and 1.4%, respectively. Overall, an enormous increase in fracture-related arthroplasty could be identified, with the number of fracture-related rTSA showing an almost ten-fold increase during that time span (Figure 2). Additionally, the overall number of osteoarthritis (OA)-related procedures also almost tripled, with rTSA becoming increasingly important compared to aTSA or HA.

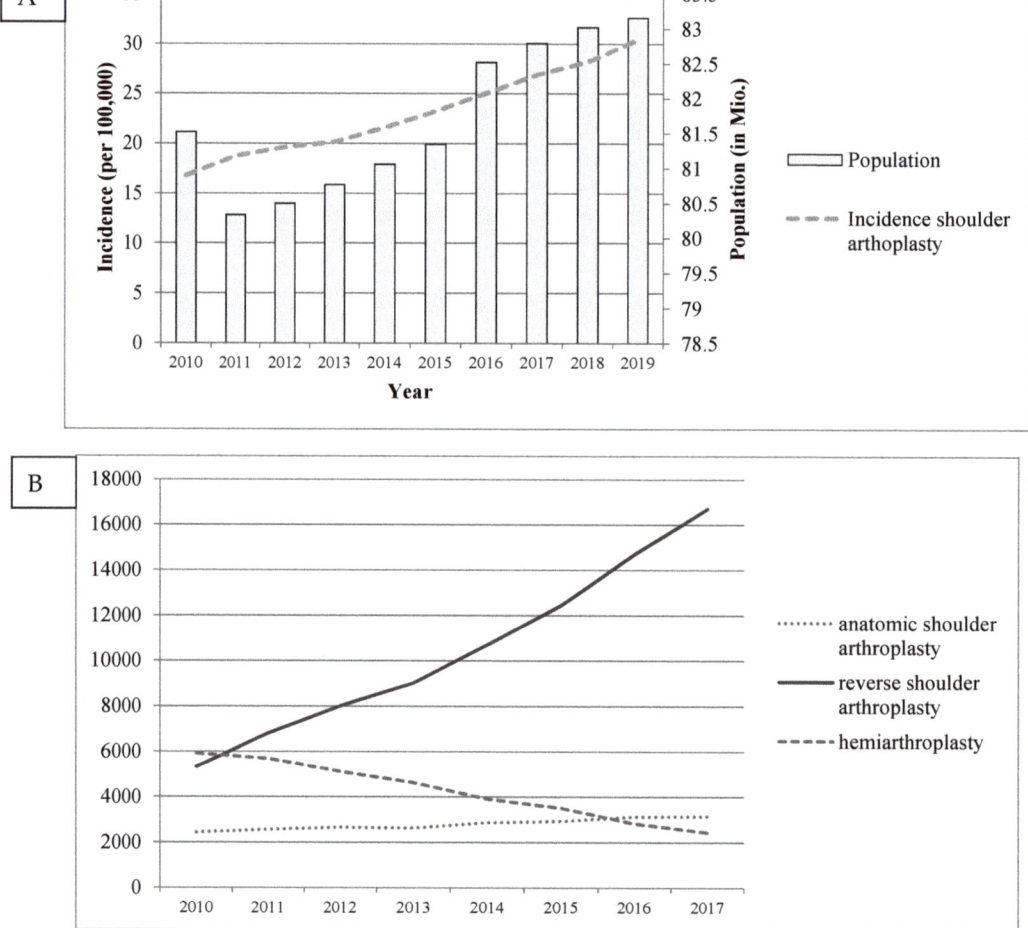

Figure 1. German population, shoulder arthroplasty incidence (**A**) and type of procedure (**B**) from 2010 to 2017.

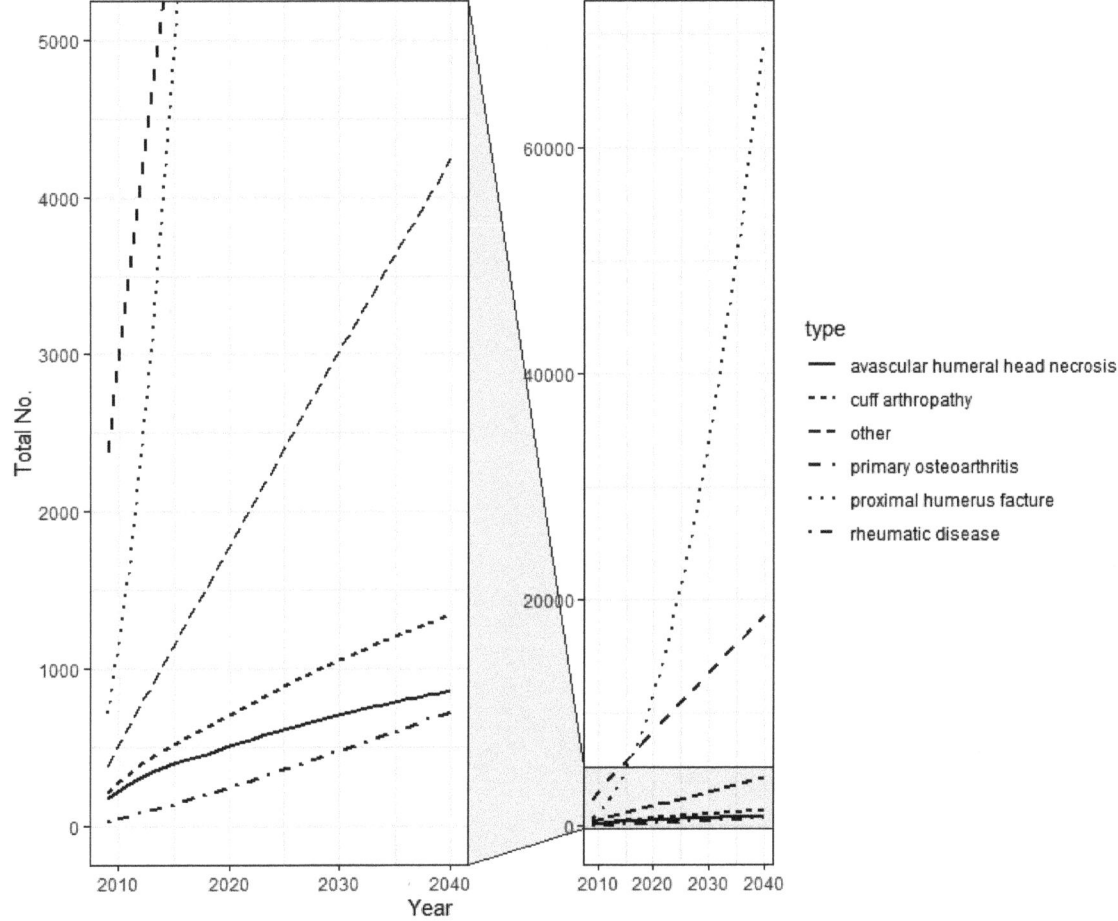

Figure 2. Historical and projected main indications for reverse shoulder arthroplasty from 2010 to 2040.

During the study period, 19,190 revision procedures (replacements or explanations) were undertaken, which included 5748 revisions for HA and 13,241 for TSA, with an overall RB of 12.9% for HA and 7.0% for TSA. However, we identified a slight RB decrease for TSA, while the RB for HA significantly increased (from 7.1% to 18.4%). For both procedure types, a 1.2-fold higher relative risk for revision was calculated for males compared with females.

3.2. Projection of Primary Shoulder Arthroplasty: Years 2020–2040

Based on our quasi-Poisson projection model, the annual number of shoulder replacements is estimated to grow to 95×10^3 (95% CI 79–112 $\times 10^3$) by 2040 (Figure 3). The forecasted incidence rate was projected to be 112 (95% CI 91–134) per 100,000 German residents, resulting in a more than seven-fold growth from 2010 to 2040. Additionally, we used a negative binomial approach with monotone B-splines to achieve a different projective view on the future demand for shoulder arthroplasty. This model projected the annual number of shoulder replacements to rise to 37×10^3 (95% CI 32–44 $\times 10^3$) by 2040, leading to an incidence rate of 47 (95% CI 41–55) per 100,000 inhabitants, which still represents a rise of approximately 175% since 2010.

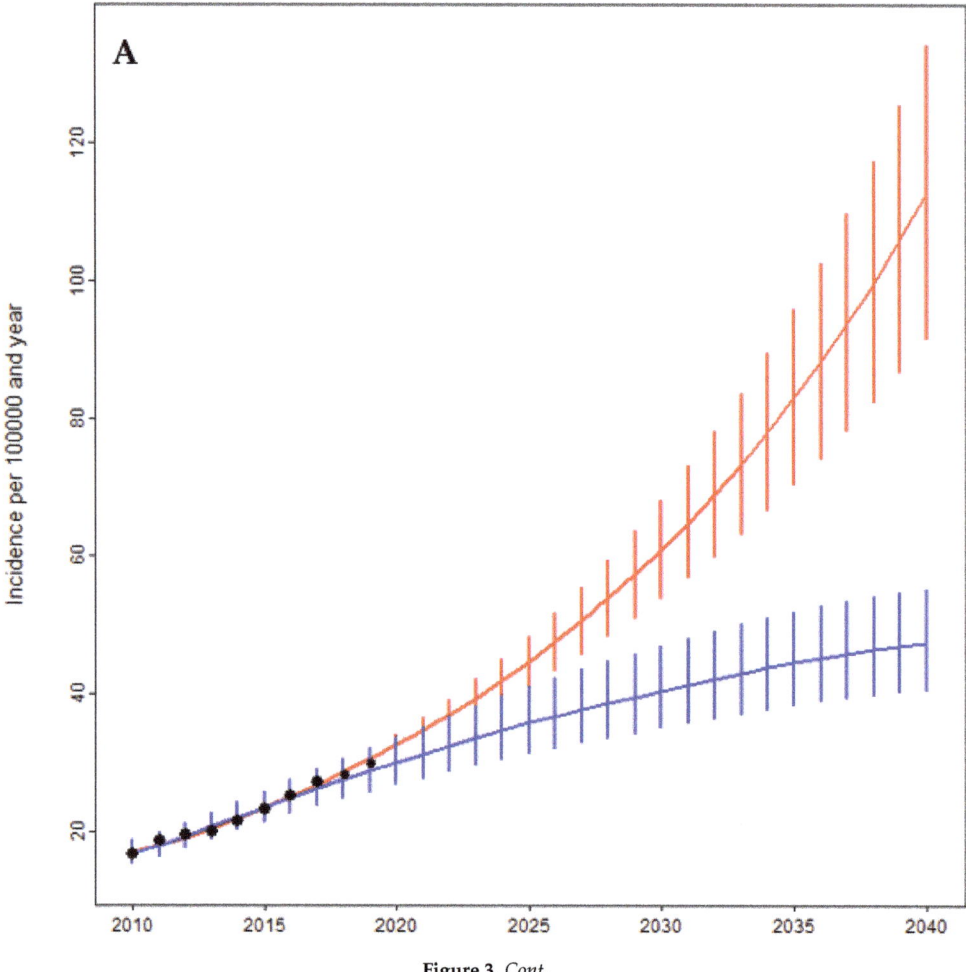

Figure 3. *Cont.*

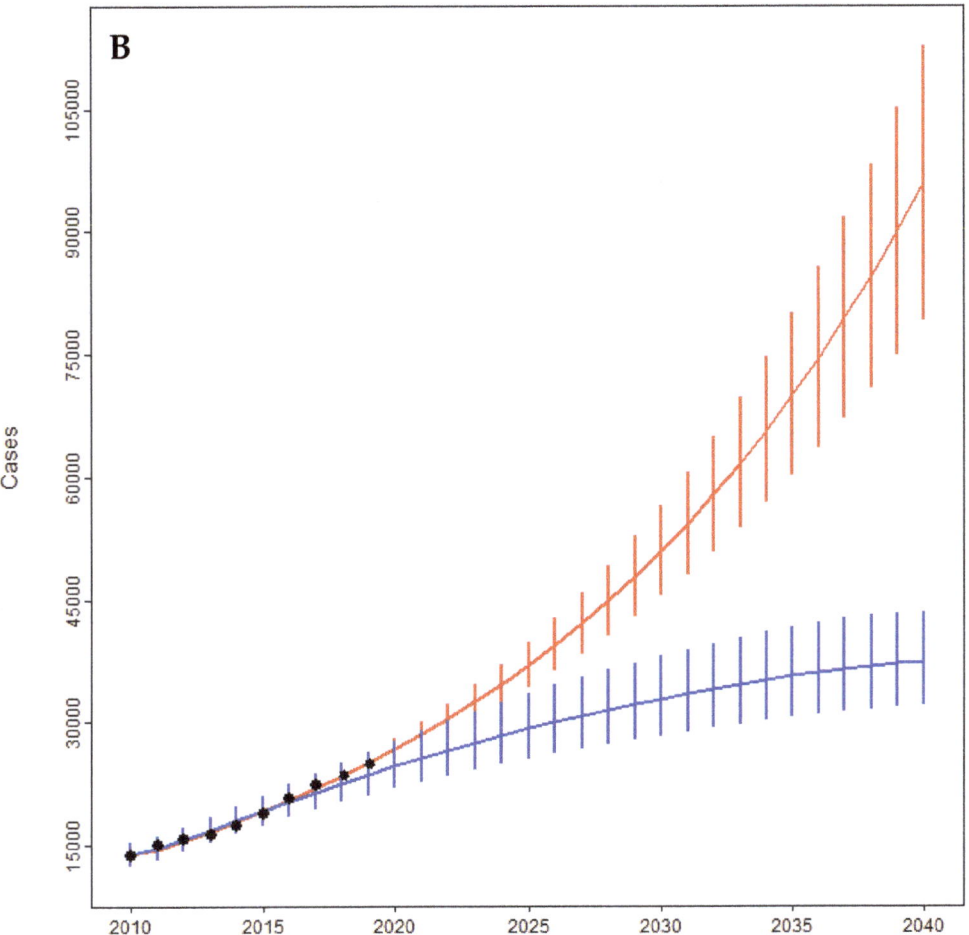

Figure 3. Projections of the incidence (**A**) and total number (**B**) of shoulder arthroplasties by the year 2040 based on a Poisson (red) and a negative binomial regression model using a monotone B-spline approach (blue). The black points represent the historical numbers.

3.3. Projections of Shoulder Arthroplasty as a Function of Age

Considering age, the incidence rates almost doubled in each age group, while the total amount of shoulder replacements showed the highest increase in older patients (Figure 4). This increase can mainly be attributed to the rising utilization of rTSA, which will be responsible for over 90% of all shoulder replacements in 2040 if our projections hold true (Figure 5). These arthroplasties will be performed due to a massive increase in fracture-related scenarios, which could reach an eight-fold increase by 2040 (Figure 2).

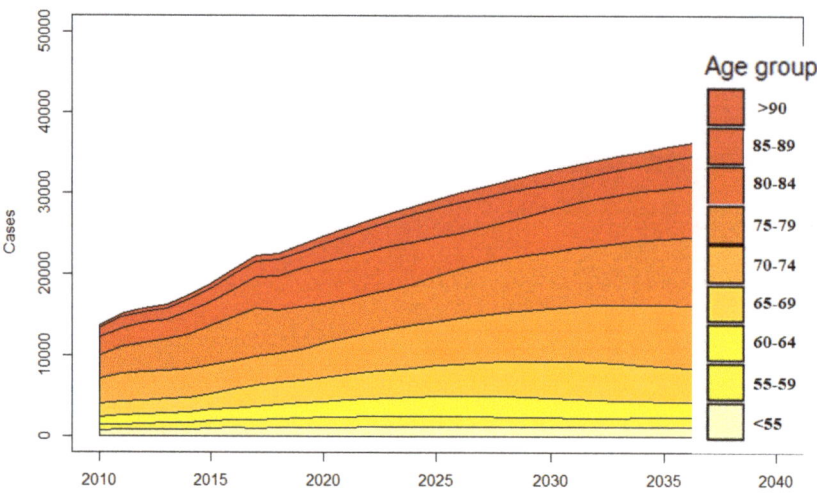

Figure 4. Reported and predicted case numbers per age group from 2010 to 2040.

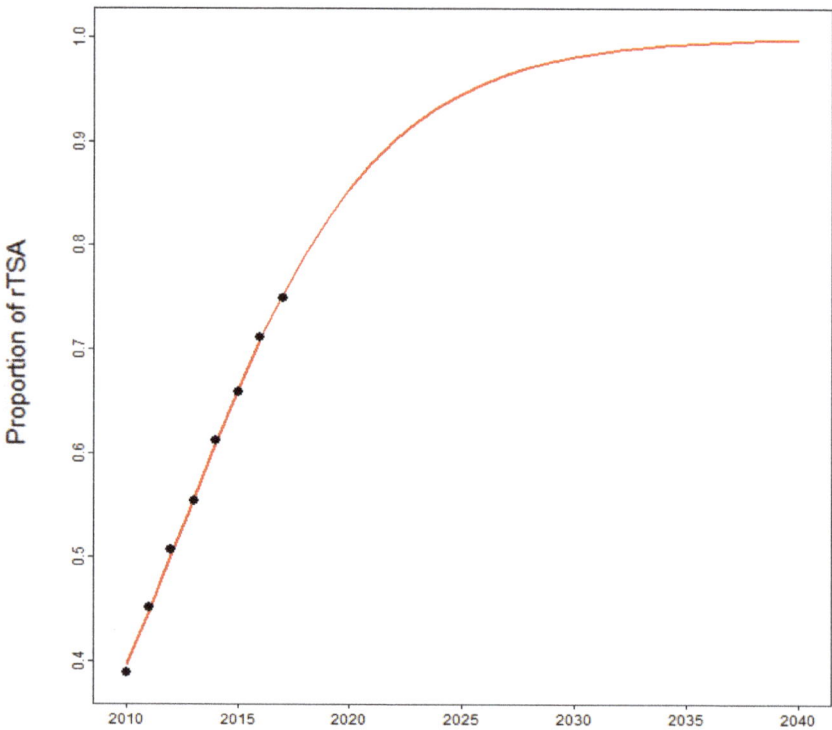

Figure 5. Projected share of reverse total shoulder arthroplasties (rTSA) in total shoulder arthroplasties from 2010 to 2040.

Despite a simultaneously rising number of TSA in younger patients, the demand for primary shoulder arthroplasties among patients aged 55 y or younger was projected to decrease from 5.2% in 2010 to 3.2% (95% CI, 2.7–3.6) of all recipients by 2040.

3.4. Projections of Revision Shoulder Arthroplasty

Along with the rising number of primary replacements, the number of revision procedures is projected to increase as well. Based on our models, this number will reach its maximum of approximately 4000 (upper 95% CI limit: 9000) procedures in 2040, which represents an increase of approximately 300%. However, because of the higher future number of rTSA, which was associated with a lower RB, the overall estimated RB will decline. For better comparison, we also calculated the number of revision procedures using a constant-rate approach. Here, we calculated the highest number of revision procedures of 4100 (95% CI 3568–4852, monotone B-spline approach) and 10,500 (95% CI 8817–12,558, Poisson modeling), respectively, which represents a 2.5 to 8.4-fold increase in revision procedures (Figure 6).

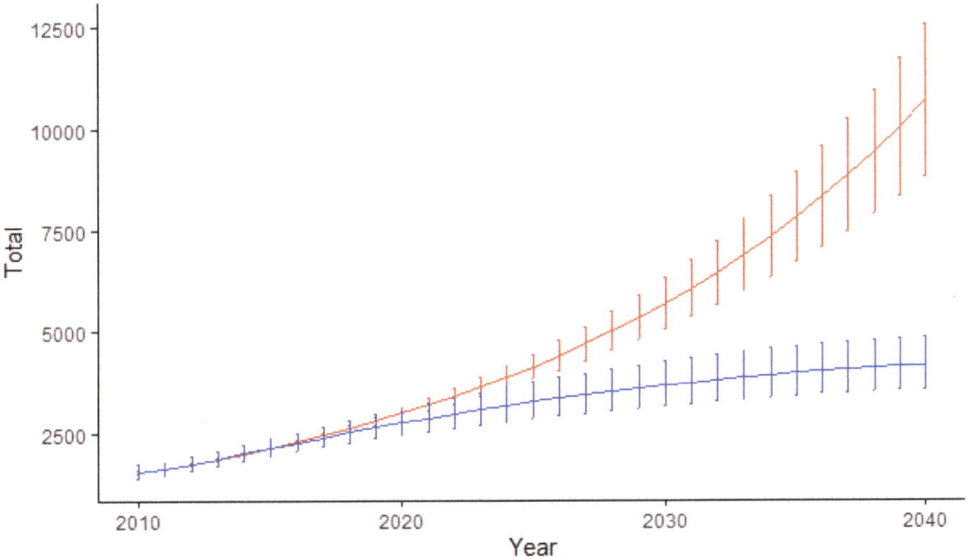

Figure 6. Projections for revision shoulder arthroplasty procedures using a "constant-rate" approach based on a Poisson (red) and a negative binomial regression model using a monotone B-spline approach (blue).

4. Discussion

Despite a rising number of projection studies for hip and knee arthroplasties in recent literature, we still lack empirical results on studies for the upper extremities. Although current growth rates for shoulder arthroplasties are reported to be comparable with, or even higher than the growth rates for total hip and knee procedures [8,10], the demand and impact of shoulder arthroplasty have been underestimated in the past. However, based on evolving scientific evidence regarding good functional outcomes and due to an expanding indication spectrum, shoulder arthroplasty has been one of the main focus in orthopedic surgery in recent years. Therefore, we opted for a data-driven model selection, by minimization of model errors to investigate the trends for primary and revision shoulder arthroplasty procedures from 2010 to 2040. Although both models predicted a slightly different total number due to their distinct intrinsic model assumptions, they showed an important trend during the upcoming decades. Using these models, the number of total shoulder replacements was estimated to grow up to 700%, mainly due to rising adoption of rTSA in fracture-related conditions of the elderly. These growth rates are substantially higher than the current rates of hip and knee arthroplasty [2,7], indicating the immense importance for orthopedic surgeons in the future.

With the total number and incidence of primary TSA procedures rising, we also modeled a rising number of revision procedures, highlighting its increasing burden in the future.

4.1. Projections of Shoulder Arthroplasty and International Comparison

When comparing our projections with other countries, we found that the trend of a rising volume of primary shoulder arthroplasties has also been reported in the United States [10,23,24]. Schwartz et al. detected an over five-fold increase in primary shoulder arthroplasty between 2001 and 2010 [24], while Wagner et al. projected even higher growth rates in upper extremity arthroplasty compared with total hip and knee procedures by the year 2025 (+235% in total volume) [25]. Padegimas et al. even projected the future volume to increase by 755% by 2030. Similar to our results, this can mainly be attributed to an exponential rise in the number of reverse shoulder arthroplasty in the upcoming years, with its prevalence already rising from 7.3 to 19.1 per 100,000 in the U.S. However, the demographic and economic characteristics of the United States cannot easily be transferred to other industrialized countries, although the global demographic pattern of an aging population is identical around the world. However, projections like those of Wagner et al. [25] tend to be overestimated due to a steep increase of procedure volume in the baseline years- a problem we also faced using a Poisson model. For this reason, we implemented an alternative methodical approach, which included a rather asymptotic development of shoulder arthroplasty in the future but still estimated an increase in incidence that is several times higher than the projected increase in hip or knee arthroplasty [2,4,5,26].

These findings are also in line with the most national recent trends for shoulder arthroplasty in Europe. Although population and economic data, as well as procedure selection for the major indications, vary between most countries, Lübbeke et al. [13] reported a strong upward trajectory in the incidence of shoulder arthroplasty in nine registries, concluding that due to growing demand, increasing health care capacity, and/or expanding indications, countries could expect to see this continuation in growth in the future. According to the most recent European study of Villate et al. derived from the French hospital discharge database, the number of total shoulder arthroplasties is projected to rise up to 322% by 2050, representing a future challenge for their healthcare system [27].

4.2. Projections as a Function of Age and Indication

Based on our data projections, this trend is mainly attributed to a considerably increasing utilization and incidence of rTSA in patients older than 80 years, although the number and incidence of procedures performed for younger patients are forecast to rise in the future as well.

While this observed trend is in line with the findings from other countries [13,28], including the United States [9], it is in contrast with the trend seen in hip and knee arthroplasties, where the incidence rate in younger and older patients remained constant over all age groups [2]. This difference may be explained by various factors. First, based on the recent population growth in Germany, the share of patients > 65 years of age is projected to increase from 21% to 30% by the year 2040, which may contribute to a rapid increase in rTSA utilization, as reverse prostheses are rarely implanted in younger patients. Second, the indications for rTSA have been expanding during the last decade, as indicated by the almost ten-fold increase in the number of proximal humerus fractures in this study. Many surgeons may also now see it as a possible solution for poor shoulder conditions, which were previously seen as unsolvable [29]. In complex proximal humerus fractures, which represent the third-most common fracture seen in patients aged > 60 years [30], rTSA was found to provide more reproducible function with better recovery, as well as lower revision rates than HA [31,32]. However, recent studies also suggest, that shoulder arthroplasty due to fracture could be associated with more inconsistent outcomes [33,34] and an increased risk of postoperative complications compared with OA and cuff arthropathy [35]. Additionally, shoulder arthroplasty for fracture seems to lead to an even higher resource utilization [36], which is especially important as we documented a massive increase in these procedures in the upcoming decades, probably affecting future healthcare costs. Against the background of moving toward the era of bundled payment models, an appropriate risk adjustment based on the indication of surgery should, therefore, be promoted to maintain the current standard of care for all patients.

Although we documented a massive increase in fracture-related rTSA in our study, current scientific evidence contrarily suggests, that non-operative treatment may be favorable in the elderly compared to surgical treatment in certain fracture patterns [37,38]. However, based on the increasing demand for self-independency in the elderly, there is still a controversial debate, on which patients may be better treated by surgical intervention. Therefore, it remains to be seen, if this trend may influence the treatment choice and amount of implantations in the future, as the number of proximal humerus fractures will be constantly rising in many European countries over the next decade [39,40].

4.3. Projections of Revision Shoulder Arthroplasty

With the total number and incidence of primary TSA procedures rising, we also modeled a rising number of revision procedures, which has globally never been performed up to date. While we were not able to calculate survival or revision rates because of the aforementioned issue, we used the RB as a surrogate parameter to assess the procedure-specific risk for revision. As a consequence, the actual revision risk, especially for TSA, appears to be underestimated by our calculations, which is why we also used a constant rate approach to estimate the number of revision surgeries based on the RB during the baseline years, which still led to an up to 8.4-fold increase by 2040.

Based on our models, revision surgery for TSA will be significant in 2040 and would be expected to increase even more over time as a direct result of the maturation of the increased number of primary surgeries being performed. This raises the concern if there will be enough resources and trained surgeons to carry out these difficult revision procedures in the future. Against the background of a rising number of fracture-related rTSA, this also highlights the enormous need for adequate fracture-prevention programs, in order to limit the number of revision surgeries in the future, as well.

4.4. Study Limitations

The current study has some limitations. First, although the German population forecasts provided rather good agreement between predicted numbers and confirmed past numbers [2,20], they are typically based on hypothetical future assumptions and are, therefore, potentially uncertain. Second, this type of study was based on the procedural growth trajectory for the years 2010–2019, as a longer time frame was not possible due to coding changes after 2009 and the occurrence of the COVID pandemic after 2019, assuming that this trend will continue. However, it is possible, that after the world has overcome all issues regarding the pandemic, new technologies, surgical innovations, or disruptive innovation techniques, such as cartilage regeneration, tissue engineering, or drug therapies that limit the progression of osteoarthritis or enhance fracture recovery or joint-preserving surgery [41]; as well as health-care reforms or reimbursement changes, will meaningfully affect the relationship between supply and demand for shoulder arthroplasty. Especially, it remains to be seen, if the demand of rTSA for proximal humerus fracture will actually see the projected rise in the future, as more and more studies suggest that non-operative treatment may be more favorable in the elderly compared to a surgical approach [37,38,42].

Overall, in contrast to clinical studies, like randomized controlled trials, which draw evidence from (allegedly) artificially generated data, large database studies, like the presented study, describe results of the actual treatment reality. The current study aims to analyze the current practice and its changes over time, giving the reader an unselected view on surgical demand, which cannot be obtained from case series or prospective studies. Therefore, it has to be seen as an important additive or complementary instrument to clinical studies, providing the possibility to examine the potential effects of current scientific evidence on the daily surgical routine on the one side and to analyze treatment trends, whose causal links can be further analyzed by randomized-controlled studies, on the other side.

5. Conclusions

The current study demonstrates that using a data-driven modeling approach, the rate of both primary and revision shoulder arthroplasty procedures is projected to rapidly increase during the next 20 years, with the rate of fracture-related rTSA, performed in elderly patients, showing the greatest impact of all procedures. In light of limited resources and healthcare budgets, this emphasizes the need for adequate prevention programs on the one side, but also for qualified surgeons to meet the demand and for future research to improve the reliability and survivorship of shoulder arthroplasties on the other side.

Author Contributions: Conceptualization, A.K.; Data curation, A.K. and Y.G.; Formal analysis, A.K. and E.H.; Investigation, A.K. and Y.G.; Methodology, A.K. and E.H.; Project administration, R.H. and Y.G.; Software, E.H.; Supervision, S.F., R.H. and Y.G.; Writing—original draft, A.K.; Writing—review & editing, A.K., S.F. and R.H. All authors have read and agreed to the published version of the manuscript.

Funding: This research received no external funding.

Institutional Review Board Statement: Not applicable.

Informed Consent Statement: Not applicable.

Acknowledgments: We thank Kristina Klug, Goethe-Universität Frankfurt, Frankfurt am Main, Institut für Psychologie, for supporting the authors with the statistical analysis.

Conflicts of Interest: None of the authors, their immediate families, and any research foundation with which they are affiliated received any financial payments or other benefits from any commercial entity related to the subject of this article.

References

1. Nowossadeck, E. Population aging and hospitalization for chronic disease in Germany. *Dtsch. Arztebl. Int.* **2012**, *109*, 151–157. [CrossRef]
2. Pilz, V.; Hanstein, T.; Skripitz, R. Projections of primary hip arthroplasty in Germany until 2040. *Acta Orthop.* **2018**, *89*, 308–313. [CrossRef]
3. Inacio, M.C.S.; Graves, S.E.; Pratt, N.L.; Roughead, E.E.; Nemes, S. Increase in Total Joint Arthroplasty Projected from 2014 to 2046 in Australia: A Conservative Local Model with International Implications. *Clin. Orthop. Relat. Res.* **2017**, *475*, 2130–2137. [CrossRef]
4. Nemes, S.; Gordon, M.; Rogmark, C.; Rolfson, O. Projections of total hip replacement in Sweden from 2013 to 2030. *Acta Orthop.* **2014**, *85*, 238–243. [CrossRef]
5. Kurtz, S.M.; Lau, E.; Ong, K.; Zhao, K.; Kelly, M.; Bozic, K.J. Future young patient demand for primary and revision joint replacement: National projections from 2010 to 2030. *Clin. Orthop. Relat. Res.* **2009**, *467*, 2606–2612. [CrossRef] [PubMed]
6. Sloan, M.; Premkumar, A.; Sheth, N.P. Projected Volume of Primary Total Joint Arthroplasty in the U.S., 2014 to 2030. *J. Bone Jt. Surg. Am.* **2018**, *100*, 1455–1460. [CrossRef] [PubMed]
7. Rupp, M.; Lau, E.; Kurtz, S.M.; Alt, V. Projections of Primary TKA and THA in Germany from 2016 through 2040. *Clin. Orthop. Relat. Res.* **2020**, *478*, 1622–1633. [CrossRef]
8. Day, J.S.; Lau, E.; Ong, K.L.; Williams, G.R.; Ramsey, M.L.; Kurtz, S.M. Prevalence and projections of total shoulder and elbow arthroplasty in the United States to 2015. *J. Shoulder Elbow Surg.* **2010**, *19*, 1115–1120. [CrossRef] [PubMed]
9. Padegimas, E.M.; Maltenfort, M.; Lazarus, M.D.; Ramsey, M.L.; Williams, G.R.; Namdari, S. Future patient demand for shoulder arthroplasty by younger patients: National projections. *Clin. Orthop. Relat. Res.* **2015**, *473*, 1860–1867. [CrossRef]
10. Kim, S.H.; Wise, B.L.; Zhang, Y.; Szabo, R.M. Increasing incidence of shoulder arthroplasty in the United States. *J. Bone Jt. Surg. Am.* **2011**, *93*, 2249–2254. [CrossRef] [PubMed]
11. Coleman, D.; Rowthorn, R. Who's afraid of population decline? A critical examination of its consequences. *Popul. Dev. Rev.* **2011**, *37*, 217–248. [CrossRef]
12. Bengtsson, T.; Scott, K. Population aging and the future of the welfare state: The example of Sweden. *Popul. Dev. Rev.* **2011**, *37*, 158–170. [CrossRef] [PubMed]

13. Lübbeke, A.; Rees, J.L.; Barea, C.; Combescure, C.; Carr, A.J.; Silman, A.J. International variation in shoulder arthroplasty. *Acta Orthop.* **2017**, *88*, 592–599. [CrossRef] [PubMed]
14. Klug, A.; Gramlich, Y.; Wincheringer, D.; Schmidt-Horlohé, K.; Hoffmann, R. Trends in surgical management of proximal humeral fractures in adults: A nationwide study of records in Germany from 2007 to 2016. *Arch. Orthop. Trauma Surg.* **2019**, *139*, 1713–1721. [CrossRef] [PubMed]
15. Luciani, P.; Farinelli, L.; Procaccini, R.; Verducci, C.; Gigante, A. Primary reverse shoulder arthroplasty for acute proximal humerus fractures: A 5-year long term retrospective study of elderly patients. *Injury* **2019**, *50*, 1974–1977. [CrossRef]
16. Ferrel, J.R.; Trinh, T.Q.; Fischer, R.A. Reverse total shoulder arthroplasty versus hemiarthroplasty for proximal humeral fractures: A systematic review. *J. Orthop. Trauma* **2015**, *29*, 60–68. [CrossRef] [PubMed]
17. Jonsson, E.Ö.; Ekholm, C.; Salomonsson, B.; Demir, Y.; Olerud, P. Reverse total shoulder arthroplasty provides better shoulder function than hemiarthroplasty for displaced 3- and 4-part proximal humeral fractures in patients aged 70 years or older: A multicenter randomized controlled trial. *J. Shoulder Elbow Surg.* **2021**, *30*, 994–1006. [CrossRef]
18. Gauci, M.-O.; Cavalier, M.; Gonzalez, J.-F.; Holzer, N.; Baring, T.; Walch, G.; Boileau, P. Revision of failed shoulder arthroplasty: Epidemiology, etiology, and surgical options. *J. Shoulder Elbow Surg.* **2020**, *29*, 541–549. [CrossRef]
19. DIMDI. *Systematisches Verzeichnis—Operationen-und Prozedurenschlüssel—Internationale Klassifikation der Prozeduren in der Medizin (OPS)*; DIMDI unter Beteiligung der Arbeitsgruppe OPS des Kuratoriums für Fragen der Klassifikation im Gesundheitswesen (KKG): Cologne, Germany, 2010–2019.
20. Pötzsch, O.R.F. *Demographic Analyses, Methods and Projections, Births and Deaths: Germany's Population by 2060—Results of the 13th Coordinated Population Projection*; Federal Statistical Office of Germany: Wiesbaden, Germany, 2015.
21. Bliemel, F. Theil's Forecast Accuracy Coefficient: A Clarification. *J. Mark. Res.* **1973**, *10*, 444. [CrossRef]
22. Hollatz, M.F.; Stang, A. Nationwide shoulder arthroplasty rates and revision burden in Germany: Analysis of the national hospitalization data 2005 to 2006. *J. Shoulder Elbow Surg.* **2014**, *23*, e267–e274. [CrossRef]
23. Harjula, J.N.E.; Paloneva, J.; Haapakoski, J.; Kukkonen, J.; Äärimaa, V. Increasing incidence of primary shoulder arthroplasty in Finland—A nationwide registry study. *BMC Musculoskelet. Disord.* **2018**, *19*, 245. [CrossRef]
24. Schwartz, B.E.; Savin, D.D.; Youderian, A.R.; Mossad, D.; Goldberg, B.A. National trends and perioperative outcomes in primary and revision total shoulder arthroplasty: Trends in total shoulder arthroplasty. *Int. Orthop.* **2015**, *39*, 271–276. [CrossRef] [PubMed]
25. Wagner, E.R.; Farley, K.X.; Higgins, I.; Wilson, J.M.; Daly, C.A.; Gottschalk, M.B. The incidence of shoulder arthroplasty: Rise and future projections compared with hip and knee arthroplasty. *J. Shoulder Elbow Surg.* **2020**, *29*, 2601–2609. [CrossRef] [PubMed]
26. Nemes, S.; Rolfson, O.; W-Dahl, A.; Garellick, G.; Sundberg, M.; Kärrholm, J.; Robertsson, O. Historical view and future demand for knee arthroplasty in Sweden. *Acta Orthop.* **2015**, *86*, 426–431. [CrossRef]
27. Villatte, G.; Erivan, R.; Barth, J.; Bonnevialle, N.; Descamps, S.; Boisgard, S. Progression and projection for shoulder surgery in France, 2012-2070: Epidemiologic study with trend and projection analysis. *Orthop. Traumatol. Surg. Res.* **2020**, *106*, 1067–1077. [CrossRef] [PubMed]
28. Bayona, C.E.A.; Somerson, J.S.; Matsen, F.A. The utility of international shoulder joint replacement registries and databases: A comparative analytic review of two hundred and sixty one thousand, four hundred and eighty four cases. *Int. Orthop.* **2018**, *42*, 351–358. [CrossRef]
29. García-Fernández, C.; Lopiz, Y.; Rizo, B.; Serrano-Mateo, L.; Alcobía-Díaz, B.; Rodríguez-González, A.; Marco, F. Reverse total shoulder arroplasty for the treatment of failed fixation in proximal humeral fractures. *Injury* **2018**, *49* (Suppl. 2), S22–S26. [CrossRef]
30. Court-Brown, C.M.; Garg, A.; McQueen, M.M. The epidemiology of proximal humeral fractures. *Acta Orthop. Scand.* **2001**, *72*, 365–371. [CrossRef]
31. Gallinet, D.; Ohl, X.; Decroocq, L.; Dib, C.; Valenti, P.; Boileau, P. Is reverse total shoulder arthroplasty more effective than hemiarthroplasty for treating displaced proximal humerus fractures in older adults? A systematic review and meta-analysis. *Orthop. Traumatol. Surg. Res.* **2018**, *104*, 759–766. [CrossRef]
32. Noguera, L.; Trigo, L.; Melero, V.; Santana, F.; Torrens, C. Reverse shoulder arthroplasty for acute proximal humeral fractures: Postoperative complications at 7 days, 90 days and 1 year. *Injury* **2019**, *50*, 371–375. [CrossRef]
33. Lindbloom, B.J.; Christmas, K.N.; Downes, K.; Simon, P.; McLendon, P.B.; Hess, A.V.; Mighell, M.A.; Frankle, M.A. Is there a relationship between preoperative diagnosis and clinical outcomes in reverse shoulder arthroplasty? An experience in 699 shoulders. *J. Shoulder Elbow Surg.* **2019**, *28*, S110–S117. [CrossRef] [PubMed]
34. Coscia, A.C.; Matar, R.N.; Espinal, E.E.; Shah, N.S.; Grawe, B.M. Does Preoperative Diagnosis Impact Patient Outcomes Following Reverse Total Shoulder Arthroplasty? A Systematic Review. *J. Shoulder Elbow Surg.* **2020**, *30*, 1458–1470. [CrossRef] [PubMed]
35. Lung, B.E.; Kanjiya, S.; Bisogno, M.; Komatsu, D.E.; Wang, E.D. Preoperative indications for total shoulder arthroplasty predict adverse postoperative complications. *JSES Open Access* **2019**, *3*, 99–107. [CrossRef]
36. Malik, A.T.; Bishop, J.Y.; Neviaser, A.S.; Beals, C.T.; Jain, N.; Khan, S.N. Shoulder Arthroplasty for a Fracture Is Not the Same as Shoulder Arthroplasty for Osteoarthritis: Implications for a Bundled Payment Model. *J. Am. Acad. Orthop. Surg.* **2019**, *27*, 927–932. [CrossRef] [PubMed]
37. Fu, B.-S.; Jia, H.-L.; Zhou, D.-S.; Liu, F.-X. Surgical and Non-Surgical Treatment for 3-Part and 4-Part Fractures of the Proximal Humerus: A Systematic Review of Overlapping Meta-Analyses. *Orthop. Surg.* **2019**, *11*, 356–365. [CrossRef] [PubMed]

38. Soler-Peiro, M.; García-Martínez, L.; Aguilella, L.; Perez-Bermejo, M. Conservative treatment of 3-part and 4-part proximal humeral fractures: A systematic review. *J. Orthop. Surg. Res.* **2020**, *15*, 347. [CrossRef] [PubMed]
39. Hemmann, P.; Ziegler, P.; Konrads, C.; Ellmerer, A.; Klopfer, T.; Schreiner, A.J.; Bahrs, C. Trends in fracture development of the upper extremity in Germany-a population-based description of the past 15 years. *J. Orthop. Surg. Res.* **2020**, *15*, 65. [CrossRef] [PubMed]
40. Martinez-Huedo, M.A.; Jiménez-García, R.; Mora-Zamorano, E.; Hernández-Barrera, V.; Villanueva-Martinez, M.; Lopez-de-Andres, A. Trends in incidence of proximal humerus fractures, surgical procedures and outcomes among elderly hospitalized patients with and without type 2 diabetes in Spain (2001-2013). *BMC Musculoskelet. Disord.* **2017**, *18*, 522. [CrossRef] [PubMed]
41. Baertl, S.; Alt, V.; Rupp, M. Surgical enhancement of fracture healing—Operative vs. nonoperative treatment. *Injury* **2020**, *52*, S12–S17. [CrossRef]
42. Gomberawalla, M.M.; Miller, B.S.; Coale, R.M.; Bedi, A.; Gagnier, J.J. Meta-analysis of joint preservation versus arthroplasty for the treatment of displaced 3- and 4-part fractures of the proximal humerus. *Injury* **2013**, *44*, 1532–1539. [CrossRef]

Article

Association of the Posterior Acromion Extension with Glenoid Retroversion: A CT Study in Normal and Osteoarthritic Shoulders

Alexandre Terrier [1,2], Fabio Becce [3], Frédéric Vauclair [2], Alain Farron [2] and Patrick Goetti [2,*]

1. Laboratory of Biomechanical Orthopedics, Ecole Polytechnique Fédérale de Lausanne, Station 19, 1015 Lausanne, Switzerland; alexandre.terrier@epfl.ch
2. Department of Orthopedics and Traumatology, Lausanne University Hospital and University of Lausanne, Avenue Pierre-Decker 4, 1011 Lausanne, Switzerland; frederic.vauclair@chuv.ch (F.V.); alain.farron@chuv.ch (A.F.)
3. Department of Diagnostic and Interventional Radiology, Lausanne University Hospital and University of Lausanne, Rue du Bugnon 46, 1011 Lausanne, Switzerland; fabio.becce@chuv.ch
* Correspondence: patrick.goetti@chuv.ch; Tel.: +41-21-314-94-03

Abstract: Posterior eccentric glenoid wear is associated with higher complication rates after shoulder arthroplasty. The recently reported association between the acromion shape and glenoid retroversion in both normal and osteoarthritic shoulders remains controversial. The three-dimensional coordinates of the angulus acromialis (AA) and acromioclavicular joint were examined in the scapular coordinate system. Four acromion angles were defined from these two acromion landmarks: the acromion posterior angle (APA), acromion tilt angle (ATA), acromion length angle (ALA), and acromion axial tilt angle (AXA). Shoulder computed tomography scans of 112 normal scapulae and 125 patients with primary glenohumeral osteoarthritis were analyzed with simple and stepwise multiple linear regressions between all morphological acromion parameters and glenoid retroversion. In normal scapulae, the glenoid retroversion angle was most strongly correlated with the posterior extension of the AA ($R^2 = 0.48$, $p < 0.0001$), which can be conveniently characterized by the APA. Combining the APA with the ALA and ATA helped slightly improve the correlation ($R^2 = 0.55$, $p < 0.0001$), but adding the AXA did not. In osteoarthritic scapulae, a critical APA > 15 degrees was found to best identify glenoids with a critical retroversion angle > 8 degrees. The APA is more strongly associated with the glenoid retroversion angle in normal than primary osteoarthritic scapulae.

Keywords: acromion morphology; glenoid retroversion; wear; osteoarthritis; computed tomography

1. Introduction

Several measures of acromion morphology, both in the sagittal and coronal planes, have been described and associated with various shoulder disorders [1]. In recent years, much research has been directed towards the characterization of the lateral extension of the acromion. The acromion index followed by the critical shoulder angle, both described on antero-posterior shoulder radiographs, have been shown to be predictors of glenohumeral osteoarthritis (OA) and rotator cuff tendon tears [2,3]. These initial findings were supported by subsequent biomechanical studies revealing increased glenohumeral joint reaction forces with decreased lateral extension of the acromion [4,5]. However, these two anatomical parameters are unable to assess the antero-posterior imbalance of the glenohumeral joint typically found in Walch type B glenoids [6].

Over the past three years, Beeler et al. analyzed shoulder computed tomography (CT) images to improve characterization of acromion roof morphology. Compared with osteoarthritic shoulders, the acromion was more externally rotated (axial plane), more downward tilted (coronal plane), and had wider posterior coverage of the glenoid (sagittal plane) in shoulders with rotator cuff tears [7]. The same research group further found a significant difference between shoulders with concentric and eccentric primary glenohumeral OA, and concluded that a flatter acromion roof with less posterior glenoid coverage could contribute to static posterior subluxation of the humeral head and posterior glenoid wear [8]. Furthermore, Meyer et al. were able to link a decreased posterior acromion slope and increased glenoid retroversion with static posterior subluxation of the humeral head and posterior glenoid wear [9]. More recently, Beeler et al. reported that the scapula of a shoulder with dynamic and static posterior instability was characterized by an increased glenoid retroversion and an acromion that was shorter posterolaterally and higher and more horizontal in the sagittal plane [10].

Static posterior subluxation of the humeral head and posterior glenoid wear are of particular interest to shoulder surgeons, as they have been related to both early glenohumeral OA in young adults [11], and higher complication rates after shoulder arthroplasty [12]. Although Walch et al. stated that static posterior subluxation of the humeral head preceded posterior glenoid wear, with glenoid retroversion as a risk factor [11,13], there is currently no consensus regarding this chicken-or-egg debate [6,14,15]. To our knowledge and despite the recent study by Beeler et al. [10], there are no published data on the correlation between the detailed three-dimensional (3D) acromion shape and glenoid retroversion.

Therefore, our objective is to investigate the potential association between the 3D acromion shape and glenoid retroversion in both normal and osteoarthritic shoulders. This could prove to be clinically useful to better understand the etiology of eccentric glenoid wear and possibly define an anatomical parameter to predict its risk of occurrence. We first examined the presence or absence of correlation between the 3D acromion shape and glenoid retroversion in normal scapulae. Then, we tested whether the same results held true in shoulders with primary glenohumeral OA.

2. Materials and Methods

2.1. Study Population

This retrospective observational study was approved by the institutional ethics committee, with a waiver of patient informed consent (CER-VD protocol number 505-15). We considered the following two patient groups, who did not need to be matched since they were analyzed separately according to the study design and primary objective (i.e., association between 3D acromion shape and glenoid retroversion).

The normal group included trauma patients aged 18 to 40, who had undergone a whole-body CT scan covering at least one of the two scapulae in full. Exclusion criteria were any radiological sign or history in medical records of disorders of the shoulder bones and joints (OA, fracture, glenoid dysplasia, or prior surgery of the upper limb), CT signs of immature skeleton (absence of fusion between any of the scapular ossification centers [16]) or CT artifacts (motion or metal). From our institutional picture archiving and communication system, an attending musculoskeletal radiologist retrospectively reviewed 221 consecutive whole-body CT scans performed over a 6-month period, and from these 112 patients met the inclusion criteria. The main characteristics of the normal subjects (79 males and 33 females) were mean age, 28.4 years (range, 18–40); mean height, 174.4 cm (range, 150–210 cm); mean weight, 75.5 kg (range, 50–120 kg); mean body mass index, 24.7 kg/m^2 (range, 18.6–38.1 kg/m^2).

The pathological group consisted of patients with glenohumeral OA who had undergone a shoulder CT scan covering the entire scapula in their preoperative planning prior to shoulder arthroplasty. Patients with any traumatic injury to the shoulder girdle, malunion or nonunion, necrosis of the humeral head, or rheumatoid arthritis were excluded. Of the 334 consecutive patients eligible from 2002 to 2016, 125 with primary glenohumeral OA met the inclusion criteria. The main characteristics of the OA patients were mean age, 71.4 (range, 46–88 years); 37 males, 88 females; mean height, 165.7 cm (range, 141–186 cm); mean weight, 78.4 kg (range, 42–129 kg); mean body mass index, 28.5 kg/m^2 (range, 17.7–43.6 kg/m^2). According to the updated Walch classification [17], the distribution of glenoid types was: A1, n = 26; A2, n = 23; B1, n = 26; B2, n = 37; B3, n = 8; C, n = 5.

2.2. CT Protocols

All CT scans were performed on multidetector-row CT systems (8–256 detector rows) from the same manufacturer (GE Healthcare), with standardized data acquisition and image reconstruction settings. For normal subjects, scapular CT images were reconstructed as follows: section thickness, 1.3 mm; section interval, 0.7–1.3 mm; kernel, sharp (bone or bone plus); pixel size, 0.4–1.0 mm. For OA patients, shoulder CT images were reconstructed as follows: section thickness, 0.6–1.3 mm; section interval, 0.3–1.0 mm; kernel, sharp (bone or bone plus; GE Healthcare); pixel size, 0.3–0.6 mm.

2.3. Scapular Coordinate System

All CT scans were analyzed in 3D using a reliable semi-automated method providing a scapular coordinate system described in detail elsewhere [18,19]. Briefly, the medio-lateral (z) axis was along the scapular axis, defined by the line fitting five points placed along the supraspinatus fossa projected in the scapular plane. The scapular (i.e., ~"coronal") plane was defined by three landmarks: the trigonum spinae (TS), the angulus inferior (AI), and the most medial of the five points defining the medio-lateral axis (Figure 1; additional illustrations on the coordinate system can be found in [19]). The postero-anterior (x) axis (i.e., ~"sagittal" plane) was then defined as being perpendicular to the scapular plane and medio-lateral axis. The infero-superior (y) axis (i.e., ~"axial" plane) was perpendicular to the other two axes. The origin of the coordinate system corresponded to the spinoglenoid notch projected on the medio-lateral scapular axis.

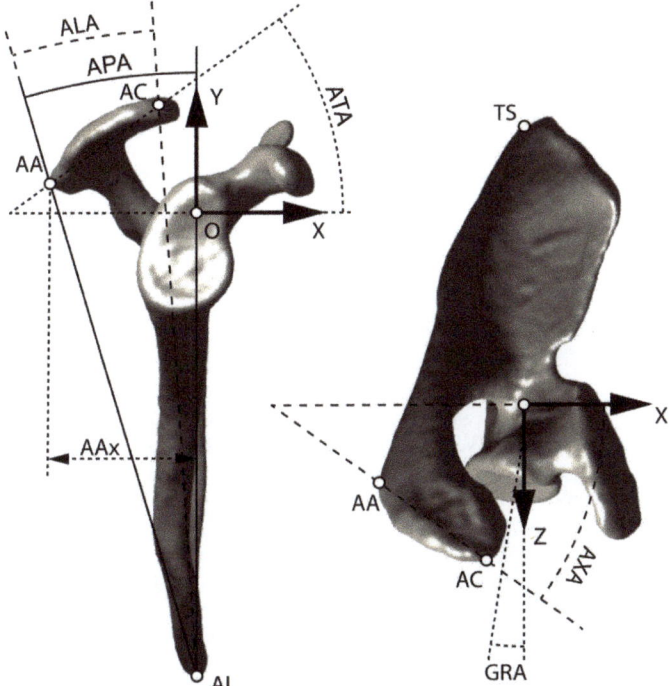

Figure 1. Anatomical description of the scapular coordinate system (OXYZ), acromion landmarks (AA, AC), trigonum spinae (TS), angulus inferior (AI), posterior extension of the acromion (AAx), acromion posterior angle (APA), acromion tilt angle (ATA), acromion length angle (ALA), and glenoid retroversion angle (GRA). The three axes (x, y, and z) correspond to postero-anterior, infero-superior, and medio-lateral, respectively.

2.4. Acromion Landmarks

Two specific acromion landmarks were placed manually on its 3D surface using the same software (Amira; Thermo Fisher Scientific) and method as above [19]: the acromion angle (AA) and the most anterior point of the acromioclavicular (AC) joint (Figure 1). These two landmarks were characterized by their three coordinates in the scapular coordinate system (AAx, AAy, AAz; and ACx, ACy, ACz). Because of the expected variability in scapular size among patients, these coordinates (distances) were normalized by the scapular height, defined by the infero-superior distance between AI (AIy) and the origin of the scapular coordinate system.

2.5. Acromion Angles

From these two acromion landmarks, we defined four specific acromion angles (Figure 1): the acromion posterior angle (APA), the acromion tilt angle (ATA), the acromion length angle (ALA), and the acromion axial tilt angle (AXA). The APA is the angle between the infero-superior axis (Y) and the axis formed by the AA landmark and AI, projected in the plane perpendicular to the medio-lateral axis (i.e., ~"sagittal" plane). The ATA is the angle between the AA-AC segment and the x-axis, in the xy plane (i.e., ~"sagittal"). The ALA corresponds to the distance between AA and AC landmarks (in the xy —i.e., ~"sagittal"plane), measured as an angle from AI. Finally, the AXA is the angle between the AA–AC segment and the x axis in the zx plane (i.e., ~"axial").

2.6. Glenoid Retroversion Angle

The glenoid retroversion angle (GRA) was measured in 3D from the CT scans using the same software (Amira) and method as above [19]: the angle between the medio-lateral axis (z) and the glenoid centerline projected in the axial plane (perpendicular to the infero-superior axis). The glenoid centerline was defined by the vector joining the center of the glenoid cavity and the center of a sphere fitting the glenoid cavity (Figure 1, right). This method has previously shown good to excellent inter- and intra-observer reliability [19]. For simplicity, we defined here retroversion as positive, and anteversion as negative. The glenoid centerline and all other 3D quantities and computations defined above were performed with Matlab (MathWorks). This script takes as input the three coordinates of all the scapular landmarks and all the points on the surface of the glenoid cavity to provide all reported measurements in the scapular coordinate system, for each case individually.

2.7. Statistical Analysis

Statistical analyses were performed in Matlab. First, for subjects with normal scapulae (i.e., trauma patients), we performed simple and stepwise multiple linear regressions to examine the correlation among all six acromion landmarks (AA and AC coordinates) and the GRA. We also evaluated the correlation among each of the four acromion angles (APA, ATA, ALA, and AXA) and the GRA. The quality of the regression was quantified by the root mean square error (RMSE), the coefficient of determination (R^2), and its p-value. We further performed a receiver operating characteristic (ROC) curve analysis to determine which critical GRA and associated morphological acromion parameter better identified the two groups (i.e., low vs. high GRA), using the area under the curve (AUC) with the Youden index. The normality of the measurement data was verified by a Shapiro–Wilk test. As an additional analysis, differences between the normal and pathological patient groups were tested by an unpaired two-tailed Student's t-test, and the effect size evaluated with Cohen's d. We also assessed the dependence on patient demographics such as gender and age, and $p < 0.05$ was considered statistically significant.

3. Results

For normal scapulae, simple linear regressions showed that AAx was the acromion landmark coordinate most strongly and significantly associated with the GRA ($R^2 = 0.480$, $p < 0.0001$), followed by ACx ($R^2 = 0.310$, $p < 0.0001$) (Table 1). Stepwise multiple linear regressions between the six acromion landmark coordinates examined here (AAx, AAy, AAz; and ACx, ACy ACz) and the GRA confirmed the importance of AAx, and the slight improvement in the model by combining AAx with AAz and ACx (R^2 = 0.530, p < 0.0001). Using this existing correlation, we were able to predict the measured GRA with an error (RMSE) of 3.6 degrees.

Table 1. Root mean square errors (RMSE), coefficients of determination (R^2), and p-values of simple and stepwise multiple linear regressions between several acromion landmark coordinates and angles and the glenoid retroversion angle (GRA), for normal scapulae.

	RMSE (Degree)	R^2	p-Value
AAx	3.73	0.480	<0.0001
AAy	5.16	0.006	0.4308
AAz	5.02	0.051	0.0096
ACx	4.31	0.310	<0.0001
Acy	5.14	0.013	0.2298
ACz	5.16	0.007	0.3739
AAx, AAz	3.66	0.505	<0.0001
AAx, AAz, ACx	3.58	0.530	<0.0001
APA	3.73	0.482	<0.0001
ALA	5.17	0.002	0.6305
ATA	5.12	0.022	0.1187
AXA	4.85	0.123	0.0001
APA, ALA	3.61	0.518	<0.0001
APA, ALA, ATA	3.50	0.551	<0.0001

Of the four acromion angles examined here (APA, ATA, ALA, and AXA in Figure 1), the APA was the most strongly and significantly associated with the GRA (R^2 = 0.482, p < 0.0001). Combining the APA with the ALA and ATA helped slightly improve the correlation, while adding the AXA did not. The APA was very strongly and significantly correlated with AAx (R^2 = 1.00, p < 0.0001) (Supplementary Material). Because of this, among the 10 morphological acromion parameters (6 landmark coordinates and 4 angles), we then focused the analysis between the acromion morphology and glenoid retroversion to the APA versus GRA (Figure 2), which can be written as follows: GRA = 1.9 × APA − 25.2 (with GRA and APA in degrees). A 1-degree increase in the APA corresponded approximately to a 2-degree increase in the GRA.

For osteoarthritic scapulae, we also observed a significant positive correlation between the APA and GRA (R^2 = 0.197, p < 0.0001), suggesting that a higher APA was associated with an increased GRA (Figure 2). While both the GRA and APA increased with the (alphabetical) progression of the updated Walch class, the increase in APA was not proportional to that of the GRA (Table 2, Figure 3). The ROC curve analysis predicted a critical GRA value of 8 degrees (AUC = 0.78) and a critical APA value of 15 degrees to best identify high GRA (>8 degrees) from low GRA (≤8 degrees).

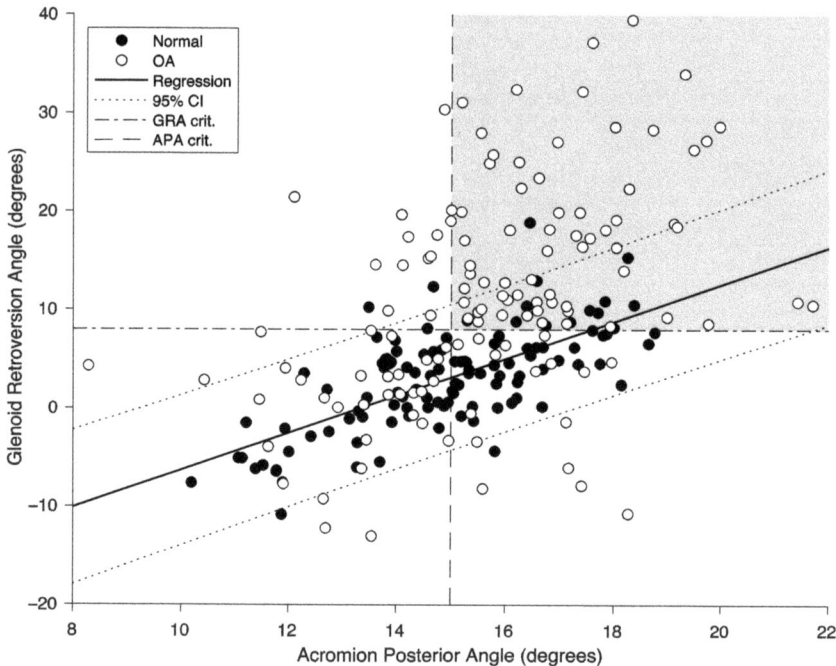

Figure 2. Measured acromion posterior angle (APA, *x* axis) vs. glenoid retroversion angle (GRA, *y* axis) for normal scapulae (black dots) and primary osteoarthritic scapulae (white dots). The continuous line represents the linear regression between the APA and GRA for normal scapulae, with its 95% confidence interval (dotted lines). The grey-shaded area (top right corner) shows the number of osteoarthritic scapulae with critical angle values (dashed lines) of APA > 15 degrees and GRA > 8 degrees.

Table 2. Glenoid retroversion angle (GRA; mean ± SD) and acromion posterior angle (APA; mean ± SD) for normal and osteoarthritic scapulae, subclassified according to the updated Walch classification.

Scapulae	GRA (Degree)	APA (Degree)
Normal (n = 112)	3.0 ± 5.2	14.9 ± 1.9
Walch type A1–A2 (n = 49)	4.5 ± 9.4	15.3 ± 2.3
Walch type B1 (n = 26)	10.1 ± 9.0	15.2 ± 1.8
Walch type B2–B3 (n = 45)	16.9 ± 8.1	16.3 ± 2.2
Walch type C (n = 5)	29.6 ± 8.4	16.9 ± 1.9

Data for the six acromion landmarks, four acromion angles, and the GRA all followed a normal distribution. Of the six acromion landmarks, AAx, AAy, ACx, and ACy differed significantly between normal and osteoarthritic scapulae ($p \leq 0.03$), but with a moderate-to-small effect size (Cohen's d ≤ 0.64). Among the four acromion angles, only APA and ALA were significantly different between normal and osteoarthritic scapulae ($p \leq 0.04$), but again with a moderate to small effect size (d ≤ 0.43). GRA was significantly more retroverted in osteoarthritic (11.1 degrees) than in normal scapulae (3.0 degrees) ($p < 0.001$). There were no significant differences in age between osteoarthritic scapulae having an APA above or below 15 degrees ($p = 0.38$). Regressions between GRA and APA were slightly different between males and females but remained within the 95% confidence intervals (CIs) of the entire datasets.

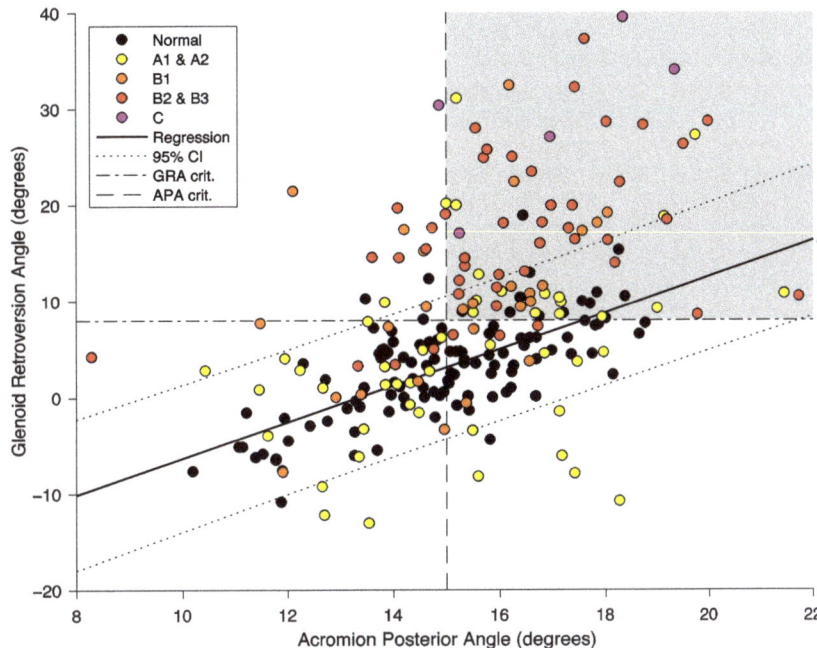

Figure 3. Measured acromion posterior angle (APA, *x* axis) vs. glenoid retroversion angle (GRA, *y* axis) for normal scapulae (black dots) and primary osteoarthritic scapulae subclassified according to the updated Walch classification (yellow, orange, red, and purple dots). The continuous line represents the linear regression between the APA and GRA for normal scapulae, with its 95% confidence interval (dotted lines). The grey-shaded area (top right corner) shows the number of osteoarthritic scapulae with critical angle values (dashed lines) of APA > 15 degrees and GRA > 8 degrees.

4. Discussion

Our objective was to test for correlations between scapular morphology and glenoid retroversion, both in patients with normal scapulae but also in those with primary glenohumeral OA. Two specific acromion landmarks were used and represented by their coordinates in the 3D scapular coordinate system. In normal (non-osteoarthritic) glenohumeral joints, we observed that the posterior extension of the acromion was strongly correlated with the GRA. This anatomical acromion measure was represented by the APA, a novel angular measure of the scapula. By comparison with the primary glenohumeral OA population, we found a critical APA value, which needs to be further investigated and might eventually be used as a predictive anatomical parameter or risk factor for posterior glenoid wear in osteoarthritic shoulders.

The two acromion landmarks used in this study characterized the acromion as a linear segment. Using the six coordinates of these two landmarks in the local scapular coordinate system, we tested all possible simple and multiple morphological associations between the defined acromion segment and GRA. These two scapular landmarks were carefully selected to be unaffected by osteoarthritic wear or osteophytes [18,19]. Bearing this in mind, the glenoid center was deliberately avoided, as its location can be modified by glenoid wear. The same logic was applied for the APA by selecting the inferior edge of the scapula (AI) as the third landmark. Although glenoid version is classically defined as negative when oriented posteriorly, we decided to use a positive value for the sake of simplicity. Hence, we used the term retroversion to avoid any confusion, and a positive correlation between the APA and GRA was reported here.

Our statistical analysis revealed that two of these six coordinates (AAx and ACx) were mainly associated with the GRA. These coordinates were therefore subsequently used to define angles that could be conveniently measured in daily clinical practice on sagittal-oblique reformats derived from preoperative shoulder CT scans. As highlighted by our results, these angles appeared to be reliable and easy-to-use alternatives to characterizing the acromion morphology. A previous analysis of the inter- and intra-observer variability in the positioning of scapular landmarks showed moderate to excellent reliability, with intraclass correlation coefficients ranging from 0.67 to 0.99 [19]. As expected, the correlation between the APA and GRA in normal scapulae was strong. The APA and AAx indeed had a strong linearly correlated since AAx is proportional to the trigonometric tangent function of the APA, which is highly linear between 0 and 20 degrees. This correlation was further enhanced after normalization of the AAx coordinate by the scapula height ($R^2 = 0.999$ and 0.830, with and without normalization by the scapula height, respectively). For normal scapulae, the more posterior the acromion extension, the wider the GRA. This was reported by the posterior extension of the AA (AAx), and by the APA. According to our regression analysis, one degree in APA related to two additional degrees in the GRA.

When secondarily looking at osteoarthritic scapulae, the correlation between AAx and the APA was still significant but weaker than in normal scapulae ($R^2 = 0.482$, $p < 0.0001$ vs. $R^2 = 0.197$, $p < 0.0001$, respectively). This meant that the correlation observed in normal scapulae seemed to be disrupted in primary glenohumeral OA patients. Our hypothesis is that this might have been related to posterior glenoid wear. Previous research identified scapulae with increased glenoid retroversion or posterior glenoid wear as a risk factor for implant failure in total shoulder arthroplasty [20,21]. In addition, posterior glenoid bone loss is known to progress over a 5- to 15-year timeframe in up to 55% of patients [22]. Our research might therefore be critical for helping council patients by defining a critical APA value related to posterior glenoid wear. We first identified a critical GRA with a ROC curve analysis. Then, by using the Youden index, we determined the optimal APA cut-off value that could distinguish between scapulae above and below this critical GRA threshold.

Glenoid retroversion also correlated with ACx, but ACx strongly correlated with AAx (see correlation matrix in Supplementary Material), meaning that the relative AP acromion length (distance between AA and AC) had a low variability. Glenoid retroversion also negatively correlated with the lateral extension of the AA (AAz), which further partly correlated with the posterior extension (Table 1). These correlations between the two acromion landmark coordinates were also present between the four tested acromion angles, and explain why they do not all appear in the multiple correlations obtained with the stepwise multiple linear regression analysis.

It appears likely that the strong correlation observed between the acromion and glenoid in normal scapulae was determined by the end of growth [23]. While several hypotheses regarding posterior glenoid wear were raised (e.g., premorbid glenoid retroversion [24], muscular imbalance [25], and lower humeral retroversion [26]), its pathophysiology remains unknown. We might reasonably assume that the acromion affected the glenoid through the action of muscles, but this remains purely conjectural. This link might also be more deeply anchored in human evolution [27].

Normalized values of the two important acromion landmarks that are the AA and AC joint have not been previously reported. However, a wide range of acromion angles have recently been described with increasing interest in characterizing the acromion morphology. The APA presents similarities with the "posterior glenoid coverage" proposed by Beeler et al. as both are based on AAx and the medio-lateral scapular plane [7,8]. However, Beeler et al. used the glenoid center as the middle point, while we used the AI instead not only because it is not affected by glenohumeral osteoarthritis, unlike the glenoid center, but also and primarily to better correlate the APA with the posterior extension of the acromion (AAx). These two angles are thus very different, and we verified that the "posterior glenoid coverage" was not correlated with the GRA in our series of normal scapulae.

The ALA corresponded to the distance between AA and AC in the sagittal (xy) plane, measured as an angle using AI as the third landmark. Again, it is similar to the "overall glenoid coverage" proposed by Beeler et al. [7,8], but uses AI instead of the glenoid center as the middle point, to better correlate with the AA–AC segment ($R^2 = 0.908$ vs. $R^2 = 0.093$, respectively). In our series of normal scapulae, these two angles were only weakly correlated ($R^2 = 0.127$), and the variability range of ALA was five times lower.

The ATA corresponds approximately to the previously defined acromion tilt [28], or 90 degrees minus the posterior acromion slope [9], or the sagittal tilt [7,8]. The ATA was 25.2 ± 8.2 (range, 5.2–46.9) degrees in our normal scapulae vs. 23.4 ± 8.7 (range, 4.5–42.5) degrees in osteoarthritic scapulae, which corresponds closely to the values in the articles referenced above.

The AXA corresponds approximately to the previously defined axial tilt angle [7,8]. The AXA was 26.1 ± 8.9 (range, 4.2–52.1) degrees in our normal scapulae vs. 29.1 ± 9.9 (range, 2.5–52.1) in osteoarthritic scapulae, which also matches the previous works mentioned above.

The main strength of the present study was the use of the 3D coordinates of two relevant acromion landmarks in a dedicated local scapular coordinate system generated from points not affected by glenoid wear that is secondary to glenohumeral osteoarthritis. This setup permitted multiple linear regression testing to identify the most significant determinants of glenoid retroversion, which was also comprehensively analyzed in 3D. A step further was taken by defining acromion angles that normalize measures to patients' height, thereby obviating the need for subsequent data processing.

The major limitation of our method was the manual identification of the two acromion landmarks, the effect of which was minimized by the good reliability in the positioning of scapular landmarks by a single experienced human observer [19]. This could be improved by using sophisticated fully automatic landmark detection methods [29]. However, even with such automated methods, the AC might still be affected by osteoarthritis, conversely to all other anatomical landmarks used to characterize the acromion morphology, the angles, and the local (i.e., scapular) coordinate system. Nevertheless, the AC is not related to the APA or the scapular coordinate system, and its variability caused by OA is supposedly weak since we found no significant difference when comparing the normal and osteoarthritic datasets. Second, patient characteristics differed between normal and osteoarthritic scapulae, as per the study design and primary objective (association between 3D acromion shape and glenoid retroversion), and considering that trauma is more common in males and shoulder OA in females. However, our aim was to assess potential morphological associations separately, first in normal and then osteoarthritic scapulae. We verified that the same correlations held true in males and females, with variations within the 95% CIs. Regarding aging, we further checked that this demographic parameter did not affect the critical APA value reported here. Finally, although trauma patients with normal scapulae and patients with glenohumeral OA were not scanned with the same CT protocols, the differences in the reconstructed geometric volumes were small (with slightly smaller voxels for OA than trauma patients) and had no impact on the positioning of scapular landmarks.

5. Conclusions

The strong correlation observed here between the posterior acromion extension, in particular the APA, and glenoid retroversion in normal scapulae suggests that the APA might be used as a predictive anatomical parameter or risk factor for the development and progression of primary glenohumeral osteoarthritis associated with posterior glenoid wear. However, the identified critical APA value at 15 degrees should now be further investigated in larger patient series with osteoarthritic scapulae/glenoids, and if possible elderly controls without any sign of glenohumeral OA. Moreover, long-term clinical studies should evaluate the impact of the APA on clinical function and surgical revision rates after shoulder arthroplasty. Finally, we should also examine whether the APA is associated with other shoulder disorders or specific treatment outcomes.

Supplementary Materials: The following are available online at https://www.mdpi.com/article/10.3390/jcm11020351/s1, Figure S1: Correlation matrix among acromion landmarks, acromion angles and glenoid retroversion angle.

Author Contributions: Conceptualization, A.T. and A.F.; methodology, A.T., F.B. and P.G.; software, A.T.; validation, F.B. and P.G.; formal analysis, A.T., F.B. and P.G.; investigation, A.T., F.B. and P.G.; resources, A.T.; data curation, F.B. and P.G.; writing—original draft preparation, A.T. and P.G.; writing—review and editing, F.B., F.V. and A.F.; funding acquisition, A.T. and A.F. All authors have read and agreed to the published version of the manuscript.

Funding: This study was funded by Wright-Tornier (Wright Medical Group, Inc., Memphis, TN, USA) and the "Lausanne Orthopedic Research Foundation".

Institutional Review Board Statement: This retrospective observational study was approved by the institutional ethics committee (CER-VD protocol number 505-15).

Informed Consent Statement: Patient informed consent was waived after study approval by the institutional ethics committee (CER-VD protocol number 505-15).

Data Availability Statement: Authors agree to make data supporting the results or analyses presented in their paper available upon reasonable request.

Conflicts of Interest: The authors declare no conflict of interest.

References

1. Nyffeler, R.W.; Meyer, D.C. Acromion and Glenoid Shape: Why Are They Important Predictive Factors for the Future of Our Shoulders? *EFORT Open Rev.* **2017**, *2*, 141–150. [CrossRef] [PubMed]
2. Nyffeler, R.W.; Werner, C.M.L.; Sukthankar, A.; Schmid, M.R.; Gerber, C. Association of a Large Lateral Extension of the Acromion with Rotator Cuff Tears. *J. Bone Jt. Surg. Am.* **2006**, *88*, 800–805. [CrossRef]
3. Moor, B.K.; Bouaicha, S.; Rothenfluh, D.A.; Sukthankar, A.; Gerber, C. Is There an Association between the Individual Anatomy of the Scapula and the Development of Rotator Cuff Tears or Osteoarthritis of the Glenohumeral Joint?: A Radiological Study of the Critical Shoulder Angle. *Bone Jt. J.* **2013**, *95-B*, 935–941. [CrossRef]
4. Engelhardt, C.; Farron, A.; Becce, F.; Place, N.; Pioletti, D.P.; Terrier, A. Effects of Glenoid Inclination and Acromion Index on Humeral Head Translation and Glenoid Articular Cartilage Strain. *J. Shoulder Elb. Surg.* **2017**, *26*, 157–164. [CrossRef]
5. Viehöfer, A.F.; Snedeker, J.G.; Baumgartner, D.; Gerber, C. Glenohumeral Joint Reaction Forces Increase with Critical Shoulder Angles Representative of Osteoarthritis-A Biomechanical Analysis. *J. Orthop. Res.* **2016**, *34*, 1047–1052. [CrossRef]
6. Jacxsens, M.; Van Tongel, A.; Henninger, H.B.; De Coninck, B.; Mueller, A.M.; De Wilde, L. A Three-Dimensional Comparative Study on the Scapulohumeral Relationship in Normal and Osteoarthritic Shoulders. *J. Shoulder Elb. Surg.* **2016**, *25*, 1607–1615. [CrossRef]
7. Beeler, S.; Hasler, A.; Getzmann, J.; Weigelt, L.; Meyer, D.C.; Gerber, C. Acromial Roof in Patients with Concentric Osteoarthritis and Massive Rotator Cuff Tears: Multiplanar Analysis of 115 Computed Tomography Scans. *J. Shoulder Elb. Surg.* **2018**, *27*, 1866–1876. [CrossRef]
8. Beeler, S.; Hasler, A.; Götschi, T.; Meyer, D.C.; Gerber, C. Different Acromial Roof Morphology in Concentric and Eccentric Osteoarthritis of the Shoulder: A Multiplane Reconstruction Analysis of 105 Shoulder Computed Tomography Scans. *J. Shoulder Elb. Surg.* **2018**, *27*, e357–e366. [CrossRef]
9. Meyer, D.C.; Riedo, S.; Eckers, F.; Carpeggiani, G.; Jentzsch, T.; Gerber, C. Small Anteroposterior Inclination of the Acromion Is a Predictor for Posterior Glenohumeral Erosion (B2 or C). *J. Shoulder Elb. Surg.* **2019**, *28*, 22–27. [CrossRef] [PubMed]
10. Beeler, S.; Leoty, L.; Hochreiter, B.; Carrillo, F.; Götschi, T.; Fischer, T.; Fürnstahl, P.; Gerber, C. Similar Scapular Morphology in Patients with Dynamic and Static Posterior Shoulder Instability. *JSES Int.* **2021**, *5*, 181–189. [CrossRef] [PubMed]
11. Walch, G.; Ascani, C.; Boulahia, A.; Nové-Josserand, L.; Edwards, T.B. Static Posterior Subluxation of the Humeral Head: An Unrecognized Entity Responsible for Glenohumeral Osteoarthritis in the Young Adult. *J. Shoulder Elb. Surg.* **2002**, *11*, 309–314. [CrossRef] [PubMed]
12. Walch, G.; Moraga, C.; Young, A.; Castellanos-Rosas, J. Results of Anatomic Nonconstrained Prosthesis in Primary Osteoarthritis with Biconcave Glenoid. *J. Shoulder Elb. Surg.* **2012**, *21*, 1526–1533. [CrossRef]
13. Domos, P.; Checchia, C.S.; Walch, G. Walch B0 Glenoid: Pre-Osteoarthritic Posterior Subluxation of the Humeral Head. *J. Shoulder Elb. Surg.* **2018**, *27*, 181–188. [CrossRef]
14. Sabesan, V.J.; Callanan, M.; Youderian, A.; Iannotti, J.P. 3D CT Assessment of the Relationship between Humeral Head Alignment and Glenoid Retroversion in Glenohumeral Osteoarthritis. *J. Bone Jt. Surg. Am.* **2014**, *96*, e64. [CrossRef]

15. Gerber, C.; Costouros, J.G.; Sukthankar, A.; Fucentese, S.F. Static Posterior Humeral Head Subluxation and Total Shoulder Arthroplasty. *J. Shoulder Elb. Surg.* **2009**, *18*, 505–510. [CrossRef]
16. Zember, J.S.; Rosenberg, Z.S.; Kwong, S.; Kothary, S.P.; Bedoya, M.A. Normal Skeletal Maturation and Imaging Pitfalls in the Pediatric Shoulder. *RadioGraphics* **2015**, *35*, 1108–1122. [CrossRef]
17. Bercik, M.J.; Kruse, K.; Yalizis, M.; Gauci, M.-O.; Chaoui, J.; Walch, G. A Modification to the Walch Classification of the Glenoid in Primary Glenohumeral Osteoarthritis Using Three-Dimensional Imaging. *J. Shoulder Elb. Surg.* **2016**, *25*, 1601–1606. [CrossRef] [PubMed]
18. Terrier, A.; Ston, J.; Farron, A. Importance of a Three-Dimensional Measure of Humeral Head Subluxation in Osteoarthritic Shoulders. *J. Shoulder Elb. Surg.* **2015**, *24*, 295–301. [CrossRef] [PubMed]
19. Terrier, A.; Ston, J.; Larrea, X.; Farron, A. Measurements of Three-Dimensional Glenoid Erosion When Planning the Prosthetic Replacement of Osteoarthritic Shoulders. *Bone Jt. J.* **2014**, *96-B*, 513–518. [CrossRef]
20. Luedke, C.; Kissenberth, M.J.; Tolan, S.J.; Hawkins, R.J.; Tokish, J.M. Outcomes of Anatomic Total Shoulder Arthroplasty with B2 Glenoids: A Systematic Review. *JBJS Rev.* **2018**, *6*, e7. [CrossRef]
21. Shapiro, T.A.; McGarry, M.H.; Gupta, R.; Lee, Y.S.; Lee, T.Q. Biomechanical Effects of Glenoid Retroversion in Total Shoulder Arthroplasty. *J. Shoulder Elb. Surg.* **2007**, *16*, S90–S95. [CrossRef]
22. Logli, A.L.; Pareek, A.; Nguyen, N.T.V.; Sanchez-Sotelo, J. Natural History of Glenoid Bone Loss in Primary Glenohumeral Osteoarthritis: How Does Bone Loss Progress over a Decade? *J. Shoulder Elb. Surg.* **2021**, *30*, 324–330. [CrossRef]
23. Kothary, P.; Rosenberg, Z.S. Skeletal Developmental Patterns in the Acromial Process and Distal Clavicle as Observed by MRI. *Skelet. Radiol.* **2015**, *44*, 207–215. [CrossRef]
24. Knowles, N.K.; Ferreira, L.M.; Athwal, G.S. Premorbid Retroversion Is Significantly Greater in Type B2 Glenoids. *J. Shoulder Elb. Surg.* **2016**, *25*, 1064–1068. [CrossRef] [PubMed]
25. Aleem, A.W.; Chalmers, P.N.; Bechtold, D.; Khan, A.Z.; Tashjian, R.Z.; Keener, J.D. Association Between Rotator Cuff Muscle Size and Glenoid Deformity in Primary Glenohumeral Osteoarthritis. *J. Bone Jt. Surg. Am.* **2019**, *101*, 1912–1920. [CrossRef] [PubMed]
26. Raniga, S.; Knowles, N.K.; West, E.; Ferreira, L.M.; Athwal, G.S. The Walch Type B Humerus: Glenoid Retroversion Is Associated with Torsional Differences in the Humerus. *J. Shoulder Elb. Surg.* **2019**, *28*, 1801–1808. [CrossRef] [PubMed]
27. Voisin, J.-L.; Ropars, M.; Thomazeau, H. The Human Acromion Viewed from an Evolutionary Perspective. *Orthop. Traumatol. Surg. Res.* **2014**, *100*, S355–S360. [CrossRef]
28. Kitay, G.S.; Iannotti, J.P.; Williams, G.R.; Haygood, T.; Kneeland, B.J.; Berlin, J. Roentgenographic Assessment of Acromial Morphologic Condition in Rotator Cuff Impingement Syndrome. *J. Shoulder Elb. Surg.* **1995**, *4*, 441–448. [CrossRef]
29. Taghizadeh, E.; Terrier, A.; Becce, F.; Farron, A.; Büchler, P. Automated CT Bone Segmentation Using Statistical Shape Modelling and Local Template Matching. *Comput. Methods Biomech. Biomed. Eng.* **2019**, *22*, 1303–1310. [CrossRef]

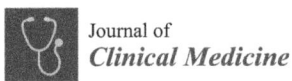

Review

Dislocation Arthropathy of the Shoulder

Ismael Coifman [1], Ulrich H. Brunner [2] and Markus Scheibel [3,4,*]

1. Department of Orthopaedic Surgery and Traumatology, IIS-Fundación Jiménez Díaz, Universidad Autónoma de Madrid (UAM), 28049 Madrid, Spain; ismael.coifman@quironsalud.es
2. Department for Traumatology and Orthopaedics, Krankenhaus Agatharied, 83734 Hausham, Germany; u.brunner@ugdb.org
3. Department of Shoulder and Elbow Surgery, Schulthess Clinic Zurich, 8008 Zurich, Switzerland
4. Center for Musculoskeletal Surgery, Campus Virchow, Charité-Universitaetsmedizin Berlin, 10117 Berlin, Germany
* Correspondence: markus.scheibel@charite.de; Tel.: +49-30-450652145

Abstract: Glenohumeral osteoarthrosis (OA) may develop after primary, recurrent shoulder dislocation or instability surgery. The incidence is reported from 12 to 62%, depending on different risk factors. The risk of severe OA of the shoulder following dislocation is 10 to 20 times greater than the average population. Risk factors include the patient's age at the first episode of instability or instability surgery, bony lesions, and rotator cuff tears. For mild stages of OA, arthroscopic removal of intraarticular material, arthroscopic debridement, or arthroscopic arthrolysis of an internal rotation contracture might be sufficient. For severe stages, mobilization of the internal rotation contracture and arthroplasty is indicated. With an intact rotator cuff and without a bone graft, results for anatomical shoulder arthroplasty are comparable to those following primary OA. With a bone graft at the glenoidal side, the risk for implant loosening is ten times greater. For the functional outcome, the quality of the rotator cuff is more predictive than the type of the previous surgery or the preoperative external rotation contracture. Reverse shoulder arthroplasty could be justified due to the higher rate of complications and revisions of non-constrained anatomic shoulder arthroplasties reported. Satisfactory clinical and radiological results have been published with mid to long term data now available.

Keywords: glenohumeral osteoarthrosis; shoulder dislocation; shoulder instability; dislocation arthropathy; arthroplasty

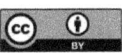

1. Introduction

Instability-mediated OA is a particular degenerative joint disease after a primary or recurrent dislocation or after instability surgery. In 1982 Neer [1] reported on 26 patients that had been treated with total shoulder arthroplasty due to severe OA after recurrent instability and anterior or posterior surgical stabilization in most cases: "recurrent dislocations and preceding surgery have tensed the capsule and thereby caused a fixed subluxation in the opposite direction of the instability". Since then, it has been discussed whether this unique type of OA is caused by the primary dislocation and thereby is predetermined, or recurrent dislocations, concomitant fractures, other risk factors, and different surgical therapies themselves worsen the prognosis or even cause it. This review clinical article deals with the following aspects: physical examination, diagnostic radiology, causes, prognostic factors, and treatments options and their results so far.

2. Physical Examinations

Typical examination finding in patients with recurrent instability and OA is an increasing loss of range of motion, particularly a restriction of external rotation. Rosenberg et al. reported a mean limitation in external rotation of 18° with the arm at the side and

15° in 90° abduction in patients evaluated 15 years after open Bankart reconstruction [2]. Pelet et al. found a mean loss of external rotation of 24° in their retrospective 29-year follow-up study following open Bankart repair [3]. Oh et al. evaluated the association between shoulder OA and functional results as determined by the DASH score, which was significantly increased according to the severity of shoulder OA [4]. As a matter of course, severe pain and joint crepitation are commonly found in patients suffering from OA [5]. A rotator cuff examination is essential to rule out tears and insufficiencies. Particular attention should be paid to the subscapularis muscle after the anterior approach, which involves its detachment if the patient presents with pain, recurrent instability, weakness in internal rotation, and increased external rotation. An essential examination should include a lift-off test, internal rotation lag sign, modified belly press test, and belly-off sign [6].

3. Diagnostic Radiology

Conventional radiographs usually confirm the diagnosis of OA in advanced stages or provide essential hints for differential diagnosis. The typical findings of OA are narrowing of joint space as an indirect sign of reduction of cartilage, subchondral sclerosis representing an adaptation reaction of the bone, and metaplastic responses known as osteophytes [7]. The extent of these changes is underestimated by plain-film radiography [8]. Computer tomography (CT) could finally increase the accuracy in diagnosis and the prevalence of OA essentially (Figure 1). In 282 patients with unilateral instability without surgery, the rate of OA was 11.3% in conventional radiographic imaging and 31.2% when CT was used. Even small osteophytes can be detected. CT can also detect the loss of the anterior and posterior part of the joint gap when it remains almost unaltered in conventional radiographic ap-projection [9]. Ogawa et al. [10] reviewed 167 joints of 163 patients undergoing the open Bankart procedure. Preoperative CT showed OA in 44 shoulders (26.3%), among which 12 shoulders (7.2%) showed OA on the preoperative radiographs. Preoperative CT-proven OA in 20 shoulders never became visible on postoperative radiographs. Recent three-dimensional computed tomography (3D CT) trends could better define the relationship between the humeral head and the glenoid [11]. Posterior wear after index surgery should be analyzed if the progression of OA is recognized to define new treatment options [12]. Ultrasound is the method to depict intra-articular effusion at early stages. Osteophytes or the degree of synovitis are also visible. Subchondral lesions, changes in cartilage volume, and concomitant soft-tissue alterations were detected earlier using MRI [7,9]. MRI also enables semi-quantitative analysis of the postoperative changes of the subscapularis muscle. The results provide indications of the causes of the clinical dysfunction of the subscapularis musculotendinous unit after open shoulder stabilization [13].

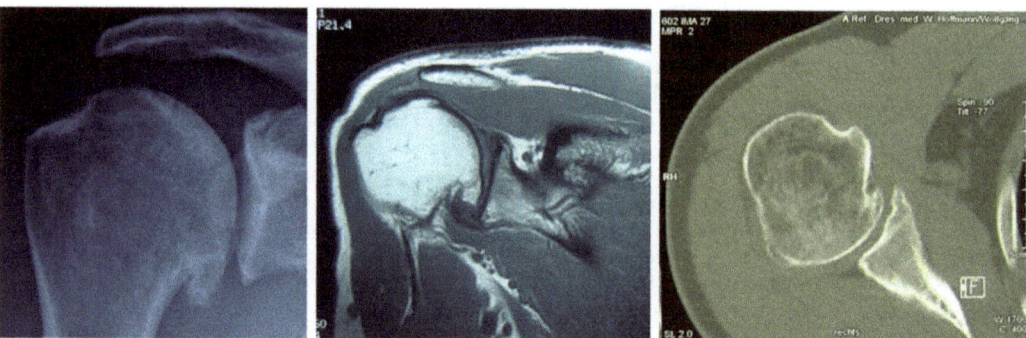

Figure 1. Imaging methods for evaluating dislocation arthropathy. Examples of conventional radiographs, MRI, and CT scan showing OA.

4. Classification

In 1983 Samilson and Prieto [14] reported 74 patients with OA after multiple dislocations or surgical stabilization. They defined the term Dislocation Arthropathy and the Samilson and Prieto Classification (SPC) and suggested three stages based on anteroposterior radiographic images:

- Mild OA: Osteophytes on the lower humeral head or the lower glenoid rim <3 mm
- Moderate OA: Osteophytes on the lower humeral head or the lower glenoid rim between 3–7 mm
- Severe OA: Osteophytes on the lower humeral head or the lower glenoid rim larger than 7 mm with slimming of the joint gap and sclerosis

To increase the classification accuracy according to Samilson and Prieto, Buscayret et al. suggested subdividing the severe OA stage into two stages: one with humeral osteophytes above 8 mm and a last one with the loss of the joint gap (Figure 2) [15].

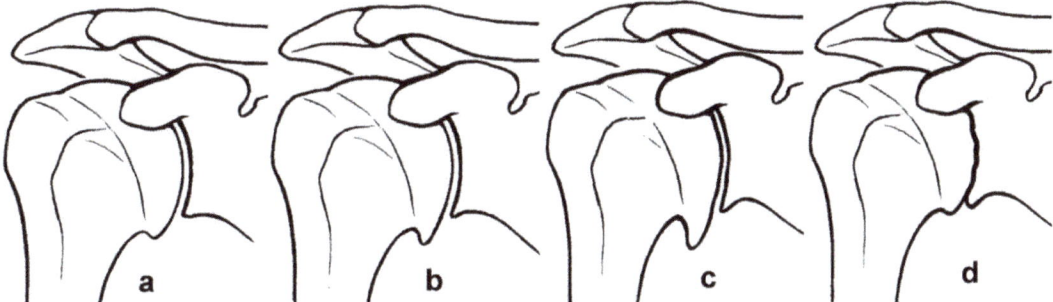

Figure 2. Image modified from Buscayret et al. [15]. (**a**): humeral osteophyte <3 mm. (**b**): humeral osteophyte >3 mm and <8 mm. (**c**): humeral osteophyte >8 mm. (**d**): obliteration of glenohumeral joint space.

The Samilson and Prieto classification is radiographic, but can it draw clinical conclusions? For example, Kircher et al. correlated pain, active and passive range of motion with OA graded according to Samilson and Prieto, finding the primary clinical feature, pain, as the main indication for surgery, not related to radiological parameters. In addition, the increasing size of the caudal humeral osteophyte was associated with a decreased functional status in all planes [16].

SPC is based only on 2D examination. Recently, Link et al. found no correlation between SPC and Walch classification for primary OA. Therefore, understanding glenoid morphology in the axial plane is mandatory in the final stage of OA for correct implant selection. However, no validated classification has been published to assess Dislocation Arthropathy in the axial plane [17].

5. Causes and Prognostic Factors

Since the first descriptions of OA after instability were carried out on patient groups that underwent surgery in most cases, it was presumed that OA results from the surgery itself [18].

5.1. Development of OA after Non-Operative Management of Shoulder Instability

Hovelius found that with a follow-up of 225 patients with first-time dislocations after 25 years, the spontaneous process after first-time dislocation accompanies OA development [19]. In a prospective study of patients with first-time dislocation after conservative therapy, 16.1% of 106 patients with a single dislocation without recurrence after ten years developed OA. With and without recurrence and operation, 11% of 208 shoulders had slight and 9% moderate or severe OA. The interesting point is that the shoulders with only one recurrence had similar rates of OA to those with recurrent dislocations or operations [20].

Hovelius [19], and Singer [21], conclude that the primary dislocation introduces the development of the OA and that later recurrences are in this regard of minor importance. Ogawa et al., however, found that the number of the dislocations/subluxations was significantly different between shoulders with and without OA [9].

Buscayret et al. analyzed the pre and postoperative radiologic processes of 570 patients that had undergone shoulder stabilization [15]. They found five factors with statistically significant influence on the development of a preoperative OA without operation: The age at the first-time dislocation and at the time of the operation, in each case with higher risk at higher age; bony defects at the front lower glenoid or at the humeral head as well as a rotator cuff tear. Kraus et al. evaluated the results of conservative treatment of acute anteroinferior glenoid fractures [22]. Intra-articular step-off amounted to 6 mm (mean 2 mm); nevertheless, no significant increase in the OA rate could be found after a mean follow-up of 26.4 months. Marquiera et al. evaluated 14 patients with large Bankart fractures (>5 mm) and dislocation >2 mm that underwent conservative treatment [23]. After a mean follow-up of 5.6 years, every shoulder was stable. Only two patients showed mild and one patient moderate radiographic signs of arthrosis. Finally, Weisser et al. recently published excellent results of nonoperative treatment of anterior glenoid rim fractures after primary traumatic anterior shoulder dislocation. In the cohort of 30 patients with a >5 mm anterior glenoid rim fracture, functional outcome was reported as excellent with a low rate of recurrent instability (3%) and a low rate of new-onset OA (23%). To achieve these outcomes well centered post-reduction humeral head was mandatory. Anterior subluxation after reduction might develop in recurrent instability and OA, and should be considered a contraindication for nonoperative treatment [23,24].

The risk of developing a severe OA for individuals that suffered a shoulder dislocation is 10–20 fold increased [25]. The risk factors after conservative and surgical therapy are partially congruent (age, extended time until operation, bony defects, alcohol, smoker, hyperlaxity, high BMI, and increased age at initial instability event) [15,26–28].

5.2. OA after Surgical Stabilization

The incidence of OA after anterior surgical stabilization is stated between 12–62% [2,4,29,30]. In a prospective study with 41 patients that had at least two anterior dislocations and underwent arthroscopic transglenoidal suture, 12% showed radiographic changes after a follow-up of 52 months. There was a significant correlation between these changes and a worse clinical outcome. Patients with Bankart and Hill–Sachs lesions or other bony alterations on the preoperative images presented with a significantly worse functional outcome [4].

In a retrospective study, 30 of 39 patients that underwent open Bankart reconstruction could be examined after a mean follow-up of 29 years. Five patients were treated with total shoulder arthroplasty, and seven presented with radiographic signs of OA. Overall, the rate of OA was 40%. The authors, therefore, concluded that even though satisfying long-term results could be attained, the development of OA could not be stopped by surgery [3].

In another retrospective study after open Bankart reconstruction 33 of 53 shoulders could be evaluated after 15 years; 87% presented with no or minor radiographic signs of OA, 14 patients with minimal, and one patient with severe signs of OA. A significant correlation between the radiographic degenerative alterations and limitation of external rotation in 90° abduction depending on the time of follow-up could be shown. An influence of the limited external rotation in developing arthrosis was discussed but could not be proved [2]. In 2010, Ogawa et al. reviewed 163 patients undergoing the open Bankart procedure, finding that the development and progression of OA cannot be prevented by surgical intervention [10]. Most postoperatively detected OA developed already before surgery; nevertheless, the progression of postoperative OA was prolonged. Recent studies with over 20 years of follow-up still report satisfying outcomes. Moroder et al., with a mean

22-year follow-up after open Bankart repair in 26 patients, reported good clinical outcomes with minimal loss in the range of motion [31]. However, OA was found in up to 50% of patients and was associated with loss of external rotation, raising the question of whether the loss of external rotation was caused by OA or by overtightening the anterior capsule.

After Latarjet stabilization, 56 of 95 patients could be evaluated after a mean follow-up of 14.3 years. Three factors could be identified to be relevant for the development of postoperative OA: rotator cuff lesions, intra- or postoperative complications, and positioning of the coracoid to lateral. This last one is the most important prognostic factor. It was discussed that even though the rate of OA is quite high, stage I OA seems not to influence the postoperative outcome even after ten years [29]. Mizuno et al. conducted a retrospective review of 68 open Latarjet patients with a mean follow-up of 20 years. Of the 60 shoulders without OA preoperatively, 12 developed OA at final follow-up [32]. Overall, postoperative OA was mild, finding stage 1 in 14.7%, stage 2 in 5.9%, and stage 3 in 8.8% of patients. On the other hand, Gordins et al. report 65% of OA in 31 patients after 33 years of follow-up open Latarjet [33]. However, the technique implemented was the one described by May, and all patients were operated on before the modified Latarjet technique by Patte et al. [34]. Coracoid dimensions and standing up "May coracoid transfer" might influence these OA outcomes.

Comparing the rate of OA after Bankart and Bristow–Latarjet procedures after ten years of follow up Hovelius found a higher incidence after the Bankart procedure (16 of 26) than after the Bristow–Latarjet procedure (9 of 30). A recent meta-analysis suggests that the Latarjet procedure has a lower OA degree than other treatments, including non-operative treatment [35].

After glenoid reconstruction of significant bony defects using a J-graft, most relevant studies showed that there was no significant correlation between the number of dislocations and the rate of OA and that a significant influence of the performed surgery could not be found [26]. A recent follow-up of the cohort published by Moroder et al. shows excellent results regarding stability and function after a mean follow-up of 18 years [36]. However, OA was present in 74% of the patients now. Therefore, the development of dislocation arthropathy may not be prevented by this procedure.

Of 34 patients that underwent Weber-osteotomy, only four (9%) had no OA, nine (26%) had been treated with total shoulder arthroplasty. The increased internal rotation and the degree of arthrosis were statistically significant [37].

The rate of OA after the Eden–Hybinette procedure is always mentioned to be one of the highest [38]. In a retrospective study including 74 shoulders with a mean follow-up of 29 years after the Eden-Hybinett procedure, a recurrence occurred in 15 cases (20%) and OA in 35 cases (47%).

The ages at the time of the primary dislocation, surgery, and follow-up were mentioned as risk factors. Shoulders with signs of OA showed significant limitations of external rotation, even though most of them were subjectively satisfied [39]. Comparing 2- and 5-years follow-ups, the degree of limitation in the external rotation was not correlated significantly to the rate of OA. The rate of arthrosis was higher after primary dislocation at a higher age (above 23) [40]. Buscaryet et al. showed in 570 patients after surgical stabilization that lower degrees of OA remain without progress more often than higher degrees; 19.9% of the patients who had no preoperative signs of OA developed postoperative OA [15]. The lengths of follow-up and the number of preoperative dislocations were found as risk factors. The time to surgery, the degree of instability (luxation or subluxation), the level of sportive activity, and especially the type of surgery were found to have no significant correlation with the development of OA. Therefore, there was no difference found between the Latarjet-procedure and soft-tissue techniques. When comparing the three groups with equal follow-up, no significant differences could be found concerning the rate of OA.

After arthroscopic stabilization, there was a lower rate of OA but a lower time of follow-up [15]. Other authors found similar rates of OA both in open and arthroscopic procedures [7]. Boileau et al. reported an increase in glenohumeral OA incidence from 4%

preoperatively to 17% postoperatively after arthroscopic stabilization [41]. Meantime, a couple of literature reports deal with the long-term appearance of OA after arthroscopic Bankart repair. Castagna et al. found mild (29%) to moderate (10%) arthrosis after a minimum of 10 years after arthroscopic Bankart repair, but degenerative changes of the glenohumeral joint had no significant effect on the clinical outcomes [42]. Kavaja et al. examined the radiologic and clinical occurrence of glenohumeral OA 13 years after arthroscopic Bankart repair [43]. OA was diagnosed radiologically in 68 percent but rarely caused subjective symptoms. Franceschi et al. found OA in 21.8% of the patients with no preoperative degenerative changes eight years after arthroscopic Bankart repair [44]. Finally, the latest arthroscopic Bankart repair cohort published by Plath et al. reports 69% of OA over a hundred patients with a mean follow-up of 13 years [45].

These studies show that postoperative OA in different degrees occurs, both in open and arthroscopic procedures. As risk factors in developing postoperative OA, bony lesions (Bankart and Hill–Sachs lesions), lengths of follow-up, concomitant lesions of the rotator cuff, intra- and postoperative complications, positioning of the coracoid to lateral, higher age at primary dislocation or surgery, and a long time to surgery are mentioned. In addition, loose or proud metal pieces (screws, staples) (Figure 3) could cause a progressive OA quickly [46]. Yeh and Kharrazi report a rare but dramatic complication following shoulder arthroscopy: post arthroscopic glenohumeral chondrolysis [47]. The articular cartilage undergoes rapid degenerative changes shortly after arthroscopic surgery. Although the etiology of post arthroscopic glenohumeral chondrolysis is not yet fully understood, the pathophysiology is likely multifactorial.

After arthroscopic stabilization using screws positioned at the glenoidal rim, Tauber et al. found only one case in 10 cases of material impingement that made the removal necessary after two years [48]. Experimental studies show that a loss of the anteroinferior labrum reduces the contact area by 7–15% and increases the contact pressure by 8–20%, concerning the anteroinferior part of the glenoid even at 53%. A bony loss of 30% of the glenoid diameter increases the contact pressure at the anteroinferior part even at 300–400% [49]. Whether such a loss or step-off formation is relevant for instability and development of arthrosis seems to be dependent on a centered or decentered humeral head.

5.3. Capsulorrhaphy Arthropathy as an Own Entity?

Matsen et al. defined the term capsulorrhaphy arthropathy for patients who develop OA due to too strongly strained anterior capsules [50]. The strong harnessing of the anterior soft tissues, e.g., a Putti–Platt, or a too strongly strained Bankart operation, leads to compression and intensified shearing stresses on the joint surface that increase if the patient goes into external rotation. It is postulated that this mechanism develops in all operations where the external rotation is excessively limited [51].

Biomechanical and anatomical studies today offer evidence that a non-anatomical strain of the anterior capsule leads to an increase in posterior joint pressure, posteroinferior subluxation of the humeral head, and thus pain and the development of arthrosis [52]. In a cadaveric comparison of a front capsule strain with an anteroinferior capsule shift, it could be shown that during the strain of the front capsule the stability decreases and the external rotation and elevation are limited. That larger shear joint forces are necessary to reach the maximum elevation. In contrast, the anteroinferior capsule shift improves stability without limiting the external rotation or elevation [53] (Figure 4).

Gerber and Werner experimentally showed the effect of selective capsulorrhaphy on the translation and the passive range of motion [54,55].

On the one hand, these studies document that capsulorrhaphy arthropathy is biomechanically justified and permits, on the other hand, developing more anatomical stabilization operations. In retrospective studies, a decreased external rotation was connected with an increased rate of OA; whether this was the cause or the effect could not be clarified [15].

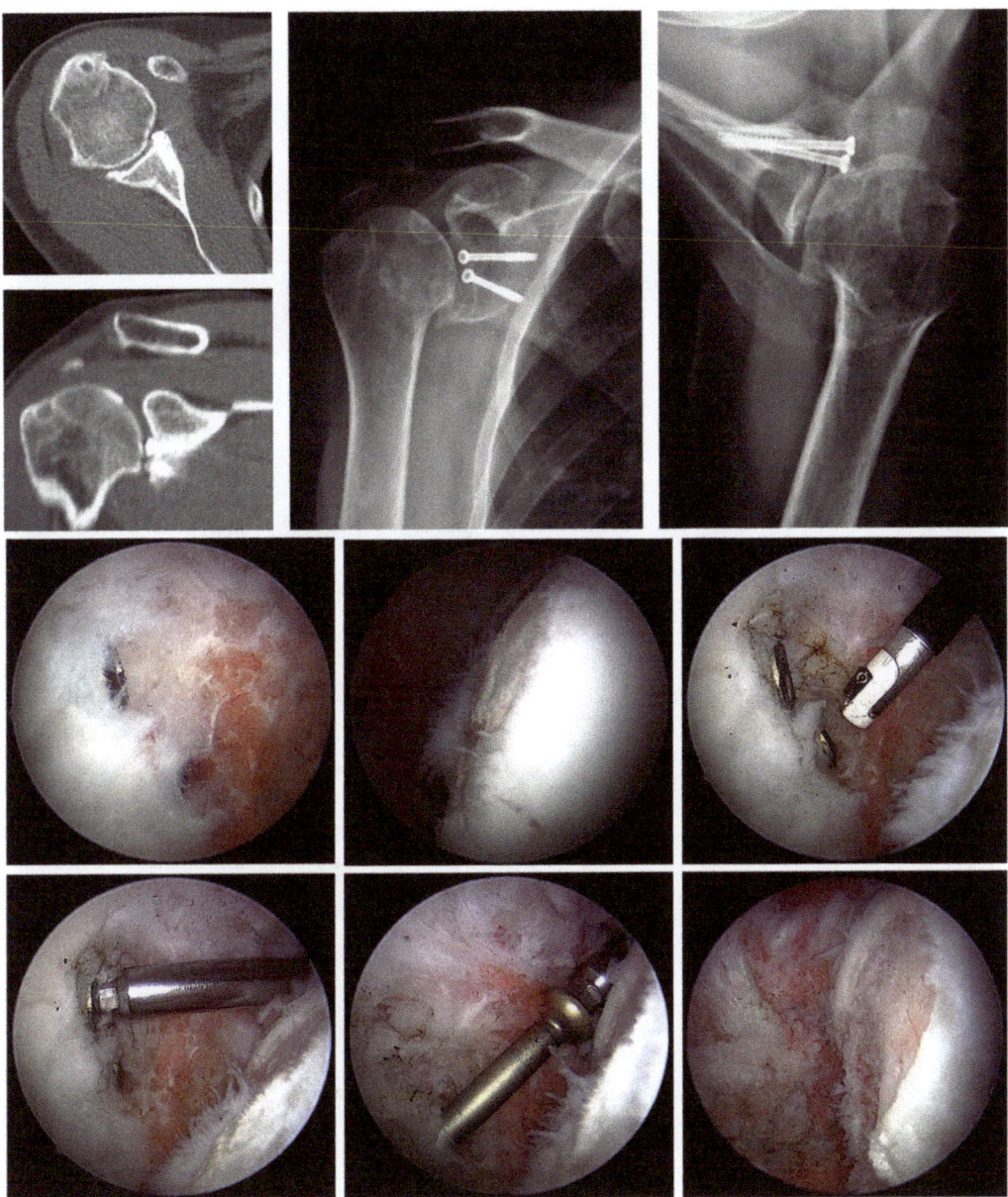

Figure 3. Details of proud screws after glenoid fracture surgery removed arthroscopically. **First row**: radiologic studies showing instability surgery performed and proud implants. **Second row**: Images of a humeral cartilage defect and debridement necessary to expose implants. **Third row**: Arthroscopic screws removal.

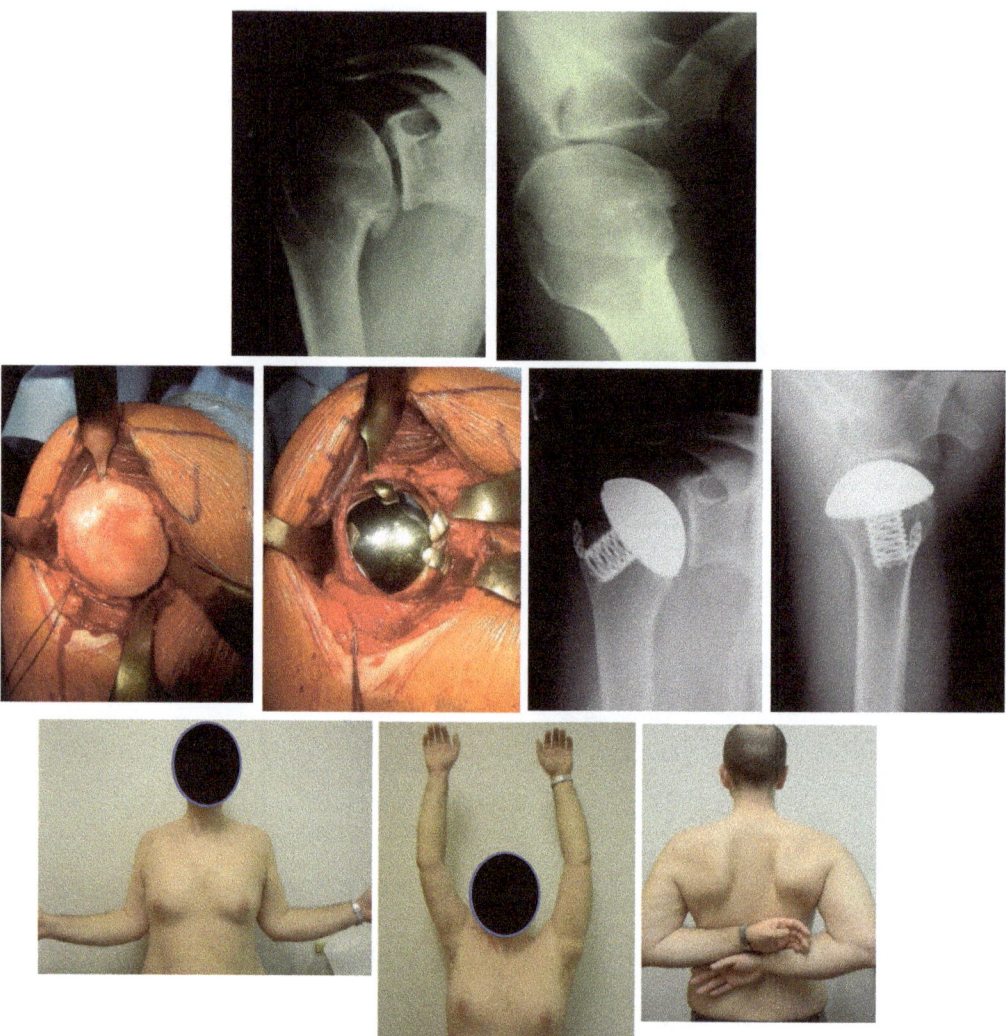

Figure 4. 43 year-old patient treated with hemiprosthesis after capsulorrhaphy arthropathy subsequent to open instability repair. **First row**: preoperative radiographs. **Second row**: intraoperative pictures of hemiprosthesis implant and postoperative radiographs. **Third row**: Physical examination and shoulder function at final follow-up.

6. Treatment Options and Results

6.1. Nonoperative Treatment

Non-operative treatment of shoulder dislocation arthropathy should be the first step of management. Classic studies have shown similar OA proportions between non-operative and operative treatment at any point of follow up [35]. There is no evidence of significant benefit in using non-steroidal anti-inflammatory drugs (oral or topic) to treat shoulder pain. Improvements could be found with oral prednisolone, but side effects should be taken into special consideration when using these medications. Intraarticular corticosteroids or hyaluronic acid are among the most popular nonoperative treatments for glenohumeral OA. While both have demonstrated sustained pain relief, difficulty in accurately administering them in the glenohumeral joint without ultrasound assistance has been pointed out. There are no efficacy studies regarding physical therapy as an isolated treatment. Several multimodal therapy plans have proven sustained improvements in pain and function [56].

6.2. Removal of Foreign Material

Metal anchors that contact the joint surface will lead to a progressive OA in the shortest time. Pain or crepitation after shoulder stabilization should, therefore, be clarified. The positions of possible metal anchors can be retraced in a thin slice CT. Without the slightest doubt, a revision arthroscopy and the removal of the anchors are necessary. The knowledge of the kind of brought-in anchors is vital to providing the right removal instrument. To approach the anchor in its centerline, percutaneous instrumenting can be helpful. Metal portions that are not visible in the joint at first sight could be covered by only a thin layer of soft tissue and should, therefore, be removed.

Implants for shoulder stabilization have evolved to suture anchors manufactured of various materials, including metal, poly-L-lactic acid, PEEK (polyether ether ketone), and all sutures. "Anchor arthropathy" could be defined as an own entity after stabilization surgery. Early-onset of pain and stiffness, usually before 10 months after index surgery, could be found. Waltz et al. found advanced imaging, such as MRI unreliable to confirm proud implants or prominent suture knots. Therefore, early arthroscopy to assess painful and stiff shoulders after instability repair should have a low threshold [57].

6.3. Arthroscopic Debridement and Arthrolysis

In the case of an early stage of OA arthroscopic, debridement with loose cartilage portions removal and partial synovectomy can improve functionality and relieve pain. The cause of arthritis, e.g., the eccentric load of the glenoid as its "engine", is not resolved by this. An arthroscopic debridement can only help if a sufficient passive range of motion with the possibility of relieving after treatment is present. Removing the osteophytes, usually within the front lower range of the anatomical neck, is technically challenging. Millet's CAM procedure was developed as a joint-preserving arthroscopic treatment approach for young, active patients with advanced shoulder OA [58]. Besides chondroplasty, synovectomy, loose body removal, and subacromial decompression, the CAM procedure also involves extensive capsular release to restore motion, humeral osteoplasty, and osteophyte excision to recontour the humeral head, restore abduction, and potentially decompress impingement on the axillary nerve; axillary nerve neurolysis when scarring is seen and biceps tenodesis when there is significant tenosynovitis, SLAP tear or a pulley lesion [59]. Arner et al. reported significant improvements in 38 patients after 10 years of follow-up of the CAM procedure. Humeral head flattening and severe joint incongruity were risk factors for CAM failure, although survivorship was 63% at a minimum 10-year follow-up [60]. A recent investigation from the same group found similar results after arthroplasty, whether a prior CAM procedure was performed before the prosthesis [61].

6.4. Arthroplasty

The problem with dislocation arthropathy is that these patients are younger than those with idiopathic OA and usually have substantial internal rotation contracture and posterior glenoid defects [62].

As with each OA, the preoperative clinical examination with determination of the rotation is essential. A limited external rotation is a prognostically negative criterion for the post-op result. The preoperative analysis of the glenoid constellation is often insufficient in the axial projection and is better investigated in the CT. The MRI is used to evaluate fatty atrophy and integrity of the subscapular muscle and the other portions of the rotator cuff.

During the approach, the mobilization with an anterior extension of the subscapular muscle is critical of particular importance. This can be achieved by completely separating the subscapular tendon and approximately 1 cm medial refixation. A medialization of around 1 cm corresponds to an external rotation gain of approximately 20°. In case of stronger contractions, a bifocal capsulotomy according to Habermeyer is preferred [63]. The incision begins at the rotator interval. After ligature of the anterior circumflex arteries and protection of the latissimus dorsi and teres major insertion, the subscapular muscle is wholly detached down to the metaphysis [64]. The medial mobilization behind the anterior margin of the coracobrachialis muscle is not recommended to preserve blood circulation and innervation and avoid secondary damage to the subscapular muscle.

The replacement on the humeral side depends on the size of the defect. In younger patients, a cup, stemless or short stem/stem prostheses are possible (Figure 5). In the cup prosthesis, the bony defect should not exceed 30%. Recent studies report comparable short-term results between a combination of humeral surface replacement with cemented glenoid component and conventional total shoulder arthroplasty [65].

Dorsal rolled out glenoids require excellent preoperative planning to define the glenoid form and version. After the good exposition, the axis and the glenoid center should be marked with, e.g., a K-wire to plan the correct inclination and version. The value of navigation still must be proven. In most cases, with sufficient bone substance, the higher edge of the glenoid is removed to create a correct version. In larger, usually posterior defects, a reconstruction by a bone graft ("contained defect") or accumulation of an iliac crest graft ("non contained defect") is necessary (Figure 6). Bone transplantation for reestablishment of the glenoid defects or correcting the version is already mentioned in small numbers by Neer [66] after introducing the unlinked prostheses. The simultaneous implantation of a cemented glenoid is problematic from a biological point of view. Here two-step procedures should be preferred. The fixation of anterior bone grafts is substantially more straightforward and unproblematic than that of posterior defects. The posterior bone grafts can be placed only sometimes from the anterior. If a dorsal defect without hold to the medial exists, the graft must be inserted from the posterior. The graft is fixed with two screws that should not affect the implantation of the glenoid (keel or pegs). If a strong posterior inclination of the glenoid is present and no sufficient correction of the version is possible, stability can be increased by adapting the version of the components against each other. If this is not possible, it is better to surrender the glenoidal component. In case of a simultaneous existing out-of-center rotator cuff lesion, the implantation of Reverse Shoulder Arthroplasty (RSA) is possible.

Results after Arthroplasty

Green and Norri [62] retrospectively evaluated 17 of 19 patients with shoulder prosthesis (15 TSA and two HSA) due to dislocation arthropathy (four Bristow, four Putti Platt, four Magnuson Stack, two Bankart, and four soft tissue operations) after 62 months; 94% had significant pain relief. Except for one, all patients received a better function. Subjectively, 16 patients judged the result as much better or better and one as worse. Three patients had to be revised.

Sperling et al. examined 31 patients (21 TSA, 10 HSA) retrospectively for at least two years and an average of 7 years postoperatively [67]. Pain, external rotation, and active abduction improved significantly without differences between HSA and TSA. The survival rate after two years was 97%, after five years 86%, and after ten years, only 61%. Nevertheless, 3/10 HSA and 8/21 TSA had to be revised.

Hill and Norris examined the results after bony glenoid reconstruction at five anterior and 12 posterior defects, five patients with arthrosis, three with capsulorrhaphy arthropathy, two with recurrent dislocations, and one after revision. All had a certain anterior or posterior instability preoperatively [68]. In 15 patients, a bone from the resected humeral head was used. The indication for transplantation of a bone graft existed, if the bone substance was not sufficient to correct the version (version >15°), to ensure the fixation of the glenoidal component (withdraw the keel when planning), or if via a version of the components no adjustment could be made. After correction, an average retroversion of 4° with an average correction angle of 33° could be seen. Three patients with graft failure (nonunion, dissolution, or graft dislocation) and five failures with glenoid revisions because of rotator cuff rupture, persisting instability, wrong component placement, or loosening of the transplant, showing unsatisfactory functional results. In 14 of 17 cases, the version and substance of the glenoid could be repaired. The patients without implant or transplant failure showed an apparent reduction in pain and good gain of function (AAE on average 107° (30–165°), i.e., satisfying functional results in nine of 17 patients. The study of Neer showed a lower failure rate (0 of 19) [66].

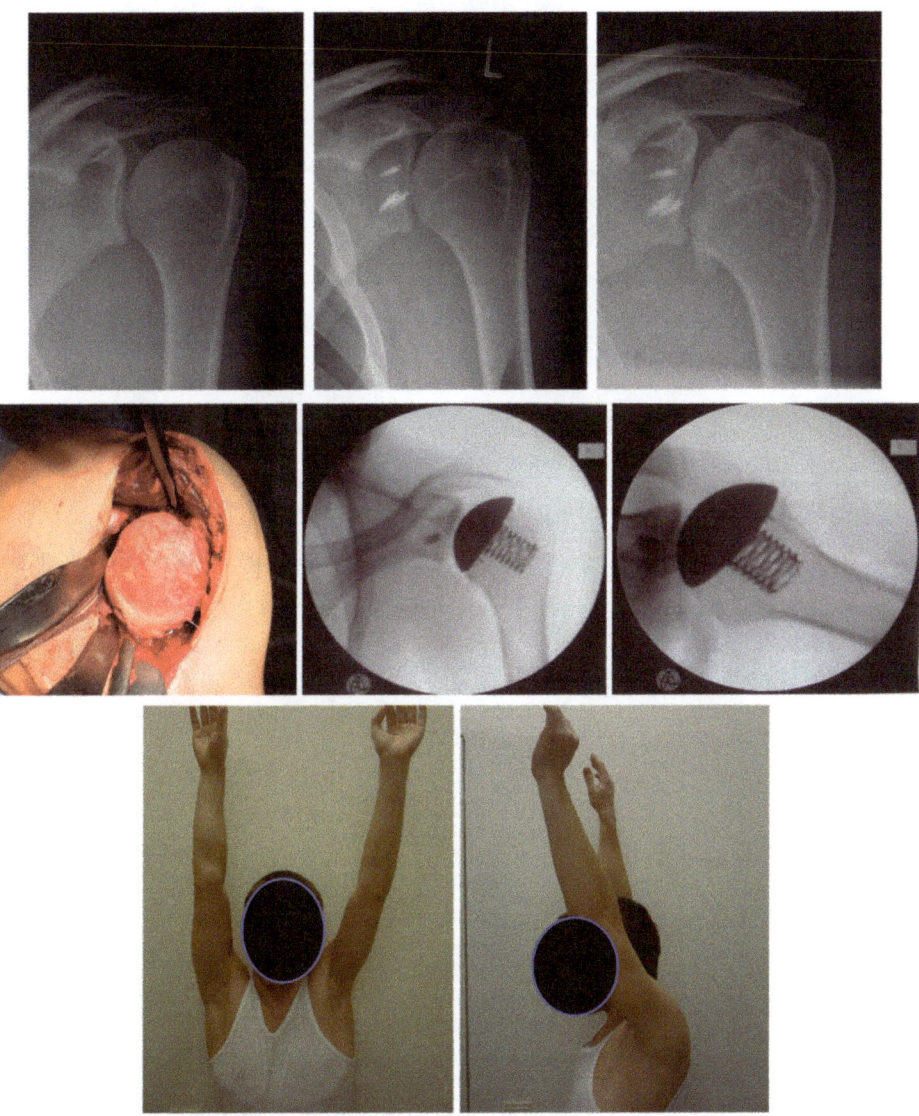

Figure 5. 22-year-old patient with dislocation arthropathy after instability surgery treated with stemless prosthesis. **First row**: radiographs showing OA after shoulder instability surgery. **Second row**: intraoperative pictures of hemiprosthesis. **Third row**: Physical examination and shoulder function at final follow-up.

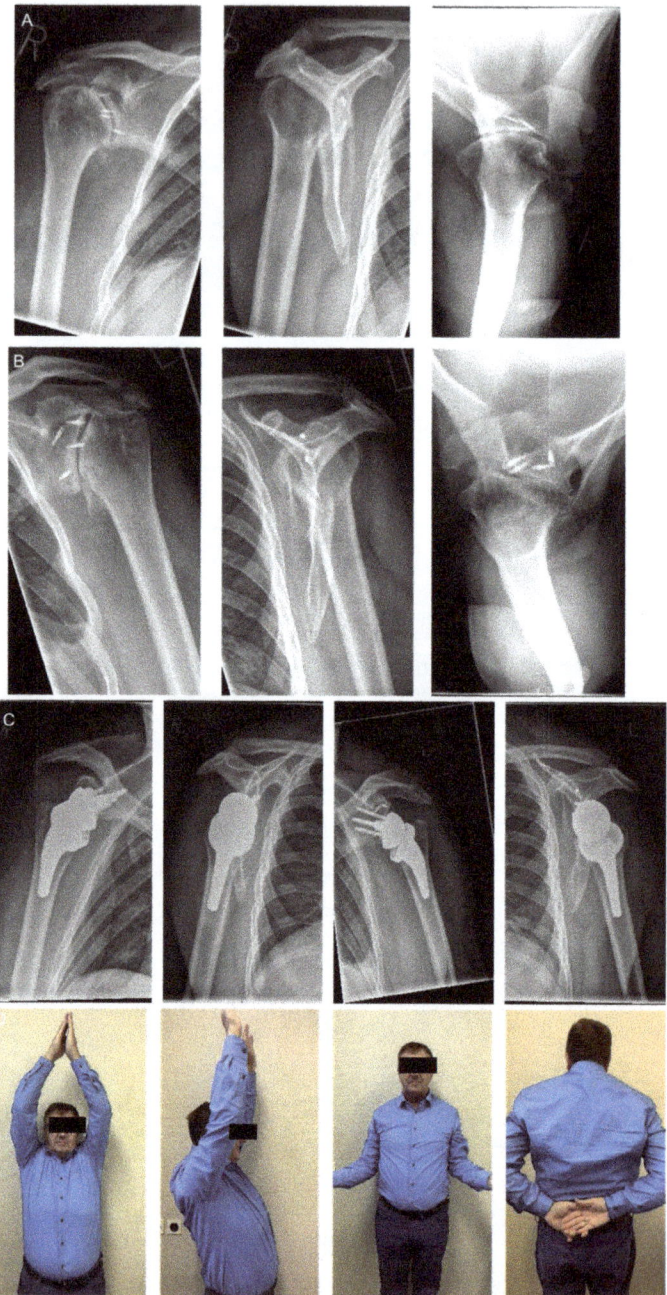

Figure 6. 61-year-old male with bilateral dislocation arthropathy. (**A**): right shoulder dislocation arthropathy after instability surgery. (**B**): left shoulder dislocation arthropathy after instability surgery. (**C**): treatment with bilateral two surgeries Reverse Shoulder Arthroplasty using full wedge. (**D**): right side 12 months follow up and left side 6 months follow up clinical results.

Primary glenoidal bone graft transplantation has a ten times higher risk of glenoidal failure than patients with primary implantation without bone transplantation. If the transplant heals sufficiently, there is no tendency for early loosening. The transplantation is suitable to lower the post-operational instability rate [68].

Matsoukis et al. examined two collectives in a multicentric study, one with and one without previous stabilization operation [69]. Twenty-eight patients without preceding operations had been seen at least for two years. One group sustained the first dislocation under and the other one over the age of 40 years. Below 40 years, the processes were longer, and there were numerous recurrences, but only one rotator cuff tear was found; 64% had an excellent or good result, similar to concentric osteoarthritis. The processes were short in the second group with patients older than 40 years. With seven rotator cuff tears, only 36% of them had an excellent or good result. Because of the rotator cuff tears, hemiprostheses had been implanted in most cases. The difference is probably due to the higher rate of rotator cuff tears.

In contrast to fatty degeneration of the rotator cuff, especially of the subscapularis muscle, the preceding operation and the preoperative external rotation did not influence the result. Altogether, prosthetics could achieve good results due to dislocation arthropathy after conservative and operational treatment. Significantly better results were shown after TSA than HSA. Adverse prognostic factors were a higher age at the initial dislocation and a rotator cuff tear. The previous surgery, e.g., bone block or soft part operation, was without significant influence (10 complications in 55 prostheses, three cases of glenoid loosening in connection with rotator cuff ruptures, four anterior instabilities, six revisions) [70]. Lehmann et al. report a significantly increased weighted average constant score following shoulder arthroplasty for OA caused by shoulder instability [63]. The authors found no significant difference between total shoulder replacements and hemiarthroplasty. Nevertheless, a relatively high rate of complications (40%) was revealed, with 20% requiring an operative revision.

Due to inconsistent results, surgeons are moving towards the implantation of RSA after dislocation arthropathy (Figure 6). There is a trend of positive results with these implants, yet follow-up is still relatively short. RSA has been used in recent years for patients with OA and rotator cuff deficiency after shoulder stabilization. Raiss et al. describe the results of 13 patients with a median follow-up of 3.5 years and a median age of 70 years that had at least one rotator cuff tendon tear in combination with an OA treated before for recurrent anterior shoulder instability. Constant score, shoulder flexion, and internal rotation significantly improved after RSA and were comparable with those of other studies reporting on the outcome of reverse shoulder arthroplasty for other conditions [71].

For Clavert et al., RSA is justified due to the higher rate of complications and revisions of non-constrained anatomic shoulder arthroplasties reported. In his cohort of 25 patients with a mean follow-up of 6.6 years, clinical results were comparable to other studies describing results of RSA, even in cases where bone grafting was mandatory [72]. Besides satisfactory clinical and radiological results have been published, and follow-up is still relatively short for this indication.

7. Conclusions

Dislocation arthropathy can be the consequence of an instability episode of the shoulder. The risk of developing OA after primary traumatic dislocation compared to the normal situation is increased up to 10–20-fold. The age at the initial dislocation, bony lesions at the glenoid, and the head or a rotator cuff tear increase the risk. The classification according to Samilson and Prieto is used. CT and MR tomographic diagnostics increase the genesis statement, the classification, and the therapeutic options. Rates of OA after stabilization range between 12 and 62%, whereby a safe designation of the operational procedures cannot be made. The Latarjet procedure seems to have a lower degree of OA than other treatments, even conservative treatments. Metal anchors and screws with joint contact lead to a rapidly progressive OA and must be removed, arthroscopically. In low-grade OA, arthroscopic debridement is helpful. Arthroscopic arthrolysis with capsulotomy can improve elevation and external rotation in cases of internal rotation contracture. If massive OA is present, prosthesis becomes inevitable. However, patients with instability arthropathy are mostly younger and suffer from a considerable internal rotation deficit and glenoid defects. The defect size determines the humeral replacement. Using Cup-prostheses, it should not exceed 30%. Results of total shoulder prosthesis are superior to those of hemiarthroplasty. Three-dimensional planning tools are becoming useful for correct implant selection. Results of RSA are promising; however, a longer follow-up is required. Significant glenoid defects need to be treated with bone grafting to provide stability. Nevertheless, bone grafting increases the risk of implant failure. The type of primary treatment and external rotation did not affect the prognosis of the prosthesis after glenohumeral stabilization, whereas fatty degeneration of the rotator cuff did.

Funding: This research received no external funding.

Institutional Review Board Statement: Not applicable.

Informed Consent Statement: Not applicable.

Conflicts of Interest: Ulrich H. Brunner and Markus Scheibel are consultant for Stryker.

References

1. Neer, C.S.; Watson, K.C.; Stanton, F.J. Recent Experience in Total Shoulder Replacement. *J. Bone Jt. Surg. Am.* **1982**, *64*, 319–337. [CrossRef]
2. Rosenberg, B.N.; Richmond, J.C.; Levine, W.N. Long-Term Followup of Bankart Reconstruction. Incidence of Late Degenerative Glenohumeral Arthrosis. *Am. J. Sports Med.* **1995**, *23*, 538–544. [CrossRef] [PubMed]
3. Pelet, S.; Jolles, B.M.; Farron, A. Bankart Repair for Recurrent Anterior Glenohumeral Instability: Results at Twenty-Nine Years' Follow-up. *J. Shoulder Elb. Surg.* **2006**, *15*, 203–207. [CrossRef] [PubMed]
4. Oh, J.H.; Chung, S.W.; Oh, C.H.; Kim, S.H.; Park, S.J.; Kim, K.W.; Park, J.H.; Lee, S.B.; Lee, J.J. The Prevalence of Shoulder Osteoarthritis in the Elderly Korean Population: Association with Risk Factors and Function. *J. Shoulder Elb. Surg.* **2011**, *20*, 756–763. [CrossRef] [PubMed]
5. Swanson, A.B.; de Groot Swanson, G.; Maupin, B.K.; Wei, J.N.; Khalil, M.A. Bipolar Implant Shoulder Arthroplasty. *Orthopedics* **1986**, *9*, 343–351. [CrossRef] [PubMed]
6. Scheibel, M.; Habermeyer, P. Subscapularis Dysfunction Following Anterior Surgical Approaches to the Shoulder. *J. Shoulder Elb. Surg.* **2008**, *17*, 671–683. [CrossRef]
7. Zacher, J.; Carl, H.D.; Swoboda, B.; Backhaus, M. Imaging of osteoarthritis of the peripheral joints. *Z. Rheumatol.* **2007**, *66*, 257–258; 260–264; 266. [CrossRef]
8. Kerr, R.; Resnick, D.; Pineda, C.; Haghighi, P. Osteoarthritis of the Glenohumeral Joint: A Radiologic-Pathologic Study. *AJR Am. J. Roentgenol.* **1985**, *144*, 967–972. [CrossRef]
9. Ogawa, K.; Yoshida, A.; Ikegami, H. Osteoarthritis in Shoulders with Traumatic Anterior Instability: Preoperative Survey Using Radiography and Computed Tomography. *J. Shoulder Elb.Surg.* **2006**, *15*, 23–29. [CrossRef]
10. Ogawa, K.; Yoshida, A.; Matsumoto, H.; Takeda, T. Outcome of the Open Bankart Procedure for Shoulder Instability and Development of Osteoarthritis: A 5- to 20-Year Follow-up Study. *Am. J. Sports Med.* **2010**, *38*, 1549–1557. [CrossRef]
11. Sabesan, V.J.; Callanan, M.; Youderian, A.; Iannotti, J.P. 3D CT Assessment of the Relationship Between Humeral Head Alignment and Glenoid Retroversion in Glenohumeral Osteoarthritis. *J. Bone Jt. Surg.* **2014**, *96*, e64. [CrossRef] [PubMed]
12. Gates, S.; Sager, B.; Khazzam, M. Preoperative Glenoid Considerations for Shoulder Arthroplasty: A Review. *EFORT Open Rev.* **2020**, *5*, 126–137. [CrossRef] [PubMed]
13. Schröder, R.-J.; Scheibel, M.; Tsynman, A.; Magosch, P.; Habermeyer, P. Magnetresonanztomographische Untersuchung des Musculus subscapularis nach offener vorderer Schulterstabilisierung. *Fortschr. Röntgenstrahlen* **2006**, *178*, 706–712. [CrossRef] [PubMed]
14. Samilson, R.L.; Prieto, V. Dislocation Arthropathy of the Shoulder. *J. Bone Jt. Surg. Am.* **1983**, *65*, 456–460. [CrossRef]
15. Buscayret, F.; Edwards, T.B.; Szabo, I.; Adeleine, P.; Coudane, H.; Walch, G. Glenohumeral Arthrosis in Anterior Instability before and after Surgical Treatment: Incidence and Contributing Factors. *Am. J. Sports Med.* **2004**, *32*, 1165–1172. [CrossRef]
16. Kircher, J.; Morhard, M.; Magosch, P.; Ebinger, N.; Lichtenberg, S.; Habermeyer, P. How Much Are Radiological Parameters Related to Clinical Symptoms and Function in Osteoarthritis of the Shoulder? *Int. Orthop.* **2010**, *34*, 677–681. [CrossRef]
17. Linke, P.M.; Zemke, K.; Ecker, N.U.; Neumann, J.; Werner, A.W. Standard Radiological Classification of Glenohumeral Osteoarthritis Does Not Correlate with the Complexity of the Arthritic Glenoid Deformity. *Arch. Orthop. Trauma Surg.* **2021**. Online ahead of print. [CrossRef]
18. Neer, C.S. *Shoulder Reconstruction*; WB Saunders: Philadelphia, PA, USA, 1990.

19. Hovelius, L.K.; Sandström, B.C.; Rösmark, D.L.; Saebö, M.; Sundgren, K.H.; Malmqvist, B.G. Long-Term Results with the Bankart and Bristow-Latarjet Procedures: Recurrent Shoulder Instability and Arthropathy. *J. Shoulder Elb. Surg.* **2001**, *10*, 445–452. [CrossRef]
20. Hovelius, L.; Augustini, B.G.; Fredin, H.; Johansson, O.; Norlin, R.; Thorling, J. Primary Anterior Dislocation of the Shoulder in Young Patients. A Ten-Year Prospective Study. *J. Bone Jt. Surg. Am.* **1996**, *78*, 1677–1684. [CrossRef]
21. Singer, G.C.; Kirkland, P.M.; Emery, R.J. Coracoid Transposition for Recurrent Anterior Instability of the Shoulder. A 20-Year Follow-up Study. *J. Bone Jt. Surg. Br.* **1995**, *77*, 73–76. [CrossRef]
22. Kraus, N.; Gerhardt, C.; Haas, N.; Scheibel, M. Conservative therapy of antero-inferior glenoid fractures. *Unfallchirurg* **2010**, *113*, 469–475. [CrossRef] [PubMed]
23. Maquieira, G.J.; Espinosa, N.; Gerber, C.; Eid, K. Non-Operative Treatment of Large Anterior Glenoid Rim Fractures after Traumatic Anterior Dislocation of the Shoulder. *J. Bone Jt. Surg. Br.* **2007**, *89*, 1347–1351. [CrossRef] [PubMed]
24. Wieser, K.; Waltenspül, M.; Ernstbrunner, L.; Ammann, E.; Nieuwland, A.; Eid, K.; Gerber, C. Nonoperative Treatment of Anterior Glenoid Rim Fractures after First-Time Traumatic Anterior Shoulder Dislocation: A Study with 9-Year Follow-up. *JBJS Open Access* **2020**, *5*, e20.00133. [CrossRef] [PubMed]
25. Marx, R.G.; McCarty, E.C.; Montemurno, T.D.; Altchek, D.W.; Craig, E.V.; Warren, R.F. Development of Arthrosis Following Dislocation of the Shoulder: A Case-Control Study. *J. Shoulder Elb. Surg.* **2002**, *11*, 1–5. [CrossRef] [PubMed]
26. Auffarth, A.; Schauer, J.; Matis, N.; Kofler, B.; Hitzl, W.; Resch, H. The J-Bone Graft for Anatomical Glenoid Reconstruction in Recurrent Posttraumatic Anterior Shoulder Dislocation. *Am. J. Sports Med.* **2008**, *36*, 638–647. [CrossRef] [PubMed]
27. Cameron, M.L.; Kocher, M.S.; Briggs, K.K.; Horan, M.P.; Hawkins, R.J. The Prevalence of Glenohumeral Osteoarthrosis in Unstable Shoulders. *Am. J. Sports Med.* **2003**, *31*, 53–55. [CrossRef] [PubMed]
28. Kruckeberg, B.M.; Leland, D.P.; Bernard, C.D.; Krych, A.J.; Dahm, D.L.; Sanchez-Sotelo, J.; Camp, C.L. Incidence of and Risk Factors for Glenohumeral Osteoarthritis after Anterior Shoulder Instability: A US Population–Based Study with Average 15-Year Follow-up. *Orthop. J. Sports Med.* **2020**, *8*, 232596712096251. [CrossRef] [PubMed]
29. Allain, J.; Goutallier, D.; Glorion, C. Long-Term Results of the Latarjet Procedure for the Treatment of Anterior Instability of the Shoulder. *J. Bone Jt. Surg. Am.* **1998**, *80*, 841–852. [CrossRef]
30. Chapnikoff, D.; Besson, A.; Chantelot, C.; Fontaine, C.; Migaud, H.; Duquennoy, A. Bankart procedure: Clinical and radiological long-term outcome. *Rev. Chir. Orthop. Reparatrice Appar. Mot.* **2000**, *86*, 558–565.
31. Moroder, P.; Odorizzi, M.; Pizzinini, S.; Demetz, E.; Resch, H.; Moroder, P. Open Bankart Repair for the Treatment of Anterior Shoulder Instability without Substantial Osseous Glenoid Defects: Results After a Minimum Follow-up of Twenty Years. *J. Bone Jt. Surg.-Am. Vol.* **2015**, *97*, 1398–1405. [CrossRef]
32. Mizuno, N.; Denard, P.J.; Raiss, P.; Melis, B.; Walch, G. Long-Term Results of the Latarjet Procedure for Anterior Instability of the Shoulder. *J. Shoulder Elb. Surg.* **2014**, *23*, 1691–1699. [CrossRef] [PubMed]
33. Gordins, V.; Hovelius, L.; Sandström, B.; Rahme, H.; Bergström, U. Risk of Arthropathy after the Bristow-Latarjet Repair: A Radiologic and Clinical Thirty-Three to Thirty-Five Years of Follow-up of Thirty-One Shoulders. *J. Shoulder Elb. Surg.* **2015**, *24*, 691–699. [CrossRef]
34. Patte, D.; Bernageau, J.; Rodineau, J.; Gardes, J.C. Epaules Douloureuses et Instables. *Rev. Chirugie Orthopédique* **1980**, *60*, 157–165.
35. Verweij, L.P.E.; Pruijssen, E.C.; Kerkhoffs, G.M.M.J.; Blankevoort, L.; Sierevelt, I.N.; van Deurzen, D.F.P.; van den Bekerom, M.P.J. Treatment Type May Influence Degree of Post-Dislocation Shoulder Osteoarthritis: A Systematic Review and Meta-Analysis. *Knee Surg. Sports Traumatol. Arthrosc.* **2021**, *29*, 2312–2324. [CrossRef] [PubMed]
36. Moroder, P.; Plachel, F.; Becker, J.; Schulz, E.; Abdic, S.; Haas, M.; Resch, H.; Auffarth, A. Clinical and Radiological Long-Term Results After Implant-Free, Autologous, Iliac Crest Bone Graft Procedure for the Treatment of Anterior Shoulder Instability. *Am. J. Sports Med.* **2018**, *46*, 2975–2980. [CrossRef] [PubMed]
37. Flury, M.P.; Goldhahn, J.; Holzmann, P.; Simmen, B.R. Does Weber's Rotation Osteotomy Induce Degenerative Joint Disease at the Shoulder in the Long Term? *J. Shoulder Elb. Surg.* **2007**, *16*, 735–741. [CrossRef] [PubMed]
38. Hindmarsh, J.; Lindberg, A. Eden-Hybbinette's Operation for Recurrent Dislocation of the Humero-Scapular Joint. *Acta Orthop. Scand.* **1967**, *38*, 459–478. [CrossRef]
39. Rahme, H.; Wikblad, L.; Nowak, J.; Larsson, S. Long-Term Clinical and Radiologic Results after Eden-Hybbinette Operation for Anterior Instability of the Shoulder. *J. Shoulder Elb. Surg.* **2003**, *12*, 15–19. [CrossRef]
40. Hovelius, L.; Sandström, B.; Saebö, M. One Hundred Eighteen Bristow-Latarjet Repairs for Recurrent Anterior Dislocation of the Shoulder Prospectively Followed for Fifteen Years: Study II-the Evolution of Dislocation Arthropathy. *J. Shoulder Elb. Surg.* **2006**, *15*, 279–289. [CrossRef]
41. Boileau, P.; Fourati, E.; Bicknell, R. Neer Modification of Open Bankart Procedure: What Are the Rates of Recurrent Instability, Functional Outcome, and Arthritis? *Clin. Orthop. Relat. Res.* **2012**, *470*, 2554–2560. [CrossRef]
42. Castagna, A.; Markopoulos, N.; Conti, M.; Delle Rose, G.; Papadakou, E.; Garofalo, R. Arthroscopic Bankart Suture-Anchor Repair: Radiological and Clinical Outcome at Minimum 10 Years of Follow-up. *Am. J. Sports Med.* **2010**, *38*, 2012–2016. [CrossRef] [PubMed]
43. Kavaja, L.; Pajarinen, J.; Sinisaari, I.; Savolainen, V.; Björkenheim, J.-M.; Haapamäki, V.; Paavola, M. Arthrosis of Glenohumeral Joint after Arthroscopic Bankart Repair: A Long-Term Follow-up of 13 Years. *J. Shoulder Elb. Surg.* **2012**, *21*, 350–355. [CrossRef] [PubMed]

44. Franceschi, F.; Papalia, R.; Del Buono, A.; Vasta, S.; Maffulli, N.; Denaro, V. Glenohumeral Osteoarthritis after Arthroscopic Bankart Repair for Anterior Instability. *Am. J. Sports Med.* **2011**, *39*, 1653–1659. [CrossRef] [PubMed]
45. Plath, J.E.; Aboalata, M.; Seppel, G.; Juretzko, J.; Waldt, S.; Vogt, S.; Imhoff, A.B. Prevalence of and Risk Factors for Dislocation Arthropathy: Radiological Long-Term Outcome of Arthroscopic Bankart Repair in 100 Shoulders at an Average 13-Year Follow-Up. *Am. J. Sports Med.* **2015**, *43*, 1084–1090. [CrossRef] [PubMed]
46. O'Driscoll, S.W.; Evans, D.C. Long-Term Results of Staple Capsulorrhaphy for Anterior Instability of the Shoulder. *J. Bone Jt. Surg. Am.* **1993**, *75*, 249–258. [CrossRef]
47. Yeh, P.C.; Kharrazi, F.D. Postarthroscopic Glenohumeral Chondrolysis. *J. Am. Acad. Orthop. Surg.* **2012**, *20*, 102–112. [CrossRef]
48. Tauber, M.; Moursy, M.; Eppel, M.; Koller, H.; Resch, H. Arthroscopic Screw Fixation of Large Anterior Glenoid Fractures. *Knee Surg. Sports Traumatol. Arthrosc.* **2008**, *16*, 326–332. [CrossRef]
49. Greis, P.E.; Scuderi, M.G.; Mohr, A.; Bachus, K.N.; Burks, R.T. Glenohumeral Articular Contact Areas and Pressures Following Labral and Osseous Injury to the Anteroinferior Quadrant of the Glenoid. *J. Shoulder Elb. Surg.* **2002**, *11*, 442–451. [CrossRef]
50. Matsen, F.; Rockwood, C. The Shoulder Matsen FA, Rockwood CA Wirth MA. Glenohumeral Arthritis and Its Management. In *The Shoulder*, 2nd ed.; WB Saunders: Philadelphia, PA, USA, 1998; pp. 870–872.
51. Hawkins, R.J.; Angelo, R.L. Glenohumeral Osteoarthrosis. A Late Complication of the Putti-Platt Repair. *J. Bone Jt. Surg. Am.* **1990**, *72*, 1193–1197. [CrossRef]
52. Ahmad, C.S.; Wang, V.M.; Sugalski, M.T.; Levine, W.N.; Bigliani, L.U. Biomechanics of Shoulder Capsulorrhaphy Procedures. *J. Shoulder Elb. Surg.* **2005**, *14*, 12S–18S. [CrossRef]
53. Thomazeau, H.; Rolland, Y.; Lucas, C.; Duval, J.M.; Langlais, F. Atrophy of the Supraspinatus Belly. Assessment by MRI in 55 Patients with Rotator Cuff Pathology. *Acta Orthop. Scand.* **1996**, *67*, 264–268. [CrossRef] [PubMed]
54. Gerber, C.; Werner, C.M.L.; Macy, J.C.; Jacob, H.A.C.; Nyffeler, R.W. Effect of Selective Capsulorrhaphy on the Passive Range of Motion of the Glenohumeral Joint. *J. Bone Jt. Surg. Am.* **2003**, *85*, 48–55. [CrossRef] [PubMed]
55. Werner, C.M.L.; Nyffeler, R.W.; Jacob, H.A.C.; Gerber, C. The Effect of Capsular Tightening on Humeral Head Translations. *J. Orthop. Res.* **2004**, *22*, 194–201. [CrossRef]
56. Ansok, C.B.; Muh, S.J. Optimal Management of Glenohumeral Osteoarthritis. *Orthop. Res. Rev.* **2018**, *10*, 9–18. [CrossRef]
57. Waltz, R.A.; Wong, J.; Peebles, A.M.; Golijanin, P.; Ruzbarsky, J.J.; Arner, J.W.; Peebles, L.A.; Godin, J.A.; Millett, P.J.; Provencher, M.T. Postoperative Stiffness and Pain After Arthroscopic Labral Stabilization: Consider Anchor Arthropathy. *Arthrosc. J. Arthrosc. Relat. Surg.* **2021**, *37*, 3266–3274. [CrossRef]
58. Ernat, J.J.; Wright, C.J.; Rakowski, D.R.; Millett, P.J. Comprehensive Arthroscopic Management for Severe Glenohumeral Arthritis in an Ultimate Fighting Championship Fighter: A Case Report. *JBJS Case Connect.* **2021**, *11*, e20. [CrossRef]
59. Millett, P.J.; Horan, M.P.; Pennock, A.T.; Rios, D. Comprehensive Arthroscopic Management (CAM) Procedure: Clinical Results of a Joint-Preserving Arthroscopic Treatment for Young, Active Patients with Advanced Shoulder Osteoarthritis. *Arthrosc. J. Arthrosc. Relat. Surg.* **2013**, *29*, 440–448. [CrossRef]
60. Arner, J.W.; Elrick, B.P.; Nolte, P.-C.; Haber, D.B.; Horan, M.P.; Millett, P.J. Survivorship and Patient-Reported Outcomes after Comprehensive Arthroscopic Management of Glenohumeral Osteoarthritis: Minimum 10-Year Follow-up. *Am. J. Sports Med.* **2021**, *49*, 130–136. [CrossRef]
61. Nolte, P.-C.; Elrick, B.P.; Arner, J.W.; Ridley, T.J.; Woolson, T.E.; Tross, A.-K.; Midtgaard, K.S.; Millett, P.J. Total Shoulder Arthroplasty After Previous Arthroscopic Surgery for Glenohumeral Osteoarthritis: A Case-Control Matched Cohort Study. *Am. J. Sports Med.* **2021**, *49*, 1839–1846. [CrossRef]
62. Green, A.; Norris, T.R. Shoulder Arthroplasty for Advanced Glenohumeral Arthritis after Anterior Instability Repair. *J. Shoulder Elb. Surg.* **2001**, *10*, 539–545. [CrossRef]
63. Lehmann, L.; Magosch, P.; Mauermann, E.; Lichtenberg, S.; Habermeyer, P. Total Shoulder Arthroplasty in Dislocation Arthropathy. *Int. Orthop.* **2010**, *34*, 1219–1225. [CrossRef] [PubMed]
64. Habermeyer, P.; Lichtenberg, S.; Magosch, P.; Baierle, T. (Eds.) *Schulterchirurgie: Mit dem Plus im Web; Zugangscode im Buch*; 4. Aufl.; Elsevier, Urban & Fischer: München, Germany, 2010; ISBN 978-3-437-22341-9.
65. Pape, G.; Raiss, P.; Aldinger, P.R.; Loew, M. Comparison of short-term results after CUP prosthesis with cemented glenoid components and total shoulder arthroplasty: A matched-pair analysis. *Z. Orthop. Unf.* **2010**, *148*, 674–679. [CrossRef] [PubMed]
66. Neer, C.S.; Morrison, D.S. Glenoid Bone-Grafting in Total Shoulder Arthroplasty. *J. Bone Jt. Surg. Am.* **1988**, *70*, 1154–1162. [CrossRef]
67. Sperling, J.W.; Antuna, S.A.; Sanchez-Sotelo, J.; Schleck, C.; Cofield, R.H. Shoulder Arthroplasty for Arthritis after Instability Surgery. *J. Bone Jt. Surg. Am.* **2002**, *84*, 1775–1781. [CrossRef] [PubMed]
68. Hill, J.M.; Norris, T.R. Long-Term Results of Total Shoulder Arthroplasty Following Bone-Grafting of the Glenoid. *J. Bone Jt. Surg. Am.* **2001**, *83*, 877–883. [CrossRef]
69. Matsoukis, J.; Tabib, W.; Guiffault, P.; Mandelbaum, A.; Walch, G.; Némoz, C.; Edwards, T.B. Shoulder Arthroplasty in Patients with a Prior Anterior Shoulder Dislocation. Results of a Multicenter Study. *J. Bone Jt. Surg. Am.* **2003**, *85*, 1417–1424. [CrossRef]
70. Matsoukis, J.; Tabib, W.; Mandelbaum, A.; Walch, G. Shoulder arthroplasty for non-operated anterior shoulder instability with secondary osteoarthritis. *Rev. Chir. Orthop. Reparatrice Appar. Mot.* **2003**, *89*, 7–18.

71. Raiss, P.; Zeifang, F.; Pons-Villanueva, J.; Smithers, C.J.; Loew, M.; Walch, G. Reverse Arthroplasty for Osteoarthritis and Rotator Cuff Deficiency after Previous Surgery for Recurrent Anterior Shoulder Instability. *Int. Orthop. (SICOT)* **2014**, *38*, 1407–1413. [CrossRef]
72. Clavert, P.; Kling, A.; Sirveaux, F.; Favard, L.; Mole, D.; Walch, G.; Boileau, P. Reverse Shoulder Arthroplasty for Instability Arthropathy. *Int. Orthop. (SICOT)* **2019**, *43*, 1653–1658. [CrossRef]

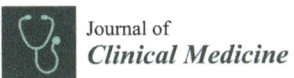
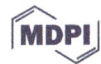

Article

Tranexamic Acid for Shoulder Arthroplasty: A Systematic Review and Meta-Analysis

Jaroslaw Pecold [1,2], Mahdi Al-Jeabory [1,2], Maciej Krupowies [2], Ewa Manka [3], Adam Smereka [4], Jerzy Robert Ladny [2,5] and Lukasz Szarpak [2,6,7,*]

1. Department of Trauma and Orthopedic Surgery, Ruda Slaska City Hospital, 41-703 Ruda Slaska, Poland; Jarekpecold@Tlen.pl (J.P.); mmahdi@interia.pl (M.A.-J.)
2. Research Unit, Polish Society of Disaster Medicine, 05-806 Warsaw, Poland; krupowiesmaciej@gmail.com (M.K.); Jerzy.r.ladny@gmail.com (J.R.L.)
3. Department of Internal Medicine, Angiology and Physical Medicine in Bytom, Faculty of Medical Sciences in Zabrze, Medical University of Silesia in Katowice, 41-800 Zabrze, Poland; ewa.irena.manka@gmail.com
4. Department of Gastroenterology and Hepatology, Faculty of Medicine, Wroclaw Medical University, 53-126 Wroclaw, Poland; adam.smereka@umw.edu.pl
5. Department of Emergency Medicine, Bialystok Medical University, 15-026 Bialystok, Poland
6. Institute of Outcomes Research, Maria Sklodowska-Curie Medical Academy, 03-411 Warsaw, Poland
7. Research Unit, Maria Sklodowska-Curie Bialystok Oncology Center, 15-027 Bialystok, Poland
* Correspondence: Lukasz.szarpak@gmail.com or Lukasz.szarpak@uczelniamedyczna.com.pl; Tel.: +48-500-186-225

Abstract: Tranexamic acid (TXA) is an antifibrinolytic agent that has been shown to decrease blood loss and transfusion rates after knee and hip arthroplasty, however with only limited evidence to support its use in shoulder arthroplasty. Therefore, we performed a systematic review and meta-analysis to evaluate the clinical usefulness of tranexamic acid for shoulder arthroplasty. A thorough literature search was conducted across four electronic databases (PubMed, Cochrane Library, Web of Science, Scopus) from inception through to 1 December 2021. The mean difference (MD), odds ratio (OR) or relative risk (RR) and 95% confidence interval (CI) were used to estimate pooled results from studies. Total of 10 studies comprising of 993 patients met the inclusion criteria and were included in the analysis. Blood volume loss in the TXA and non-TXA group was 0.66 ± 0.52 vs. 0.834 ± 0.592 L (MD= -0.15; 95%CI: -0.23 to -0.07; $p < 0.001$). Change of hemoglobin levels were 2.2 ± 1.0 for TXA group compared to 2.7 ± 1.1 for non-TXA group (MD= -0.51; 95%CI: -0.57 to -0.44; $p < 0.001$) and hematocrit change was $6.1 \pm 2.7\%$ vs. $7.9 \pm 3.1\%$, respectively; (MD= -1.43; 95%CI: -2.27 to -0.59; $p < 0.001$). Tranexamic acid use for shoulder arthroplasty reduces blood volume loss during and after surgery and reduces drain output and hematocrit change.

Keywords: tranexamic acid; TXA; shoulder; arthroscopy; bleeding; systematic review; meta-analysis

Citation: Pecold, J.; Al-Jeabory, M.; Krupowies, M.; Manka, E.; Smereka, A.; Ladny, J.R.; Szarpak, L. Tranexamic Acid for Shoulder Arthroplasty: A Systematic Review and Meta-Analysis. *J. Clin. Med.* **2022**, *11*, 48. https://doi.org/10.3390/jcm11010048

Academic Editors: Markus Scheibel, Alexandre Lädermann and Laurent Audigé

Received: 8 December 2021
Accepted: 23 December 2021
Published: 23 December 2021

Publisher's Note: MDPI stays neutral with regard to jurisdictional claims in published maps and institutional affiliations.

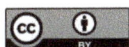

Copyright: © 2021 by the authors. Licensee MDPI, Basel, Switzerland. This article is an open access article distributed under the terms and conditions of the Creative Commons Attribution (CC BY) license (https://creativecommons.org/licenses/by/4.0/).

1. Introduction

Tranexamic acid (TXA) is an antifibrinolytic that inhibits fibrin's plasmin-mediated degradation and is used to stabilize clots and reduce active bleeding. In orthopaedic surgery, tranexamic acid is most notably involved in the elective orthopaedic procedures necessitating transfusion [1,2]. The use of tranexamic acid has become widely accepted in total knee and hip arthroplasty to prevent extensive blood loss and lower transfusion rates, but it can be also beneficial for patients who undergo total shoulder arthroplasty [3]. A significant benefit of TXA in several types of orthopaedic surgery may also be a reduction in the need for blood product transfusions, reduced hospital costs, laboratory costs and shorter hospital stays [3]. When considering the benefits of TXA, it is also essential to consider the risk for increased thromboembolic events and provide post-operative thromboprophylaxis [4].

Shoulder-scapular-joint alloplasty procedures have become increasingly popular in recent years. Modern implants provide various surgical options, depending on the indications and anatomical conditions. Although the number of possible complications is still high, the results of revision surgery are improving [5]. Shoulder alloplasty can be divided into the partial and total shoulder [5]. Total shoulder arthroplasty is divided into anatomic total shoulder arthroplasty (ATSA) and reverse total shoulder arthroplasty (RTSA) [6]. One method used to improve the procedure's effectiveness and reduce possible bleeding complications and the need for blood transfusions is the perioperative use of tranexamic acid [7]. Importantly, perioperative use of TXA does not appear to significantly increase the risk of incident embolic and thrombotic events [8], including patients with a history of similar incidents [9]. Additionally, perioperative use of tranexamic acid at a dose of 20 mg/kg body weight shortens the recovery time of patients and contributes to shorter hospitalizations [10].

We already know that TXA reduces blood loss in shoulder arthroplasty, but the benefits and risks of using tranexamic acid are still unclear. Meta-analysis of data from different studies may facilitate clinical decision-making regarding the use of TXA, including support for accurate assessment of some rare complications and their clinical significance.

Therefore, we performed a systematic review and meta-analysis to evaluate the clinical usefulness of tranexamic acid of the shoulder arthroplasty.

2. Materials and Methods

2.1. Search Strategy

The study was designed as a systematic review and meta-analysis and was performed in accordance with the Preferred Reporting Items for Systematic Reviews and Meta-Analysis (PRISMA) statement [11].

In this systematic review and meta-analysis, we searched PubMed, Cochrane Library, Web of Science, Scopus from the databases' inception to 1 December 2021 for original, peer-reviewed primary research articles, including observational or interventional studies, that describe the clinical usefulness of tranexamic acid for shoulder arthroplasty. We searched the following terms: "tranexamic acid" OR "TXA" AND "shoulder". Additionally, the reference lists of retrieved articles were also reviewed to identify additional eligible studies. To avoid double data counting, when there were multiple publications from the same trial sample, the one with the largest sample size was included.

2.2. Inclusion Criteria

Studies that were included in this meta-analysis had to fulfil the following PICOS criteria: (1) Participants, patients with 18 years old or older requiring shoulder arthroplasty; (2) Intervention, tranexamic acid treatment; (3) Comparison, non-TXA treatment; (4) Outcomes, operative data and adverse events occurrence; (5) Study design, randomized controlled trials and retrospective trials comparing TXA and non-TXA care for their effects in patients with shoulder arthroplasty. Studies were excluded if they were reviews, animal studies, case reports, letters, conference or poster abstracts, or articles not containing original data.

2.3. Data Extraction

Data extraction was performed by two reviewers (J.P. and M.A.-J.). From the studies that met the inclusion eligibility criteria, the following data were extracted into a predefined Microsoft Excel spreadsheet (Microsoft Corp., Redmond, WA, USA): (a) study characteristic (i.e., first author, year of publication, country, study design, inclusion and exclusion criteria, primary outcomes, findings; intervention and control group); (b) participant characteristics (i.e., number of participants, age, sex); (c) main study outcomes (i.e., blood volume loss, operative time, adverse events, hospital length of stay). Potential disagreements were resolved by discussion with a third reviewer (L.S.).

2.4. Quality Assessment

Two reviewers (J.P. and M.A.-J.) evaluated the quality of each study. Potential disagreements were discussed and resolved in a consensus meeting with the third reviewer

(L.S.). The RoB 2 tool (revised tool for risk of bias in randomized trials) was used to assess the quality of randomized studies [12], and the ROBINS-I tool (tool to determine the risk of bias in non-randomized studies of interventions) was used to assess the quality of non-randomized trials [13]. The risk of bias assessments was visualized using the Robvis application [14].

2.5. Statistical Analysis

The meta-analysis was conducted using the Review Manager, version 5.4EN (RevMan; The Cochrane Collaboration, Oxford, UK). The significance level was set at 0.05 for all analyses. When the continuous outcomes were reported in a study as median, range, and interquartile range, we estimated means and standard deviations using the formula described by Hozo et al. [15]. The mean difference (MD), odds ratio (OR) or relative risk (RR) and 95% confidence interval (CI) were used to estimate pooled results from studies. The Q and I^2 statistic were used to investigate heterogeneity among the studies. A fixed model effect was used when $I^2 < 50\%$, and a random model effect was used in other cases.

3. Results

3.1. Eligible Studies and Study Characteristics

The database search identified 240 citations (Figure 1). After excluding duplicates, reviews, editorials, letters, case reports and meta-analysis, a total of ten studies [10,16–24] met the inclusion and exclusion criteria and were included in the analysis, comprising 993 patients.

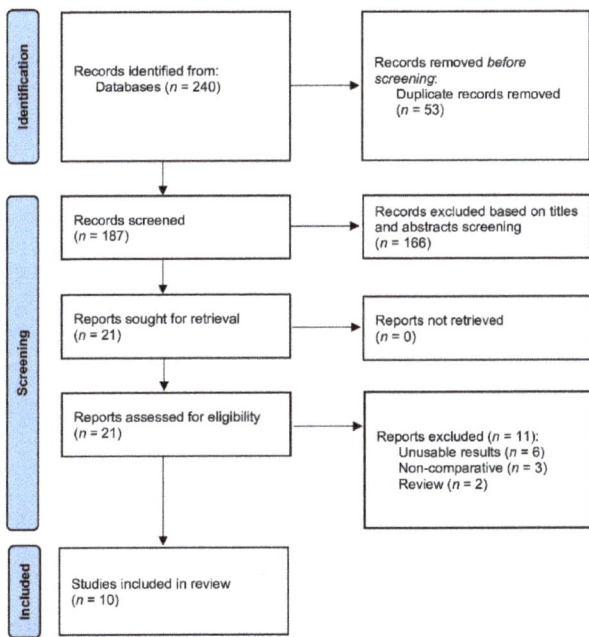

Figure 1. Forest plot of blood volume loss among TXA and non-TXA groups. The centre of each square represents the weighted mean differences for individual trials, and the corresponding horizontal line stands for a 95% confidence interval. The diamonds represent pooled results.

The mean age of participants in TXA and non-TXA groups was 59.6 ± 21.5 and 60.3 ± 21.3 years, respectively. The men constituted 51.5% vs 49.4%, respectively, for TXA and non-TXA groups. Baseline characteristics for all included studies are shown in Table 1 and Table S1. Studies were published from 2015 to 2021. Seven studies were designed as randomized controlled trials [17–21,23,24]. The results of the assessment of risk of bias among included studies are provided in Figures S1–S4.

Table 1. Study characteristics.

Study	Country	Study Design	TXA Group				Non-TXA Group		
			No	Age	Sex, Male	TXA Dose	No	Age	Sex, Male
Abildgaard et al. 2016	USA	Retrospective	77	71.6 ± 10.2	49 (63.6%)	1 g	94	72.9 ± 9.4	51 (54.3%)
Cunningham et al. 2021	Switzerland	RCT	31	72 ± 8	11 (35.5%)	2 g	29	73 ± 9	6 (20.7%)
Cvetanovich et al. 2018	USA	RCT	52	67.7 ± 10.9	23 (44.2%)	1 g	56	65.2 ± 9.2	28 (50.0%)
Friedman et al. 2016	USA	Retrospective	106	NS	46 (43.4%)	20 mg/kg	88	NS	33 (37.5%)
Garcia et al. 2021	Portugal	RCT	23	76.7 ± 7.1	4 (17.4%)	1 g	22	75.7 ± 5.7	3 (13.6%)
Gillespie et al. 2015	USA	RCT	61	67.59	25 (40.9%)	2 g	57	66.45	27 (47.4%)
Hurley et al. 2020	Ireland	RCT	50	25.1 ± 6.5	48 (96.0%)	1 g	50	23.8 ± 3.4	48 (96.0%)
Kim et al. 2017	Republic of Korea	Retrospective	24	73.2 ± 4.4	3 (12.5%)	0.5 g	24	74.2 ± 4.4	6 (25.0%)
Pauzenberger et al. 2017	Austria	RCT	27	70.3 ± 9.3	20 (74.1%)	1 g	27	71.3 ± 7.9	18 (66.7%)
Vara et al. 2017	USA	RCT	53	67 ± 9	20 (37.7%)	20 mg/kg	49	66 ± 9	22 (44.9%)

Legend: NS = not specified; RCT = randomized controlled trial; TXA = tranexamic acid.

3.2. Meta-Analysis

Blood volume loss in the TXA and non-TXA group varied and amounted to 0.66 ± 0.52 vs. 0.834 ± 0.592 L (MD = -0.15; 95%CI: -0.23 to -0.07; $I^2 = 84\%$; $p < 0.001$; Figure 2).

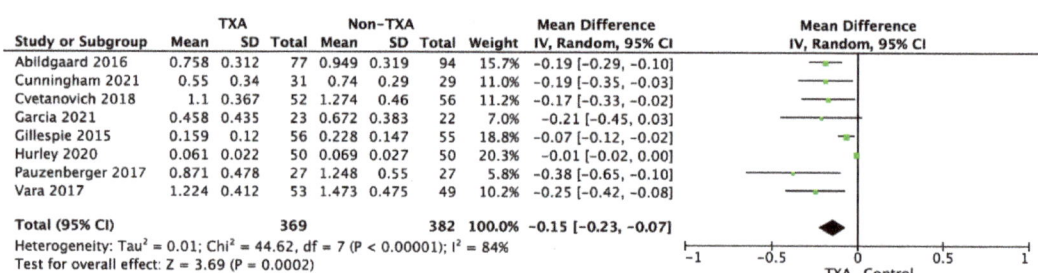

Figure 2. Forest plot of blood volume loss among TXA and non-TXA groups. The centre of each square represents the weighted mean differences for individual trials, and the corresponding horizontal line stands for a 95% confidence interval. The diamonds represent pooled results. Legend: CI = confidence interval; SD = standard deviation.

Drain output was reported in six studies. Polled analysis of drain output was 110.5 ± 100.4 mL for TXA group, and 222.9 ± 187.2 mL for non-TXA group (MD = -92.51; 95%CI: -141.09 to -43.93; $I^2 = 92\%$; $p < 0.001$).

Change of hemoglobin levels form preoperatively to postoperatively periods were reported in six trials and were 2.2 ± 1.0 for TXA group compared to 2.7 ± 1.1 for non-TXA group (MD = −0.51; 95%CI: −0.57 to −0.44; I^2 = 0%; p < 0.001).

Hematocrit change was reported in five studies and was statistically smaller in TXA group (6.1 ± 2.7%), compared to non-TXA group (7.9 ± 3.1%); MD= −1.43; 95%CI: −2.27 to −0.59; I^2 = 95%; p < 0.001).

Operation time was reported in six trials and was 89.5 ± 33.0 min for TXA group compared to 88.5 ± 32.2 min for non-TXA group (MD = −2.25; 95%CI: −4.54 to 0.05; I^2 = 0%; p = 0.06; Figure 3). Length of hospital stay in TXA and non-TXA (control) groups was 2.1 ± 1.7 vs. 2.2 ± 1.6 days, respectively (MD = −0.15; 95%CI: −0.32 to 0.01; I^2 = 0%; p = 0.07).

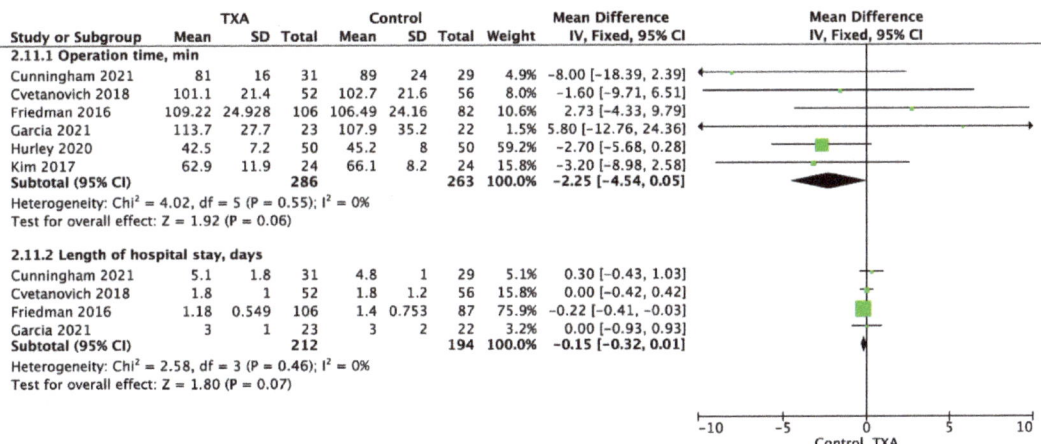

Figure 3. Forest plot of (**2.11.1**) operation time; (**2.11.2**) length of hospital stay among TXA and non-TXA groups. The centre of each square represents the weighted mean differences for individual trials, and the corresponding horizontal line stands for a 95% confidence interval. The diamonds represent pooled results.

Polled analysis of three studies showed that 3.0% of patients in the TXA group and 3.5% in the non-TXA group required transfusion (RR = 0.56; 95%CI: 0.20 to 1.59; p = 0.28). Revision was no required in TXA compared to 0.9% of cases in non-TXA group (RR = 0.33; 95%CI: 0.01 to 7.99; p = 0.50). Hematoma was observed in 20.4% in the TXA group and 53.8% in non-TXA group (RR = 0.39; 95%CI: 0.27 to 0.57; p < 0.001). Thromboembolic complications were not noted in any of the groups.

4. Discussion

TXA is currently a commonly used perioperative antifibrinolytic agent. The antifibrinolytic is used in surgery but also in various other bleeding manifestations in congenital coagulopathies, such as fibrinogen deficiency [25]. With the increase in the number of TSAs performed, and the constant expansion of the indications qualifying for the procedure, there is a need to reduce postoperative complications and improve the procedure's results.

In this study, we evaluate results from three retrospective studies [10,16,22] and seven RCTs that compared outcomes in the TXA group and non-TXA group [17–21,23,24]. The main findings of this meta-analysis relate to nine factors, which we have sorted out for clarity: blood volume loss, hematocrit change, length of hospitalization, operation time, hematoma, drain output, need for revision and thromboembolic complications. In a retrospective study including an analysis of 155 complications after TSA, Anthony et al. highlights that the most common complication is bleeding-requiring transfusion [26].

Our study identified a notably increased blood volume loss in the non-TXA group of 0.834 ± 0.592 L compared to 0.66 ± 0.52 L in the TXA group, which is also reflected in the change in hematocrit values, whose change for the described groups was 7.9 ± 3.1% for the non-TXA group compared to TXA group 6.1 ± 2.7%, respectively. TXA successfully prevents perioperative blood loss. This decreases postoperative pain and reduces complications, postoperative mortality, and the length of hospitalization. At the same time, TXA has side effects limited to nausea and diarrhoea, making it a well-tolerated drug [27]. These benefits also carry a reduction in costs associated with postoperative care. As reported by Kandil et al. in 2016, the hospitalization time for patients after TSA who required a blood transfusion is 1.8 days longer which is $11,794 more, compared to patients who did not receive a transfusion [28]. In our meta-analysis results, the hospitalization time of patients in the TXA group is 2.1 ± 1.7 vs. 2.2 ± 1.6 in the non-TXA group. This emphasizes the need for further in-depth analyses of the available studies due to the discrepancy with the reports mentioned above of Kandil et al., especially considering the difference we also showed in the duration of the operation itself. These times differed slightly (TXA 89.5 ± 33.0 min vs non-TXA 89.1 ± 32.2 min) but in the study by Friedman et al. performed on a group of 194 patients, the time in the recovery room in the TXA group was shorter on average by as much as 24 min [10].

Wang et al. in a 2021 study showed that patients with moderate to severe preoperative anemia were at increased risk of cardiac and pulmonary complications, postoperative blood transfusion, prolonged length of stay, reoperation, and death [29]. In our assessment, these results are transferable to the postoperative situation because it has been proven that TSA without antifibrinolytics is associated with high blood loss. According to studies, the volume of blood lost in the first postoperative day ranges from 159 to 1473 mL [10,16–21,23,24].

The reduction in postoperative pain is also associated with a significant difference in the incidence of postoperative hematoma. In our meta-analysis, the occurrence rate in the TXA group was 20.4%, while hematoma formation in non-TXA patients occurred 53.8%. Hematomas which result from continuous blood loss cause painful swelling, which contributes to the use of opioid medications and may even result in the need for surgical drainage, which directly delays hospital discharge time [17,21]. Moreover, persistent postoperative drainage may increase the risk of tissue contamination and deep infection, which prolongs the time and cumulates the costs of treatment [30,31].

Among the studies we analyzed that used drain output, only Cvetanovich et al. reported no statistically significant difference in drainage volume [18]. The other studies show a reduced volume in the TXA group (109.9 ± 104.3 mL) versus the non-TXA group (254.4 ± 200.5 mL). This difference shows the need for additional large randomized controlled trials. Additionally, in the two studies we analyzed, the TSA requiring revision surgery percentage was 0.9% in the non-TXA group, whereas patients after TXA application did not require revision. This may be related to the reported lower complications resulting from less blood loss in patients who received an antifibrinolytic agent.

Our meta-analysis also highlighted the finding of Cvetanovich et al. [18]. As indicated in the study, thromboembolic complications were not noted in any of the groups. This aspect is particularly relevant given that deep vein thrombosis and pulmonary embolism are considered the leading complications of orthopedic surgery [31,32]. This is consistent with other meta-analyses and RCTs that evaluated the safety of TXA in total joint arthroplasty. No increase in the risk of thromboembolic complications was demonstrated.

It is worth pointing out that in five analyzed studies, TXA was administered intravenously, only Gillespie et al. used in the treatment group 100 mL of normal saline infused with 2 g of TXA poured into the surgical wound and left in place for 5 min. To the best of our knowledge, there have not been many studies comparing these two methods of TXA application. Budge et al. in 2019 conducted a retrospective review on a group of only three patients comparing whether Intravenous and topical TXA are equivalent in improving postoperative hemoglobin in TSA [33]. However, Li et al., in a meta-analysis, evaluated the efficiency and safety of combined use of intravenous and topical versus single intravenous TXA [34]. The meta-analysis concerns total primary knee and hip arthroplasty. The study team shows a statistically significant reduction in total blood loss with the combined application with no increase in the risk of thromboembolic complications [35]. The findings from our statistics and the described studies demonstrate the need to compare TXA application methods further.

In performed statistical analysis, we reported significant benefits for TXA in all described aspects. However, significant heterogeneity between the compared studies was demonstrated in terms of total blood loss or drain output. This phenomenon cannot be sufficiently explained by possible differences in the anaesthetic protocol used, the thromboembolic prophylaxis plan or the way TXA was applied. In the opinion of our research team, these differences may be due to individual variability of patients, inclusion or exclusion criteria, differences in surgical protocols and different methods of measuring outcomes.

This study has limitations related to the relatively small number of studies included and to its retrospective nature. However, the data collected indicate statistically and clinically significant findings regarding the manner and safety of TXA application. Because of the limited high-quality evidence currently available, there is a need for further in-depth analysis of the available studies in terms of the most beneficial way of TXA application.

5. Conclusions

Tranexamic acid use for shoulder arthroplasty reduces blood volume loss during and after surgery and reduces drain output and hematocrit change.

Supplementary Materials: The following supporting information can be downloaded at: https://www.mdpi.com/article/10.3390/jcm11010048/s1, Table S1: Methodology characteristics among included trials, Figure S1: A summary table of review authors' judgements for each risk of bias item for each randomized study, Figure S2: A plot of the distribution of review authors' judgements across randomized studies for each risk of bias item, Figure S3: A summary table of review authors' judgements for each risk of bias item for each non-randomized study, Figure S4: A plot of the distribution of review authors' judgements across non-randomized studies for each risk of bias item.

Author Contributions: Conceptualization, J.P. and L.S.; methodology, J.P.; software, J.P. and L.S.; validation, J.P., L.S. and M.A.-J.; formal analysis, J.P. and L.S.; investigation, J.P., A.S., M.A.-J. and L.S.; resources, L.S.; data curation, J.P. and L.S.; writing—original draft preparation, J.P., M.K., E.M., M.A.-J. and L.S.; writing—review and editing, all authors; visualization, L.S.; supervision, J.P. and L.S.; project administration, J.P. and L.S.; funding acquisition, A.S. All authors have read and agreed to the published version of the manuscript.

Funding: This research received no external funding.

Institutional Review Board Statement: Not applicable.

Informed Consent Statement: Not applicable.

Data Availability Statement: Not applicable.

Acknowledgments: The study was supported by the ERC Research Net and by the Polish Society of Disaster Medicine.

Conflicts of Interest: The authors declare no conflict of interest.

References

1. Ashkenazi, I.; Schermann, H.; Gold, A.; Lin, R.; Pardo, I.; Steinberg, E.; Sternheim, A.; Snir, N. Tranexamic acid in hip hemiarthroplasty. *Injury* **2020**, *51*, 2658–2662. [CrossRef]
2. Heyns, M.; Knight, P.; Steve, A.K.; Yeung, J.K. A Single Preoperative Dose of Tranexamic Acid Reduces Perioperative Blood Loss: A Meta-analysis. *Ann. Surg.* **2021**, *273*, 75–81. [CrossRef]
3. Lin, Z.X.; Woolf, S.K. Safety, Efficacy, and Cost-effectiveness of Tranexamic Acid in Orthopedic Surgery. *Orthopedics* **2016**, *39*, 119–130. [CrossRef]
4. Fillingham, Y.A.; Ramkumar, D.B.; Jevsevar, D.S.; Yates, A.J.; Shores, P.; Mullen, K.; Bini, S.A.; Clarke, H.D.; Schemitsch, E.; Johnson, R.L.; et al. The Efficacy of Tranexamic Acid in Total Knee Arthroplasty: A Network Meta-Analysis. *J. Arthroplast.* **2018**, *33*, 3090–3098.e1. [CrossRef] [PubMed]
5. Sanchez-Sotelo, J. Total shoulder arthroplasty. *Open Orthop. J.* **2011**, *5*, 106–114. [CrossRef] [PubMed]
6. Wicha, M.; Tomczyk-Warunek, A.; Jarecki, J.; Dubiel, A. Total shoulder arthroplasty, an overview, indications and prosthetic options. *Wiad. Lek* **2020**, *73*, 1870–1873. [CrossRef]
7. Kuo, L.T.; Hsu, W.H.; Chi, C.C.; Yoo, J.C. Tranexamic acid in total shoulder arthroplasty and reverse shoulder arthroplasty: A systematic review and meta-analysis. *BMC Musculoskelet. Disord.* **2018**, *19*, 60. [CrossRef] [PubMed]
8. Sun, C.X.; Zhang, L.; Mi, L.D.; Du, G.Y.; Sun, X.G.; He, S.W. Efficiency and safety of tranexamic acid in reducing blood loss in total shoulder arthroplasty: A systematic review and meta-analysis. *Medicine* **2017**, *96*, e7015. [CrossRef]
9. Carbone, A.; Poeran, J.; Zubizarreta, N.; Chan, J.; Mazumdar, M.; Parsons, B.O.; Galatz, L.M.; Cagle, P.J. Administration of tranexamic acid during total shoulder arthroplasty is not associated with an increased risk of complications in patients with a history of thrombotic events. *J. Shoulder Elb. Surg.* **2021**, *30*, 104–112. [CrossRef]
10. Friedman, R.J.; Gordon, E.; Butler, R.B.; Mock, L.; Dumas, B. Tranexamic acid decreases blood loss after total shoulder arthroplasty. *J. Shoulder Elb. Surg.* **2016**, *25*, 614–618. [CrossRef] [PubMed]
11. Page, M.J.; McKenzie, J.E.; Bossuyt, P.M.; Boutron, I.; Hoffmann, T.C.; Mulrow, C.D.; Shamseer, L.; Tetzlaff, J.M.; Akl, E.A.; Brennan, S.E.; et al. The PRISMA 2020 statement: An updated guideline for reporting systematic reviews. *BMJ* **2021**, *372*, n71. [CrossRef]
12. Sterne, J.A.C.; Savović, J.; Page, M.J.; Elbers, R.G.; Blencowe, N.S.; Boutron, I.; Cates, C.J.; Cheng, H.Y.; Corbett, M.S.; Eldridge, S.M.; et al. RoB 2: A revised tool for assessing risk of bias in randomized trials. *BMJ* **2019**, *366*, l4898. [CrossRef] [PubMed]
13. Sterne, J.A.; Hernán, M.A.; Reeves, B.C.; Savović, J.; Berkman, N.D.; Viswanathan, M.; Henry, D.; Altman, D.G.; Ansari, M.T.; Boutron, I.; et al. ROBINS-I: A tool for assessing risk of bias in non-randomized studies of interventions. *BMJ* **2016**, *355*, i4919. [CrossRef] [PubMed]
14. McGuinness, L.A.; Higgins, J.P.T. Risk-of-bias VISualization (robvis): An R package and Shiny web app for visualizing risk-of-bias assessments. *Res. Synth. Methods* **2021**, *12*, 55–61. [CrossRef] [PubMed]
15. Hozo, S.P.; Djulbegovic, B.; Hozo, I. Estimating the mean and variance from the median, range, and the size of a sample. *BMC Med. Res. Methodol.* **2005**, *5*, 13. [CrossRef]
16. Abildgaard, J.T.; McLemore, R.; Hattrup, S.J. Tranexamic acid decreases blood loss in total shoulder arthroplasty and reverse total arthroplasty. *J. Shoulder Elb. Surg.* **2016**, *25*, 1643–1648. [CrossRef] [PubMed]
17. Cunningham, G.; Hughes, J.; Borner, B.; Mattern, O.; Taha, M.E.; Smith, M.M.; Young, A.A.; Cass, B. A single dose of tranexamic acid reduces blood loss after reverse and anatomic shoulder arthroplasty: A randomized controlled trial. *J. Shoulder Elb. Surg.* **2021**, *30*, 1553–1560. [CrossRef]
18. Cvetanovich, G.L.; Fillingham, Y.A.; O'Brien, M.; Forsythe, B.; Cole, B.J.; Verma, N.N.; Romeo, A.A.; Nicholson, G.P. Tranexamic acid reduces blood loss after primary shoulder arthroplasty: A double-blind, placebo-controlled, prospective, randomized controlled trial. *JSES Open Access* **2018**, *2*, 23–27. [CrossRef]
19. Garcia, T.; Fragão-Marques, M.; Pimentão, P.; Pinto, M.; Pedro, I.; Martinsa, C. Tranexamic acid in total shoulder arthroplasty under regional anesthesia: A randomized, single blinded, controlled trial. *Braz. J. Anesthesiol.* **2021**, 2–17. [CrossRef]
20. Gillespie, R.; Shishani, Y.; Joseph, S.; Streit, J.J.; Gobezie, R. Neer Award 2015: A randomized, prospective evaluation on the effectiveness of tranexamic acid in reducing blood loss after total shoulder arthroplasty. *J. Shoulder Elb. Surg.* **2015**, *24*, 1679–1684. [CrossRef]
21. Hurley, E.T.; Lim Fat, D.; Pauzenberger, L.; Mullett, H. Tranexamic acid for the Latarjet procedure: A randomized controlled trial. *J. Shoulder Elb. Surg.* **2020**, *29*, 882–885. [CrossRef]
22. Kim, S.H.; Jung, W.I.; Kim, Y.J.; Hwang, D.H.; Choi, Y.E. Effect of Tranexamic Acid on Hematologic Values and Blood Loss in Reverse Total Shoulder Arthroplasty. *Biomed. Res. Int.* **2017**, *2017*, 9590803. [CrossRef] [PubMed]
23. Pauzenberger, L.; Domej, M.A.; Heuberer, P.R.; Hexel, M.; Grieb, A.; Laky, B.; Blasl, J.; Anderl, W. The effect of intravenous tranexamic acid on blood loss and early post-operative pain in total shoulder arthroplasty. *Bone Jt. J.* **2017**, *99*, 1073–1079. [CrossRef] [PubMed]
24. Vara, A.D.; Koueiter, D.M.; Pinkas, D.E.; Gowda, A.; Wiater, B.P.; Wiater, J.M. Intravenous tranexamic acid reduces total blood loss in reverse total shoulder arthroplasty: A prospective, double-blinded, randomized, controlled trial. *J. Shoulder Elb. Surg.* **2017**, *26*, 1383–1389. [CrossRef] [PubMed]

25. Simurda, T.; Asselta, R.; Zolkova, J.; Brunclikova, M.; Dobrotova, M.; Kolkova, Z.; Loderer, D.; Skornova, I.; Hudecek, J.; Lasabova, Z.; et al. Congenital Afibrinogenemia and Hypofibrinogenemia: Laboratory and Genetic Testing in Rare Bleeding Disorders with Life-Threatening Clinical Manifestations and Challenging Management. *Diagnostics* **2021**, *11*, 2140. [CrossRef]
26. Anthony, C.A.; Westermann, R.W.; Gao, Y.; Pugely, A.J.; Wolf, B.R.; Hettrich, C.M. What Are Risk Factors for 30-day Morbidity and Transfusion in Total Shoulder Arthroplasty? A Review of 1922 Cases. *Clin. Orthop. Relat. Res.* **2015**, *473*, 2099–2105. [CrossRef]
27. Oremus, K.; Sostaric, S.; Trkulja, V.; Haspl, M. Influence of tranexamic acid on postoperative autologous blood retransfusion in primary total hip and knee arthroplasty: A randomized controlled trial. *Transfusion* **2014**, *54*, 31–41. [CrossRef]
28. Kandil, A.; Griffin, J.W.; Novicoff, W.M.; Brockmeier, S.F. Blood transfusion after total shoulder arthroplasty: Which patients are at high risk? *Int. J. Shoulder Surg.* **2016**, *10*, 72–77. [CrossRef]
29. Wang, K.Y.; Quan, T.; Gu, A.; Best, M.J.; Stadecker, M.; Srikumaran, U. Increased severity of anaemia is associated with postoperative complications following primary total shoulder arthroplasty. *J. Shoulder Elb. Surg.* **2021**, *30*, 2393–2400. [CrossRef]
30. Ryan, D.J.; Yoshihara, H.; Yoneoka, D.; Zuckerman, J.D. Blood transfusion in primary total shoulder arthroplasty: Incidence, trends, and risk factors in the United States from 2000 to 2009. *J. Shoulder Elb. Surg.* **2015**, *24*, 760–765. [CrossRef]
31. Cheung, E.V.; Sperling, J.W.; Cofield, R.H. Infection associated with hematoma formation after shoulder arthroplasty. *Clin. Orthop. Relat. Res.* **2008**, *466*, 1363–1367. [CrossRef] [PubMed]
32. Saleh, J.; El-Othmani, M.M.; Saleh, K.J. Deep Vein Thrombosis and Pulmonary Embolism Considerations in Orthopedic Surgery. *Orthop. Clin. N. Am.* **2017**, *48*, 127–135. [CrossRef] [PubMed]
33. Budge, M. Topical and Intravenous Tranexamic Acid Are Equivalent in Decreasing Blood Loss in Total Shoulder Arthroplasty. *J. Shoulder Elb Arthroplast.* **2019**, *3*, 2471549218821181. [CrossRef]
34. Li, J.F.; Li, H.; Zhao, H.; Wang, J.; Liu, S.; Song, Y.; Wu, H.F. Combined use of intravenous and topical versus intravenous tranexamic acid in primary total knee and hip arthroplasty: A meta-analysis of randomised controlled trials. *J. Orthop. Surg. Res.* **2017**, *12*, 1–10. [CrossRef] [PubMed]
35. Zhang, P.M.M.; Li, J.M.M.; Wang, X.M.M. Combined versus single application of tranexamic acid in total knee and hip arthroplasty: A meta-analysis of randomized controlled trials. *Int. J. Surg.* **2017**, *43*, 171–180. [CrossRef]

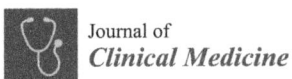

Article

Implant Sizing and Positioning in Anatomical Total Shoulder Arthroplasty Using a Rotator Cuff-Sparing Postero-Inferior Approach

Philipp Moroder [1], Lucca Lacheta [2], Marvin Minkus [2], Katrin Karpinski [2], Frank Uhing [3], Sheldon De Souza [3], Michael van der Merwe [3] and Doruk Akgün [2,*]

1. Schulthess Clinic, 8008 Zürich, Switzerland; philipp.moroder@kws.ch
2. Arthrex GMBH, D-81249 Munich, Germany; lucca.lacheta@charite.de (L.L.); marvin.minkus@charite.de (M.M.); katrin.karpinski@charite.de (K.K.)
3. Center for Musculoskeletal Surgery, Charité—University Medicine Berlin, Charitéplatz 1, D-10117 Berlin, Germany; frank.uhing@arthrex.de (F.U.); sheldon.desouza@arthrex.de (S.D.S.); michael.vandermerwe@arthrex.de (M.v.d.M.)
* Correspondence: doruk.akguen@charite.de; Tel.: +49-304-5065-2319; Fax: +49-304-5051-5905

Citation: Moroder, P.; Lacheta, L.; Minkus, M.; Karpinski, K.; Uhing, F.; De Souza, S.; van der Merwe, M.; Akgün, D. Implant Sizing and Positioning in Anatomical Total Shoulder Arthroplasty Using a Rotator Cuff-Sparing Postero-Inferior Approach. J. Clin. Med. 2022, 11, 3324. https://doi.org/10.3390/jcm11123324

Academic Editors: Alexandre Lädermann, Markus Scheibel, Laurent Audigé and Mariano Menendez

Received: 3 April 2022
Accepted: 8 June 2022
Published: 10 June 2022

Publisher's Note: MDPI stays neutral with regard to jurisdictional claims in published maps and institutional affiliations.

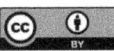

Copyright: © 2022 by the authors. Licensee MDPI, Basel, Switzerland. This article is an open access article distributed under the terms and conditions of the Creative Commons Attribution (CC BY) license (https://creativecommons.org/licenses/by/4.0/).

Abstract: Background: The goal of this study was to compare the effectiveness of a rotator cuff-sparing postero-inferior (PI) approach with subdeltoidal access to the traditional subscapularis-takedown deltopectoral approach, in terms of implant sizing and positioning in anatomical total shoulder arthroplasty (aTSA). **Methods:** This study involved 18 human cadaveric shoulders with intact rotator cuffs and no evidence of head deforming osteoarthritis. An Eclipse stemless aTSA (Arthrex, Naples, FL, USA) was implanted in nine randomly selected specimens using a standard subscapularis-tenotomy deltopectoral approach, and in the other nine specimens using the cuff-sparing PI approach. Pre- and postoperative antero-posterior (AP) and axillary fluoroscopic radiographs were analyzed by two independent, blinded raters for the following parameters: (1) anatomic and prosthetic neck-shaft angle (NSA); (2) the shift between the anatomic and prosthetic center of rotation (COR); (3) anatomical size matching of the prosthetic humeral head; (4) the calculated Anatomic Reconstruction Score (ARS); (5) glenoid positioning; as well as (6) glenoid inclination and version. **Results:** While the COR was slightly but significantly positioned ($p = 0.031$) to be more medial in the PI approach group (3.7 ± 3.4%, range: −2.3 to 8.7%) than in the deltopectoral approach group (−0.2 ± 3.6%, range: −6.9 to 4.1%), on average, none of the remaining measured radiographic parameters significantly differed between both groups (PI approach group vs. deltopectoral group: NSA 130° vs. 127°, $p = 0.57$; COR supero-inferior, 2.6% vs. 1.0%, $p = 0.35$; COR antero-posterior, 0.9% vs. 1.7%, $p = 0.57$; head size supero-inferior, 97.3% vs. 98.5%, $p = 0.15$; head size antero-posterior, 101.1% vs. 100.6%, $p = 0.54$; ARS, 8.4 vs. 9.3, $p = 0.13$; glenoid positioning supero-inferior, 49.1% vs. 51.1%, $p = 0.33$; glenoid positioning antero-posterior, 49.3% vs. 50.4%, $p = 0.23$; glenoid inclination, 86° vs. 88°, $p = 0.27$; and glenoid retroversion, 91° vs. 89°, $p = 0.27$). **Conclusions:** A PI approach allows for sufficient exposure and orientation to perform rotator-cuff sparing aTSA with acceptable implant sizing and positioning in cadaveric specimens.

Keywords: anatomical total shoulder arthroplasty; posteroinferior approach; rotator cuff-sparing; anatomical study

1. Introduction

One of the main failure modes after anatomical total shoulder arthroplasty (aTSA) is rotator cuff insufficiency [1]. While reverse total shoulder arthroplasty (rTSA) can function without an intact rotator cuff, aTSA depends on rotator cuff integrity and its ability to center the humeral head on the glenoid, due to the low constraint of the anatomical design itself.

Traditionally, aTSA is performed via an anterior deltopectoral approach that offers good exposure of the humeral head and sufficient exposure of the glenoid via takedown of the subscapularis (SSC). Different types of SSC management are being employed in an effort to simultaneously improve healing and to maintain surgical feasibility at the same time, albeit, without any clear evidence of superiority of one over the other [2–5]. Regardless of the refixation type, a takedown of the SSC poses a threat to future rotator cuff integrity, and at the same time, warrants postoperative immobilization with the associated discomfort for the patient and risk for stiffness.

Due to these concerns, different types of less cuff-jeopardizing approaches for performing aTSA have been proposed, including an anterior deltopectoral approach with only partial take-down of the inferior subscapularis [6], a superior approach through the deltoid and the rotator interval [7], and an anterior deltopectoral approach through the rotator interval [8]. While the clinical outcome for the complete rotator-cuff sparing interval approaches were comparable to the results obtained with traditional approaches, there was concern regarding non-anatomical neck osteotomies, head sizing, and neck-shaft angle, as well as increased superior decentering and an inability to resect inferior osteophytes in the calcar area, due to limited exposure [7–10].

Amirthanayagam et al., examined the anatomical feasibility and achievable exposure of the humeral head and glenoid of different anterior and posterior rotator-cuff sparing approaches [11]. They propagated the postero-inferior subdeltoid approach according to Brodsky [12] for implanting an aTSA, because it provides the greatest access while minimizing the damage to the rotator cuff [11]. It seems that anterior cuff-sparing approaches are a trade-off between limited exposure and damage of the crucial anterosuperior aspect of the rotator cuff.

While no clinical reports of aTSA via a posteroinferior subdeltoid approach have been published, Gagey et al., described a posterolateral transdeltoid approach with osteotomy of the external rotators, which allows for a wide exposure that is suitable for primary or revision of total shoulder arthroplasty [13]. Greiwe et al., reported 6-month results for aTSA implanted using a transdeltoid posterior approach with rotator cuff-sparing internervous access to the joint between the infraspinatus and the teres minor, lateral T-shaped capsulotomy, as well as an in-situ osteotomy of the humeral head. The authors conclude that this approach is a safe and effective method for performing aTSA [14]. In an anatomical study of the same approach, on average, 89% of the glenoid and 95% of the humeral cut surface could be visualized, and the stem could be reliably implanted in neutral angulation. However, the authors also stress the point that it is a challenging technique that should not be attempted in clinical practice without proper training [15].

In this anatomical study, we explored the possibility of a rotator cuff-sparing implantation of an anatomical total shoulder arthroplasty (aTSA) via the postero-inferior (PI) approach with subdeltoidal access and the posterior dislocation of the humeral head through an internervous split between the infraspinatus and the teres minor, for improved exposure and the precise osteotomy of the humeral head. The goal of this study was to compare the effectiveness of this PI approach to the traditional subscapularis takedown deltopectoral approach, in terms of sizing and positioning, when implanting an aTSA.

2. Materials and Methods

Prior to the beginning of this study, institutional ethical committee approval was obtained (EA1/026/21). 20 fresh frozen right-sided cadaveric shoulders (Science Care Inc., Phoenix, AZ, USA) were obtained. Only specimens with intact rotator cuffs and no evidence of head deforming osteoarthritis were employed for this study, leaving 18 shoulders from 13 female and 5 male donors, with a mean age at the time of death of 72 years (range: 56–93 years), for further evaluation. The cadavers were randomly divided into 2 groups of 9 specimen each. An Eclipse stemless anatomical shoulder arthroplasty (Arthrex, Naples, FL, USA) was implanted in the first group, using a standard deltopectoral approach, and in the second group, using a PI approach. True anteroposterior (AP) and axillary fluoroscopic radiographs were obtained from each specimen, pre- and postoperatively. On the postoperative images, care was taken to gather perfectly orthogonal images of the arthroplasty without any overlap between the metallic trunion and the bony surface of the osteotomy.

2.1. Surgical Technique

All surgeries were performed by the first author (PM), who was assisted by the senior author (DA).

2.1.1. Deltopectoral Approach

In the first group, a standard deltopectoral approach with subscapularis tenotomy was performed. After dislocation of the humeral head, resection was obtained at the level of the anatomic neck. The trunion size was then determined using a template, and the length of the cage screw was measured using a special cage screw sizer. Then, a complete exposure of the glenoid articular surface was obtained by releasing the labrum and the capsule. The size of the glenoid (small, medium, or large) was assessed by choosing the glenoid guide that best matched the glenoid surface area. The guide pin was then inserted through the guide into the glenoid vault until it reached the medial cortical bone. After removal of the guide, the inserted pin was cut at the level of the glenoid surface, leaving the rest of the pin in the glenoid vault to allow for later radiological evaluation of the appropriate pin positioning, as well as the pin version and inclination. No glenoid implantation was performed; however, prior to cutting the pin, a reamer was inserted in order to evaluate the theoretical level of difficulty to ream the glenoid without actually reaming the bony surface. The definitive trunion was then implanted onto the resection plane, and the definitive cage screw was inserted followed by the appropriate size humeral head. The sizing and positioning of the implant was performed in a manner representative of the current standard of care in clinical practice.

2.1.2. Posterior Approach

A subdeltoid approach, previously described by Brodsky et al. [12], was used in all cases. A 10–12 cm vertical skin incision was made on the posterior aspect of the shoulder, beginning at the posterior border of the acromion around 2 cm medial of the lateral aspect and extending inferiorly slightly lateral to the posterior axillary fold. After identifying and mobilizing the inferior border of the spinal part of the deltoid, the deltoid was retracted superiorly and laterally facilitated by the abduction of the arm. No splitting of the deltoid muscle was performed. Next, the internervous interval between the infraspinatus and the teres minor was visually identified, and its distance to the axillary nerve was measured and documented (Figure 1). A fat line between the infraspinatus and teres minor could be identified in two-thirds of the specimen to aid in identifying the internervous interval. A split between the teres minor and infraspinatus was performed with a subsequent lateral "T-shaped" capsular incision in the first three consecutive cases, and a medial "T-shaped" capsular incision in the subsequent six cases, as the latter offered a better visualization and exposure of the humerus and the glenoid. The humeral head was then dislocated posteroinferiorly through the created interval via flexion, horizontal adduction, and internal rotation (Figure 2). The humeral cut was performed at the level of the anatomic neck, while carefully protecting the rotator cuff with retractors. The trunion size was then determined using a template, and the length of the cage screw was measured using a cage screw sizer. Next, the glenoid was exposed, the labrum excised, and the capsule released around the glenoid (Figure 3). The size of the glenoid was then measured, and the guide pin was inserted and cut at the level of the glenoid surface, as previously described for the deltopectoral approach, along with the simulated glenoid reaming without actually removing bone.

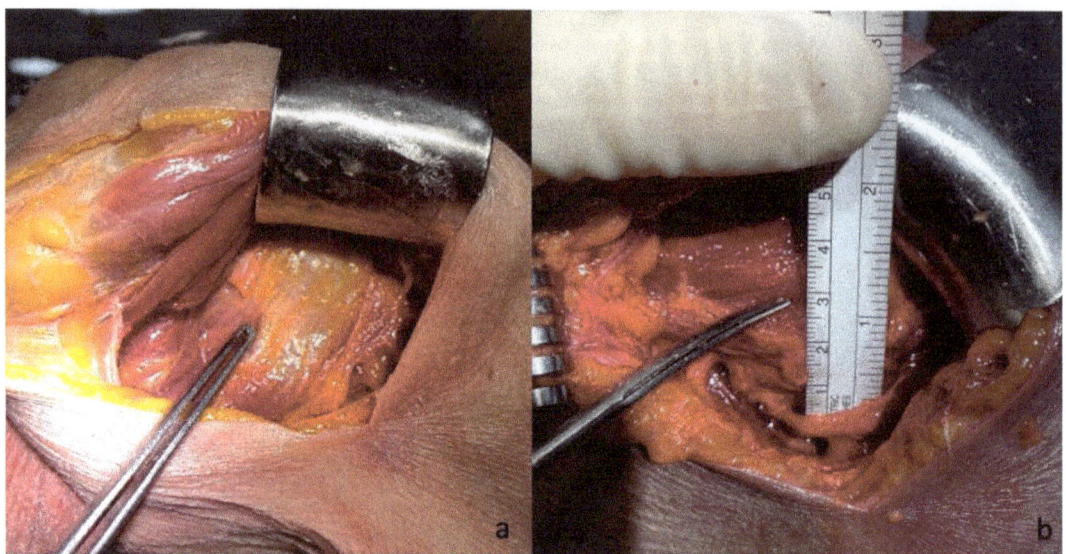

Figure 1. Identification of the internervous interval between the infraspinatus and the teres minor (**a**) and measurement of its distance to axillary nerve (**b**) in a postero-inferior approach.

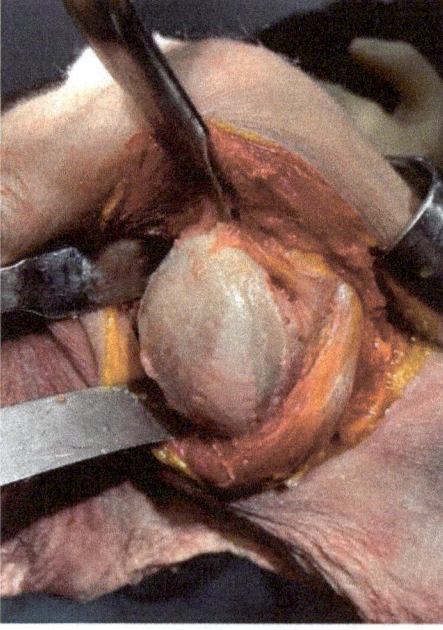

Figure 2. Humeral head exposure via the postero-inferior approach after posteroinferior dislocation through the internervous interval and below the deltoid muscle.

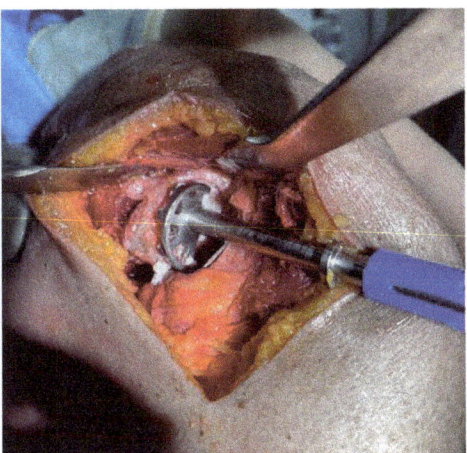

Figure 3. Glenoid exposure and simulated reaming through the postero-inferior approach.

While performing the procedure, the surgeon had to grade the difficulty (poor, acceptable, or excellent) to achieve a certain surgical step, including identification of the internervous interval between infraspinatus and teres minor, exposure of the humeral head, humeral head resection, and exposure of the glenoid, as well as glenoid reaming. At the end of the surgery, the surgeon's satisfaction score (0–100%) was noted for each case prior to taking the postoperative radiographs and revealing the quality of the implant sizing and placement.

2.2. Radiographic Analysis

Radiographic analysis was performed by two independent reviewers (LC and MM) who were not involved in the surgeries performed, and who were blinded to which case had performed, utilizing a deltopectoral or a PI approach. All measurements were performed with the image analysis software Visage 7.1 (Visage Imaging, Berlin, Germany). The preoperative and postoperative neck-shaft angle (NSA) was determined on pre- and postoperative AP radiographs, as previously described by Flurin et al. [16] (Figure 4). For the determination of the native center of rotation (COR) on the postoperative AP radiographs, a best-fit circle was placed based on three preserved bony landmarks, as previously described [17,18]: (1) the lateral cortex of the greater tuberosity; (2) the medial calcar at the inflection point; and (3) the medial footprint of the rotator cuff on the greater tuberosity. A second implant-matched circle was then placed to fit the curvature of the prosthetic humeral head. The COR from each circle was then identified, and a coordinate system was generated from the native COR, with the y-axis aligned parallel to the intramedullary axis of the shaft, and the x-axis as perpendicular to the shaft. The deviation between the pre- and postoperative COR was then determined in the x- and y-axis [18]. In the x-coordinate plane, a shift of postoperative COR medially considered as positive, and a shift laterally negative, while in the y-coordinate plane, a superior shift was considered as positive, and an inferior shift, negative. The measured distance between the native and the postoperative COR in the medio-lateral and the supero-inferior directions were then each divided by the diameter of the native best-fit circle, and were reported as a percentage (Figure 5a). In addition, the shift between the pre- and postoperative COR in anteroposterior direction was determined on axillary radiographs in a similar fashion. A best-fit circle was fitted on the two edges of the humeral resection plane, with its COR corresponding to the middle of the resection plane. A second implant matched circle was then placed to fit the curvature of the prosthetic humeral head. The COR was then identified from each circle, and a coordinate system was generated from the anatomic COR, with the y-axis aligned parallel to the intramedullary axis of the shaft, and the x-axis perpendicular to this line, to measure the distance between both COR in the anteroposterior direction. In the x-coordinate plane, a shift of postoperative COR anterior was considered positive, and a shift posterior, negative. The measured distance between the native and postoperative COR in an anteroposterior direction was then divided by the diameter of the native best-fit circle, and was given as a percentage (Figure 5b).

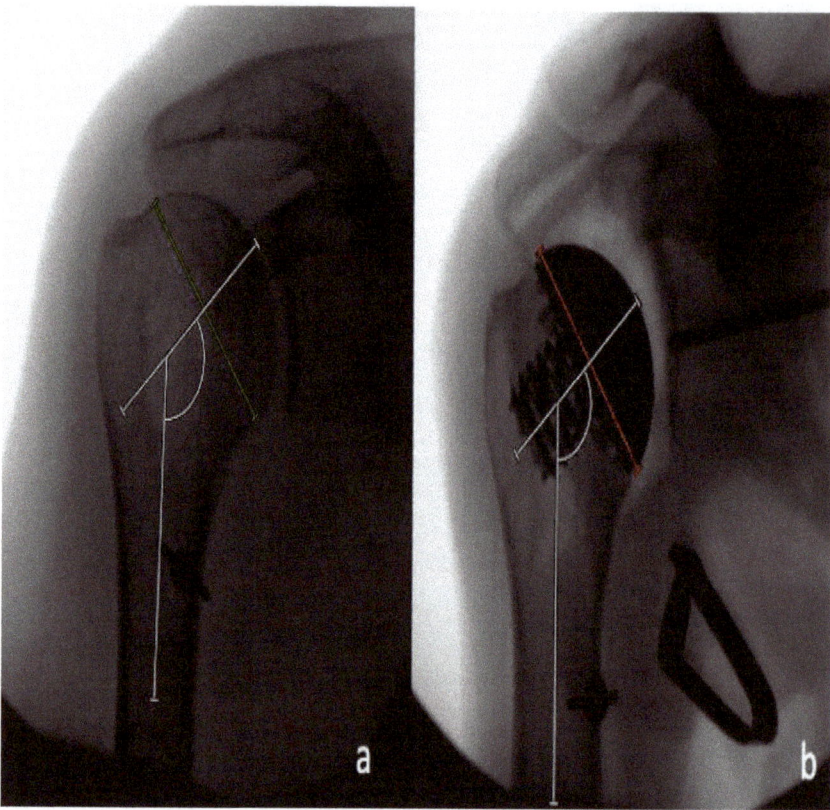

Figure 4. (**a**) Determination of the pre-operative neck-shaft angle between the line perpendicular to the anatomic neck axis (green line) and the intramedullary axis. (**b**) Determination of the post-operative neck-shaft angle between the line perpendicular to the backsurface of the trunion (red line) and the intramedullary axis.

Furthermore, the supero-inferior and antero-posterior size matching between the humeral resection plane and prosthetic humeral head diameter were determined and expressed as percentages by dividing the prosthetic head diameter by the length of the humeral resection plane in the AP and axillary radiographs, respectively (Figure 5c,d).

Each radiographic parameter obtained for the humeral component was rated based on the scoring system described in Table 1. The single scores were then summed to yield the anatomic reconstruction score (ARS) for each case, to objectively quantify and to assess the quality of the anatomical humeral head reconstruction.

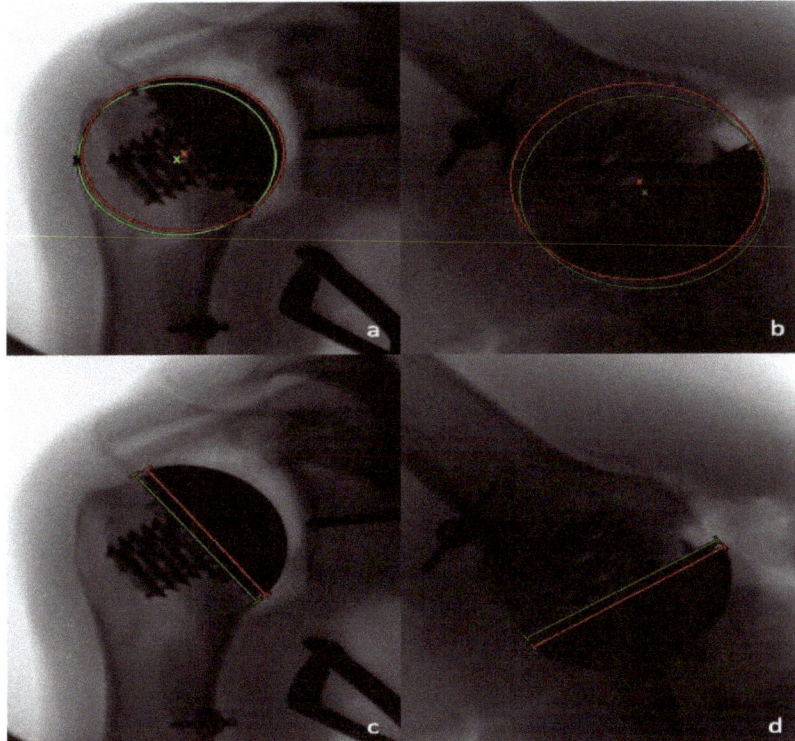

Figure 5. A best-fit anatomic circle (green circle) with its center of rotation (COR) (green x), and a best-fit implant circle (red circle) with its COR (red x) are placed on the AP (**a**) and axillary (**b**) views to determine the differences in the positioning of the COR. The length of the resection plane (green line) and the prosthetic humeral head (red line) were compared on the AP radiographs (**c**) and the axillary radiographs (**d**).

The pin positioning for the glenoid preparation was assessed in the supero-inferior and the antero-posterior directions by dividing the distance between the pin and inferior glenoid rim by the length of the glenoid, as well as the distance between the pin and the posterior glenoid rim and the width of the glenoid on the AP and the axillary radiographs, respectively (Figure 6a,b). These values were then displayed as percentages. In addition, the inclination and the version of the theoretical glenoid implantation were measured by determining the angle between the native glenoid surface and the glenoid guide pin on the AP and axillary radiographs, respectively (Figure 7a,b).

Table 1. Parameters used to calculate the Anatomic Reconstruction Score (ARS).

Neck-Shaft Angle	Pre and Post Difference
Rating of 0 points	>10°
Rating of 1 points	>5° and ≤10°
Rating of 2 points	≤5°
COR medio-lateral	Pre and post difference
Rating of 0 points	>10%
Rating of 1 points	>5% and ≤10%
Rating of 2 points	≤5%

Table 1. *Cont.*

Neck-Shaft Angle	Pre and Post Difference
COR supero-inferior	Pre and post difference
Rating of 0 points	>10%
Rating of 1 points	>5% and ≤10%
Rating of 2 points	≤5%
COR antero-posterior	Pre- and postoperative difference
Rating of 0 points	>10%
Rating of 1 points	>5% and ≤10%
Rating of 2 points	≤5%
Head size supero-inferior	
Rating of 0 points	<95% or >105%
Rating of 1 points	≥95% and ≤105%
Head size antero-posterior	
Rating of 0 points	<95% or >105%
Rating of 1 points	≥95% and ≤105%

COR, center of rotation.

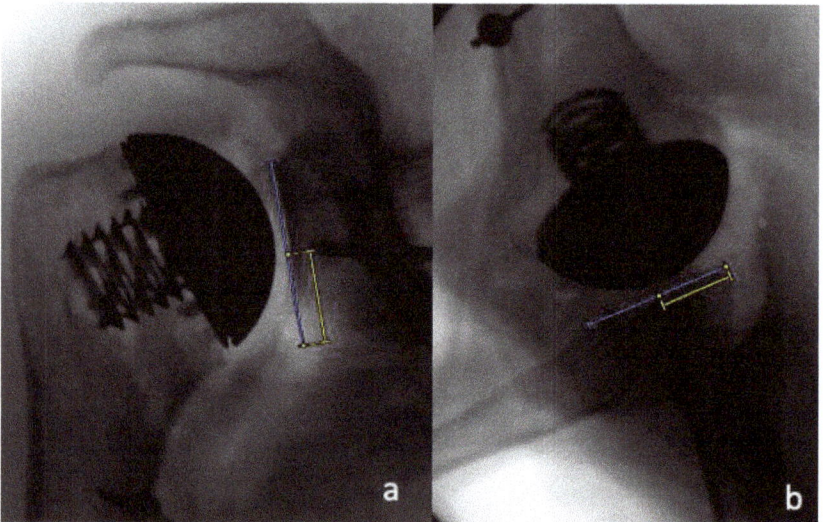

Figure 6. Pin placement was determined (**a**) by dividing the distance of the pin to the inferior glenoid rim (yellow line) by the supero-inferior extent of the glenoid (blue line) on the AP radiographs, and (**b**) the distance of the pin to the posterior glenoid rim (yellow line) by the antero-posterior extent of the glenoid (blue line) on the axillary radiographs.

2.3. Statistical Analysis

Intraclass correlation coefficients (ICC) with a 95% confidence interval (CI) were calculated for all measurements. As recommended by Landis and Koch, an ICC < 0.20 resembles slight agreement, 0.21 to 0.40, fair agreement, 0.41 to 0.60, moderate agreement, 0.61 to 0.80, substantial agreement, and >0.81, almost perfect agreement [19]. After a reliability assessment, the values of both raters were averaged for further analysis. The Kolmogorov–Smirnov test was used to test for normal distribution. The two-sample *t*-test (for parametric distribution) or the Mann–Whitney U test (for nonparametric distribution) were used to compare continuous variables between groups. For statistical analyses, IBM

SPSS Statistics 25.0 software (IBM, Armonk, NY, USA) was employed. A p-value < 0.05 was considered significant.

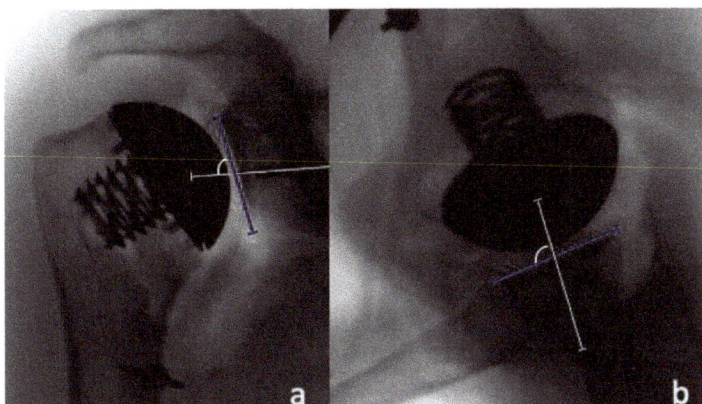

Figure 7. Measurements of theoretical glenoid component inclination (**a**) and version (**b**) by determining the angle between the native glenoid surface and the glenoid guide pin. A guide pin placed with more inclination or retroversion leads to a larger recorded angle.

3. Results

The average head and trunion size in the deltopectoral group was 42, with a range from 39 to 47; and the mean size in the PI group was 41, with a range from 39 to 43. In the deltopectoral group, six small, two medium, and one large screw were implanted, while in the PI group, three small, four medium, and two large screws were used. In both groups, five small, three medium, and one large glenoid component were trialed.

While performing the PI approach, the identification of the internervous plane was poor in four cases, acceptable in three cases, and excellent in two cases. The average distance of the internervous plane to the axillary nerve was 33 mm, with a minimum distance of 25 mm and a maximum distance of 45 mm. The posteroinferior dislocation of the humeral head through the internervous interval and inferior to the posterior deltoid was possible in all cases. The exposure of the humeral head was excellent in five cases, acceptable in three cases, and poor in one case. The possibility of resection of the humeral head was excellent in three cases, acceptable in three cases, and poor in three cases. In all cases, with a medial T-shaped incision of the capsule instead of a lateral T-shaped incision, an acceptable or excellent exposure and resection opportunity were identified. The exposure of the glenoid and simulated reaming was excellent in four cases, acceptable in three cases, and poor in two cases. The surgeon satisfaction rating with the procedure when performing the PI approach displayed a learning curve with a positive impact of the switch from a lateral T-shaped to a medial T-shaped incision of the capsule between cases 3 and 4 (Figure 8).

The intraclass correlation coefficients for the radiographic measurements of the two independent observers was almost perfect for six parameters, substantial for two parameters, moderate for two parameters, and fair for two parameters (Table 2).

While the COR was positioned significantly ($p = 0.031$) more medial in the PI approach group (3.7 ± 3.4%, range: −2.3% to 8.7%) than in the deltopectoral approach group (−0.2 ± 3.6%, range: −6.9% to 4.1%) on average, none of the remaining measured radiographic parameters were significantly different between both groups (Table 3).

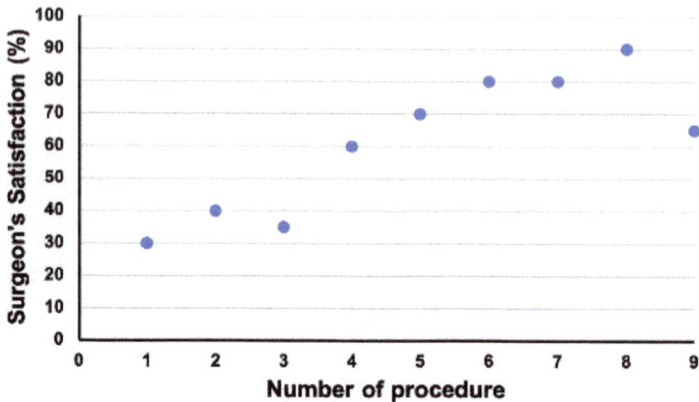

Figure 8. Change in surgeon's satisfaction from the first case to the ninth case when performing total shoulder arthroplasty via a posteroinferior approach. Between cases 3 and 4, a switch from a lateral T-shaped to a medial T-shaped incision of the capsule was made.

Table 2. Intra-class correlation coefficients (ICC) of the radiographic measurement parameters.

Measurement Parameter	ICC
Neck-Shaft Angle native (°)	0.289
Neck-Shaft Angle post-operative (°)	0.961
COR medio-lateral (%)	0.823
COR supero-inferior (%)	0.484
COR antero-posterior (%)	0.303
Head size supero-inferior (%)	0.765
Head size antero-posterior (%)	0.898
Glenoid positioning supero-inferior (%)	0.868
Glenoid positioning antero-posterior (%)	0.506
Glenoid Inclination (°)	0.938
Glenoid Retroversion (°)	0.980

Table 3. Comparison of the postoperative radiographic parameters between the anatomical arthroplasties performed via a deltopectoral approach and a postero-inferior approach.

Measurement Parameter	Deltopectoral ($n = 9$)	Postero-Inferior ($n = 9$)	p-Value
Neck-Shaft Angle post-operative (°)	127 ± 4 (range 121 to 134)	130 ± 8 (range 120–143)	0.566
COR medio-lateral (%)	−0.2 ± 3.6 (range −6.9 to 4.1)	3.7 ± 3.4 (range −2.3 to 8.7)	**0.034**
COR supero-inferior (%)	1.0 ± 2.1 (range −1.8 to 4.0)	2.6 ± 2.0 (range 0.6 to 5.4)	0.354
COR antero-posterior (%)	1.7 ± 1.5 (range −0.1 to 4.4)	0.9 ± 2.1 (range −3.9 to 3.8)	0.566
Head size supero-inferior (%)	98.5 ± 0.9 (range 96.5 to 99.6)	97.3 ± 2.6 (range 92.4 to 101.8)	0.145
Head size antero-posterior (%)	100.6 ± 2.1 (range 97.2 to 103.9)	101.1 ± 2.2 (range 98.4 to 105.6)	0.536

Table 3. Cont.

Measurement Parameter	Deltopectoral (n = 9)	Postero-Inferior (n = 9)	p-Value
Anatomic Reconstruction Score	9.3 ± 1.1 (range 7 to 10)	8.4 ± 1.2 (range 7 to 10)	0.129
Glenoid positioning supero-inferior (%)	51.1 ± 3.9 (range 44.6 to 56.1)	49.1 ± 4.6 (range 40.4 to 57.7)	0.331
Glenoid positioning antero-posterior (%)	50.4 ± 1.4 (range 48.8 to 52.4)	49.3 ± 2.1 (range 44.3 to 51.6)	0.233
Theoretical glenoid inclination (°)	88 ± 4 (range 83 to 95)	86 ± 6 (range 78 to 94)	0.270
Theoretical glenoid retroversion (°)	89 ± 2 (range 86 to 93)	91 ± 6 (range 82 to 103)	0.269

4. Discussion

The investigated PI approach involves a subdeltoidal access and an internervous split between the infraspinatus and the teres minor, as described by Brodsky et al. in 1987 [12]. Furthermore, it includes a medial T-shaped incision of the capsule with iuxtaglenoidal posterior to inferior capsular release to allow for the posteroinferior dislocation of the humeral head, and thus extended exposure for precise humeral head osteotomy. The study results show that the implantation of an anatomical total shoulder arthroplasty with acceptable implant sizing and positioning can be performed via a PI approach in a cadaveric shoulder.

While no statistically significant difference was observed regarding the neck-shaft angle, the variation and range seemed to be a little wider in the PI approach group, with a tendency towards more valgus positioning of the head in some cases. This can be explained by the fact that after postero-inferior dislocation of the humeral head through the internervous interval, the calcar tends to be covered by the teres minor, which needs to be pushed inferiorly, while the superior insertion of the rotator cuff is more easily exposed (Figure 2).

The COR was slightly but statistically significantly more medial in cases with the PI approach than with the deltopectoral approach, indicating a risk of lateral overstuffing due to insufficient resection of the humeral head. While this could be explained by a lack of exposure, it may also be caused by the presence of the bare area on the posterior side of the humerus, which makes identification of the anatomical neck more difficult. Since the neck-shaft angle is above 90°, a lack of resection of the anatomical neck tendentially also leads to a superior translation of the COR, which however, was only slightly observable in this study, and did not yield statistically significant differences. The anteroposterior positioning of the COR showed no difference between the groups.

No differences in terms of sizing of the prosthetic head were observed, with slight supero-inferior undersizing but good antero-posterior matching in both groups, as the resection plane is usually oval shaped with a smaller antero-posterior than supero-inferior diameter [20]. The larger variation in the PI approach group is likely explained by the learning curve.

While the Anatomic Reconstruction Score was not statistically different in both groups, there was a trend towards slightly lower scores in the PI group, mostly explained by the larger variation of the neck-shaft angle and the lack of sufficient resection of the humeral head.

Due to the anterior tilt of the scapula, the described approach offers a postero-inferior direct view of the glenoid, which can be changed to an e-face view when the humeral head is retracted anteriorly. This may lead to a tendency of postero-inferior placement and an increased retroversion of the glenoid guide pin in cases with poor exposure. Greiwe et al. point at different advantages of the posterior approach, including easier access to the retroverted glenoids, as well as facilitated posterior soft tissue balancing [14]. However, it remains unclear as to whether posterior approaches may also weaken the posterior soft tissues, including the posterior capsule and rotator cuff, and therefore, this may possibly aggravate the posterior humeral subluxation in patients with posterior eccentric glenoid wear.

Posterior approaches have already been used in the clinical setting to implant shoulder arthroplasties. Gagey et al., were able to implant 53 hemiarthroplasties through a posterolateral approach with subperiosteal detachment of the posterior part of the deltoid muscle and osteotomy of the external rotator muscles [13]. Although this approach provides a wide range of exposure of the glenoid and humeral head, deltoid release and detachment of the external rotators by means of an osteotomy are the main limitations, as they warrant postoperative immobilization of the arm and pose the risk for deltoid atrophy [13] and the insufficiency of external rotators. In contrast, the PI approach used in this study spares the deltoid and external rotators, and therefore, it allows for immediate postoperative mobilization. Greiwe et al., performed a total shoulder arthroplasty in 31 patients using a posterior rotator cuff-sparing approach, which uses a split of the middle and posterior heads of the deltoid muscle, a lateral based T-shaped capsular incision, and an in-situ humeral osteotomy [14]. Short-term follow up was available for 26 patients, with a significant improvement in clinical scores.

The authors also conducted an anatomic feasibility study to evaluate their approach, and this showed good access to glenoid and humerus, despite the mentioned technical difficulties [15]. While the deltoid split does not seem to affect deltoid integrity [14], the in-situ osteotomy of the humeral head, which is performed without dislocation of the head and via the internervous split, poses a surgical challenge, due to limited exposure and few bony landmarks for reference. As the identification of the anatomic neck for a precise humeral osteotomy may be difficult, there is a risk for an improper humeral cut, which can lead to malpositioning of the prosthetic humeral head, and potentially cause asymmetric loading of the glenoid, resulting in glenoid erosion and loosening [21–23]. According to the present anatomical study, a medial T-shaped incision of the capsule, with iuxtaglenoidal posterior to inferior capsular release, instead of a lateral T-shaped incision, may facilitate posteroinferior dislocation of the humeral head through the internervous interval, and thus allow for a precise identification of the anatomic neck, and easier humeral head osteotomy. However, great attention must be given not to stretch and harm the axillary nerve with the retractors placed inferiorly between the dislocated humeral head and the teres minor. Finally, it must be mentioned that even though the step of posterior dislocation of the humeral head can quite easily be obtained in cadaveric specimens, it might not be achievable in patients with severe joint stiffness due to advanced osteoarthritis.

A limitation of this study is the fact that the implantation of arthroplasties in cadaveric shoulders is typically easier, due to the reduced tension of the soft tissues. This might have facilitated the exposure and the implantation, especially in the PI approach group, as even in the cadaveric setting, only limited exposure could be obtained in some cases. Furthermore, not whole-body, but rather mere shoulder specimens were used for this study, making the placement easier to handle than what could be expected in clinical practice. While most measurement parameters have proven to be reliable, with acceptable ICCs, two parameters (pre-operative neck-shaft angle and the antero-posterior COR) showed only fair ICCs, thus limiting their interpretabilities. Finally, no conclusions regarding the risk of damage to the axillary nerve when performing the PI approach can be drawn from this study. Despite the apparently sufficient distance to the interval between the teres minor and the infraspinatus, no information on the changes in position and tension on the nerve during the posterior dislocation of the humeral head, humeral and glenoid exposure, as well as motion of the arm were collected.

5. Conclusions

The investigated postero-inferior approach with subdeltoidal access and posterior dislocation of the humeral head through an internervous split between the infraspinatus and the teres minor with a medial T-shaped incision of the capsule allows for sufficient exposure and orientation to perform rotator-cuff sparing anatomical total shoulder arthroplasty with acceptable implant sizing and positioning in cadaveric specimens. This approach tends to medialize the COR that needs to be taken into account when performing aTSA. Further research should focus on the radiological and clinical outcomes of the PI approach in daily practice.

Author Contributions: Conceptualization, D.A. and P.M.; methodology, D.A. and L.L.; formal analysis, P.M. and M.M.; data curation, D.A. and K.K.; writing—original draft preparation, D.A. and L.L.; writing—review and editing, F.U., S.D.S., M.M., M.v.d.M. and P.M.; supervision, P.M. All authors have read and agreed to the published version of the manuscript.

Funding: Funding was received from Arthrex Inc. in terms of material sources.

Institutional Review Board Statement: The study was conducted in accordance with the Declaration of Helsinki, and approved by the Institutional Review Board (or Ethics Committee) of Charite Universitätsmedizin (EA1/026/21).

Informed Consent Statement: Not applicable.

Data Availability Statement: Data available on request due to restrictions, e.g., privacy or ethical.

Conflicts of Interest: Author P.M. receives royalties from Arthrex Inc. and consultant payments from Arthrex Inc., Medacta and Depuy/Synthes. Authors F.U., S.S. and M.W. are employed by Arthrex Inc. The authors D.A., M.M., L.L. and K.K. declare they have no financial interests.

References

1. Somerson, J.S.; Hsu, J.E.; Neradilek, M.B.; Matsen, F.A. Response to Weber and McFarland regarding: "Analysis of 4063 complications of shoulder arthroplasty reported to the US Food and Drug Administration from 2012 to 2016". *J. Shoulder Elb. Surg.* **2020**, *29*, e322–e323. [CrossRef]
2. Aibinder, W.R.; Bicknell, R.T.; Bartsch, S.; Scheibel, M.; Athwal, G.S. Subscapularis management in stemless total shoulder arthroplasty: Tenotomy versus peel versus lesser tuberosity osteotomy. *J. Shoulder Elb. Surg.* **2019**, *28*, 1942–1947. [CrossRef]
3. Del Core, M.A.; Cutler, H.S.; Ahn, J.; Khazzam, M. Systematic Review and Network Meta-Analysis of Subscapularis Management Techniques in Anatomic Total Shoulder Arthroplasty. *J. Shoulder Elb. Surg.* **2020**, *30*, 1714–1724. [CrossRef]
4. Lapner, P.; Pollock, J.W.; Zhang, T.; Ruggiero, S.; Momoli, F.; Sheikh, A.; Athwal, G.S. A randomized controlled trial comparing subscapularis tenotomy with peel in anatomic shoulder arthroplasty. *J. Shoulder Elb. Surg.* **2019**, *29*, 225–234. [CrossRef]
5. Levine, W.N.; Munoz, J.; Hsu, S.; Byram, I.R.; Bigliani, L.U.; Ahmad, C.S.; Kongmalai, P.; Shillingford, J.N. Subscapularis tenotomy versus lesser tuberosity osteotomy during total shoulder arthroplasty for primary osteoarthritis: A prospective, randomized controlled trial. *J. Shoulder Elb. Surg.* **2019**, *28*, 407–414. [CrossRef]
6. Savoie, F.H., 3rd; Charles, R.; Casselton, J.; O'Brien, M.J.; Hurt, J.A., 3rd. The subscapularis-sparing approach in humeral head replacement. *J. Shoulder Elb. Surg.* **2015**, *24*, 606–612. [CrossRef]
7. Lafosse, L.; Schnaser, E.; Haag, M.; Gobezie, R. Primary total shoulder arthroplasty performed entirely thru the rotator interval: Technique and minimum two-year outcomes. *J. Shoulder Elb. Surg.* **2009**, *18*, 864–873. [CrossRef]
8. Ding, D.Y.; Mahure, S.A.; Akuoko, J.A.; Zuckerman, J.D.; Kwon, Y. Total shoulder arthroplasty using a subscapularis-sparing approach: A radiographic analysis. *J. Shoulder Elb. Surg.* **2015**, *24*, 831–837. [CrossRef]
9. Ransom, E.F.; Adkison, D.P.; Woods, D.P.; Pinto, M.C.; He, J.K.; Worthen, J.V.; Brabston, E.W.; Ponce, B.A. Subscapularis sparing total shoulder arthroplasty through a superolateral approach: A radiographic study. *J. Shoulder Elb. Surg.* **2019**, *29*, 814–820. [CrossRef]
10. Kwon, Y.W.; Zuckerman, J. Subscapularis-Sparing Total Shoulder Arthroplasty: A Prospective, Double-Blinded, Randomized Clinical Trial. *Orthopedics* **2019**, *42*, 1–7. [CrossRef]
11. Amirthanayagam, T.D.; Amis, A.A.; Reilly, P.; Emery, R.J. Rotator cuff–sparing approaches for glenohumeral joint access: An anatomic feasibility study. *J. Shoulder Elb. Surg.* **2017**, *26*, 512–520. [CrossRef] [PubMed]
12. Brodsky, J.W.; Tullos, H.S.; Gartsman, G.M. Simplified posterior approach to the shoulder joint. A technical note. *J. Bone Jt. Surg.* **1987**, *69*, 773–774. [CrossRef]
13. Gagey, O.; Spraul, J.; Vinh, T. Posterolateral approach of the shoulder: Assessment of 50 cases. *J. Shoulder Elb. Surg.* **2001**, *10*, 47–51. [CrossRef]

14. Greiwe, R.M.; Hill, M.A.; Boyle, M.S.; Nolan, J. Posterior Approach Total Shoulder Arthroplasty: A Retrospective Analysis of Short-term Results. *Orthopedics* **2020**, *43*, e15–e20. [CrossRef] [PubMed]
15. Greiwe, R.M.; Witzig, S.A.; Kohrs, B.J.; Hill, M.A.; Harm, R.G.; Bahk, M.S. Posterior approach shoulder arthroplasty: A cadaveric study assessing access. *J. Shoulder Elb. Surg.* **2020**, *30*, 1471–1476. [CrossRef] [PubMed]
16. Flurin, P.-H.; Roche, C.P.; Wright, T.W.; Zuckerman, J.D. Correlation Between Clinical Outcomes and Anatomic Reconstruction with Anatomic Total Shoulder Arthroplasty. *Bull. Hosp. Jt. Dis. (2013)* **2015**, *73* (Suppl. 1), S92–S98.
17. Youderian, A.R.; Ricchetti, E.T.; Drews, M.; Iannotti, J.P. Determination of humeral head size in anatomic shoulder replacement for glenohumeral osteoarthritis. *J. Shoulder Elb. Surg.* **2014**, *23*, 955–963. [CrossRef]
18. Alolabi, B.; Youderian, A.R.; Napolitano, L.; Szerlip, B.W.; Evans, P.J.; Nowinski, R.J.; Ricchetti, E.T.; Iannotti, J.P. Radiographic assessment of prosthetic humeral head size after anatomic shoulder arthroplasty. *J. Shoulder Elb. Surg.* **2014**, *23*, 1740–1746. [CrossRef]
19. Landis, J.R.; Koch, G.G. The measurement of observer agreement for categorical data. *Biometrics* **1977**, *33*, 159–174. [CrossRef]
20. Harrold, F.; Wigderowitz, C. Humeral head arthroplasty and its ability to restore original humeral head geometry. *J. Shoulder Elb. Surg.* **2013**, *22*, 115–121. [CrossRef]
21. Von Eisenhart-Rothe, R.; Muller-Gerbl, M.; Wiedemann, E.; Englmeier, K.H.; Graichen, H. Functional malcentering of the humeral head and asymmetric long-term stress on the glenoid: Potential reasons for glenoid loosening in total shoulder arthroplasty. *J. Shoulder Elb. Surg.* **2008**, *17*, 695–702. [CrossRef] [PubMed]
22. Ammarullah, M.I.; Afif, I.Y.; Maula, M.I.; Winarni, T.I.; Tauviqirrahman, M.; Akbar, I.; Basri, H.; van der Heide, E.; Jamari, J. Tresca Stress Simulation of Metal-on-Metal Total Hip Arthroplasty during Normal Walking Activity. *Materials* **2021**, *14*, 7554. [CrossRef] [PubMed]
23. Jamari, J.; Ammarullah, M.; Saad, A.; Syahrom, A.; Uddin, M.; van der Heide, E.; Basri, H. The Effect of Bottom Profile Dimples on the Femoral Head on Wear in Metal-on-Metal Total Hip Arthroplasty. *J. Funct. Biomater.* **2021**, *12*, 38. [CrossRef] [PubMed]

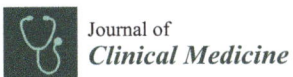
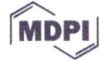

Article

COVID-19 as a Catalyst for Same-Day Discharge Total Shoulder Arthroplasty

Mariano E. Menendez [1], Noah Keegan [1], Brian C. Werner [2] and Patrick J. Denard [1,*]

[1] Oregon Shoulder Institute at Southern Oregon Orthopedics, Medford, OR 97504, USA; marianofurrer@gmail.com (M.E.M.); noahtkeegan@gmail.com (N.K.)
[2] Department of Orthopaedic Surgery, University of Virginia, Charlottesville, VA 22903, USA; BCW4X@hscmail.mcc.virginia.edu
* Correspondence: pjdenard@gmail.com

Abstract: The COVID-19 pandemic caused major disruptions to the healthcare system, but its impact on the transition to same-day discharge shoulder arthroplasty remains unexplored. This study assessed the effect of COVID-19 on length of stay (LOS), same-day discharge rates, and other markers of resource use after elective total shoulder arthroplasty. A total of 508 consecutive patients undergoing elective primary total shoulder arthroplasty between 2019 and 2021 were identified and divided into 2 cohorts: "pre-COVID" (March 2019–March 2020; n = 263) and "post-COVID" (May 2020–March 2021; n = 245). No elective shoulder arthroplasties were performed at our practice between 18 March and 11 May 2020. Outcome measures included LOS, same-day discharge, discharge location, and 90-day emergency department (ED) visits, readmissions and reoperations. There were no significant differences in baseline preoperative patient characteristics. Shoulder arthroplasty performed post-COVID was associated with a shorter LOS (12 vs. 16 h, p = 0.017) and a higher rate of same-day discharge (87.3 vs. 79.1%, p = 0.013). The rate of discharge to skilled nursing facilities was similarly low between the groups (1.9 vs. 2.0%, p = 0.915). There was a significant reduction in the rate of 90-day ED visits post-COVID (7.4 vs. 13.3%, p = 0.029), while there were no differences in 90-day reoperation (2.0 vs. 1.5%, p = 0.745) or readmission rates (1.2 vs. 1.9%, p = 0.724). The COVID-19 pandemic seems to have accelerated the shift towards shorter stays and more same-day discharge shoulder arthroplasties, while reducing unexpected acute health needs (e.g., ED visits) without adversely affecting readmission and reoperation rates.

Keywords: shoulder arthroplasty; COVID; coronavirus; length of stay; same-day discharge; pandemic

Citation: Menendez, M.E.; Keegan, N.; Werner, B.C.; Denard, P.J. COVID-19 as a Catalyst for Same-Day Discharge Total Shoulder Arthroplasty. *J. Clin. Med.* **2021**, *10*, 5908. https://doi.org/10.3390/jcm10245908

Academic Editors: Markus Scheibel, Alexandre Lädermann and Laurent Audigé

Received: 8 November 2021
Accepted: 15 December 2021
Published: 16 December 2021

Publisher's Note: MDPI stays neutral with regard to jurisdictional claims in published maps and institutional affiliations.

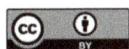

Copyright: © 2021 by the authors. Licensee MDPI, Basel, Switzerland. This article is an open access article distributed under the terms and conditions of the Creative Commons Attribution (CC BY) license (https://creativecommons.org/licenses/by/4.0/).

1. Introduction

The coronavirus (COVID-19) pandemic caused drastic disruptions to the provision of elective orthopedic surgery services in the United States [1]. This crisis also presented an opportunity for value optimization by promoting collaboration and creative thinking. One well-documented disruptive change has been the swift adoption of telehealth services [2,3]. The COVID outbreak may have also catalyzed the shift towards more resource-efficient outpatient joint arthroplasty, but this remains speculation [4].

Elective shoulder arthroplasty is an increasingly popular and highly standardized procedure that has been classically performed as inpatient [5–7]. It is unclear whether COVID has changed any of this. Patients may now be more inclined to go home shortly after surgery to minimize risk of contagion [8], and to rely more on technology (e.g., email, telehealth) to address postoperative concerns that would traditionally warrant a visit to the emergency department (ED). Hospitals may also be incentivized to more expeditiously discharge elective surgery patients to ensure continued bed capacity for potential COVID surges.

This study sought to determine the impact of the COVID-19 pandemic on length of stay (LOS) and same-day discharge rates after elective total shoulder arthroplasty.

Additionally, we examined discharge disposition patterns, ED visits, readmissions and reoperations. The hypothesis was that LOS decreased post-COVID, despite no change in patient characteristics.

2. Methods

2.1. Study Design

A retrospective study was conducted of a consecutive series of shoulder arthroplasties performed at a single private practice institution. Institutional review board approval was obtained for this study. Our registry was queried to identify all patients who underwent elective primary total shoulder arthroplasty (anatomic (ATSA) or reverse (RTSA)) between March 2019 and March 2021 by a single fellowship-trained shoulder surgeon. The inclusion criteria were: (1) an ATSA or RTSA and (2) minimum follow-up of 90 days. To achieve a homogenous sample of patients at low surgical risk, an a priori decision was made to exclude patients whose indication for surgery was traumatic, and those undergoing revision surgery.

Following the 18 March 2020 recommendation by the Centers for Medicare and Medicaid Services to postpone non-essential surgeries in response to the COVID-19 virus, no elective shoulder arthroplasties were performed at our practice until 11 May 2020. As such, the study sample was divided into two cohorts: the "pre-COVID" group for surgeries performed before 18 March 2020, and the "post-COVID" group for cases performed on or after 11 May 2020. Notably, the treating surgeon had nearly 10 years of experience at the beginning of the study period. During the study period there was no change in postoperative protocols or in the design of the implants used by the primary surgeon.

2.2. Outcomes Measures and Explanatory Variables

The main outcomes of interest included LOS (measured in hours after surgery) and same-day discharge. Discharge disposition (home versus skilled nursing facility (SNF)) was also recorded. Electronic medical records linked to the local hospital were reviewed to collect data on ED visits, readmissions, and reoperations within 90 days of surgery.

Several patient characteristics that might affect the influence of the COVID-19 pandemic on resource allocation after shoulder arthroplasty were recorded. Specifically, data were collected on age, sex, body mass index (BMI), and the presence of co-morbidities including diabetes, chronic obstructive pulmonary disease (COPD), and tobacco use. Surgical location (hospital versus ambulatory surgery center) data were also collected.

2.3. Statistical Analysis

To compare both baseline patient characteristics and postoperative outcomes between the pre- and post-COVID cohorts, Pearson chi-square tests were used for categorical variables and independent samples T-tests were used for continuous variables. Continuous variables were presented in terms of the mean and standard deviation (SD), and categorical variables were reported with frequencies and percentages. Statistical tests were 2-sided with $p < 0.05$ denoting statistical significance.

3. Results

A total of 508 patients met the study criteria. The study population consisted of 241 (47%) women and 267 men, with a mean (SD) age of 71 (8) years and BMI of 30 (6). Overall, 63% of patients underwent RTSA, while the remaining 37% had ATSA. There were no significant differences in any of the baseline patient characteristics between the pre- and post-COVID groups (Table 1). There was no difference in the rate of procedures performed in the hospital versus surgery center setting between the two groups (Table 1).

Shoulder arthroplasty performed in the post-COVID cohort was associated with a shorter LOS (12 vs. 16 h, $p = 0.017$) and higher rate of same-day discharge to home (87.3 vs. 79.1%; Figure 1, Table 2). Figure 2 is a more granular representation of the decline in the proportion of surgeries with overnight stays.

Table 1. Characteristics of the study population.

Parameter	All Patients	Period		p
		Pre-COVID	Post-COVID	
Total †	508 (100)	263 (51.8)	245 (48.2)	
Age * (year)	70.5 ± 8.2	70.7 ± 7.9	70.3 ± 8.6	0.603
Sex †				
Female	241 (47.4)	119 (45.2)	122 (49.8)	0.305
Male	267 (52.6)	144 (54.8)	123 (50.2)	
BMI *	30.2 ± 6.4	30.5 ± 6.3	29.9 ± 6.5	0.329
Diabetes †	83 (16.3)	50 (19.0)	33 (13.5)	0.091
Chronic obstructive pulmonary disease †	38 (7.5)	23 (8.7)	15 (6.1)	0.262
Tobacco use †	23 (4.5)	8 (3.0)	15 (6.1)	0.095
Total shoulder arthroplasty type †				
Anatomic	190 (37.4)	95 (36.1)	95 (38.8)	0.537
Reverse	318 (62.6)	168 (63.9)	150 (61.2)	
Surgical location †				
Hospital	409 (80.5)	213 (81.0)	196 (80.0)	0.779
Ambulatory surgery center	99 (19.5)	50 (19.0)	49 (20.0)	

BMI = body mass index. * The values are given as the mean and the standard deviation. † The values are given as the number of patients, with the percentage in parentheses.

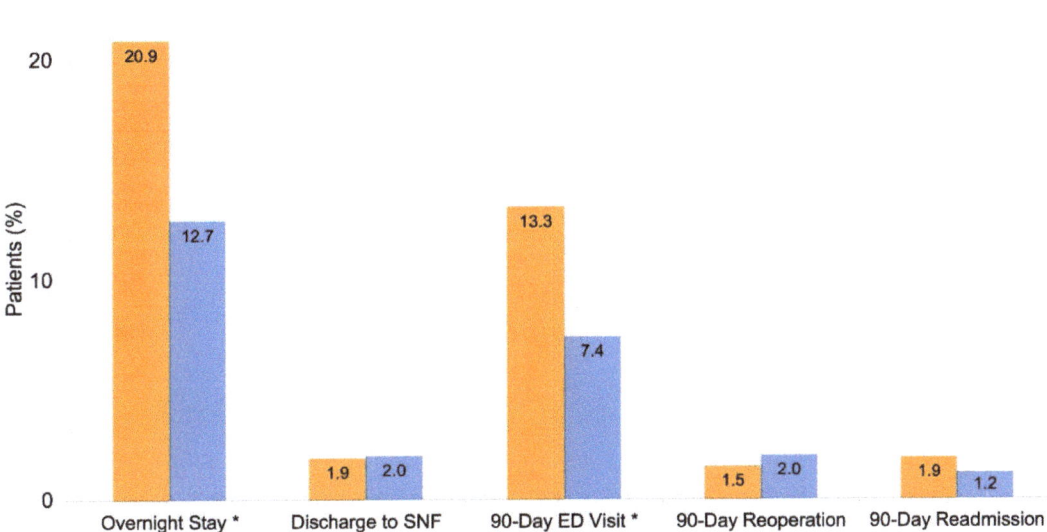

Figure 1. Outcomes after total shoulder arthroplasty in the pre- and post-COVID groups. Asterisks denote statistical significance ($p < 0.05$).

The rate of discharge to SNFs was similar between the groups (1.9 vs. 2.0%, $p = 0.915$). There was a significant reduction in the rate of 90-day ED visits in the post-COVID cohort (7.4 vs. 13.3%, $p = 0.029$), while there was no difference with regard to 90-day reoperation (2.0 vs. 1.5%, $p = 0.745$) and readmission rates (1.2 vs. 1.9%, $p = 0.724$; Table 2).

Table 2. Outcomes after total shoulder arthroplasty.

Parameter	All Patients	Period		p
		Pre-COVID	Post-COVID	
Same-day discharge †	422 (83.1)	208 (79.1)	214 (87.3)	0.013
Length of stay * (hours)	14 (3 to 192)	16 (3 to 120)	12 (3 to 192)	0.017
Discharge to skilled nursing facility †	10 (2.0)	5 (1.9)	5 (2.0)	0.915
ED visit within 90 days of surgery †	53 (10.5)	35 (13.3)	18 (7.4)	0.029
Postoperative pain	7 (1.4)	4 (1.5)	3 (1.2)	-
Wound issue	10 (2.0)	7 (2.7)	3 (1.2)	-
Medical issue	28 (5.5)	21 (8.0)	7 (2.9)	-
Musculoskeletal trauma and injury	8 (1.6)	3 (1.1)	5 (2.0)	-
Reoperation within 90 days of surgery †	9 (1.8)	4 (1.5)	5 (2.0)	0.745
Readmission within 90 days of surgery †	8 (1.6)	5 (1.9)	3 (1.2)	0.724

ED = emergency department. * The values are given as the mean, with the range in parentheses. † The values are given as the number of patients, with the percentage in parentheses.

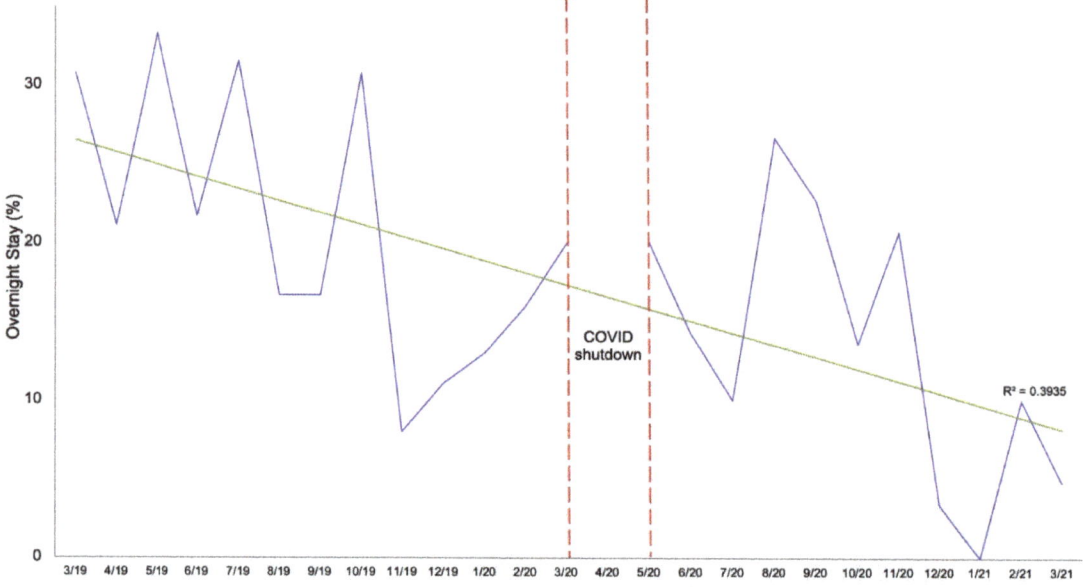

Figure 2. Rate of shoulder arthroplasties requiring overnight hospital stays over time.

4. Discussion

The COVID-19 outbreak upended traditional health system practices amid an environment that demanded an accelerated pace of innovation. Health systems were faced with difficult decisions as to how to safely resume margin-producing elective orthopedic surgery in the midst of the pandemic. Many have suggested transitioning more joint arthroplasty procedures to the outpatient setting [4,9,10], but whether this actually has taken place is unclear. This study showed that shoulder arthroplasty following the resumption of elective surgery during the COVID-19 pandemic was associated with a shorter LOS and higher rate of same-day discharge.

The finding that baseline preoperative patient characteristics remained unchanged compared to before the outbreak suggests that the observed changes in discharge patterns may indeed be a direct consequence of COVID. There is recent evidence that sociodemographic and psychological factors may have more influence than patient infirmity and technical issues in the variation in LOS and discharge disposition after shoulder arthroplasty [11]. Although this requires formal investigation, it is possible that patients may be more motivated to go home after surgery during the pandemic to minimize risk of contagion [8]. Indeed, it has been our experience during the pandemic that patients are more invested in making arrangements for going home the same day of surgery. Health systems may also be pushing for early elective surgery discharges to limit exposure and reallocate resources to sicker patients [9].

The observation that 90-day readmissions, reoperations, and ED visits did not increase following the resumption of elective surgery during the pandemic is reassuring. This is consistent with the growing realization that shorter postoperative stays after shoulder arthroplasty are safe. Shorter LOS and/or same-day discharge following shoulder arthroplasty do not seem to increase the risk of postoperative mortality and morbidity [12,13]. The important addition of the current study to this literature is the fact that both cohorts represented the majority of the shoulder arthroplasty population in the surgeon's practice. The near 90% utilization of same day discharge in the post-COVID cohort indicates that there was limited potential for patient selection bias. In other words, outpatient shoulder arthroplasty is safe in not only selected patients, but in the majority of cases based on the findings of the current study.

Interestingly, we found that the rate of ED visits decreased significantly from 13.3% (pre-pandemic) to 7.4%. It may be that patients are now more likely to use and rely on technology (e.g., emails with image exchange, telehealth) to address postoperative concerns that would traditionally warrant a visit to the ED. The observed reduction in ED visits may indicate that some of them are preventable with the use of technology and improved postoperative care coordination. This subject deserves further study. Although another explanation could be that patients were more fearful of postoperative ED visits, this is not supported by the lack of change in the 90-day complication or re-operation rate.

The principal strengths of our study include its relatively large sample size and the fact that all procedures were performed by the same experienced surgeon, thus reducing surgeon variation in perioperative protocols. Nonetheless, our analysis was subject to several shortcomings that might be addressed in future research. First, the retrospective nature of this study does not allow causal inference. Therefore, we can only determine associations between COVID and the outcomes of interest. Second, because this study was performed at a private practice with a high pre-COVID rate of same day discharge shoulder arthroplasty, the results may lack generalizability. However, one might expect an even greater increase in the rate of outpatient shoulder arthroplasty among practices with traditionally higher rates of inpatient procedures. Future studies should evaluate and compare shoulder arthroplasty discharge patterns pre- and post-COVID across different practices and regions. Third, while we collected data on multiple markers of postoperative resource use (e.g., LOS, discharge disposition, ED visits, readmissions, reoperations), we did not assess patient experience and functional outcomes to better define the value equation. Fourth, there was a trend towards a potentially clinically relevant (+5.5% difference) higher rate of diabetes in the pre-COVID cohort compared to the post-COVID cohort which, while not yet significant, may affect results in larger samples. Finally, our study was limited in follow-up duration (90 days) due to the recency of the pandemic.

5. Conclusions

This study provides evidence that the COVID-19 pandemic may have accelerated the shift towards shorter stays and more same-day discharge shoulder arthroplasties, while reducing unexpected acute health needs (e.g., ED visits) without adversely affecting readmission and reoperation rates. These findings may be generalizable to other discretionary orthopedic procedures. Additional research should evaluate and compare the patient experience and functional outcomes following elective shoulder arthroplasty before and during the pandemic.

Author Contributions: Conceptualization, M.E.M., N.K., B.C.W. and P.J.D.; methodology, M.E.M., N.K. and P.J.D.; formal analysis, M.E.M.; resources, P.J.D. and N.K.; data curation, M.E.M. and P.J.D.; writing—original draft preparation, M.E.M.; writing—review and editing, N.K., B.C.W. and P.J.D.; supervision, P.J.D. All authors have read and agreed to the published version of the manuscript.

Funding: This research received no external funding.

Institutional Review Board Statement: The study was conducted according to the guidelines of the Declaration of Helsinki, and determined exempt from review by the Southern Oregon Institutional Review Board on 8 August 2021.

Informed Consent Statement: Informed consent was obtained from all subjects involved in the study.

Data Availability Statement: Details regarding where data supporting reported results can be requested at the following e-mail address: pjdenard@gmail.com.

Conflicts of Interest: M.E.M.—American Shoulder and Elbow Surgeons: Board or committee member, Journal of Shoulder and Elbow Surgery: Editorial or governing board; N.K.—No conflict of interest to disclose; B.C.W.—Arthrex: consultant, Research support: Arthrex, Zimmer Biomet and Flexion Therapeutics; P.J.D.—Arthrex: consultant, IP royalties.

References

1. Brown, T.S.; Bedard, N.A.; Rojas, E.O.; Anthony, C.A.; Schwarzkopf, R.; Barnes, C.L.; Stambough, J.B.; Mears, S.C.; Edwards, P.K.; Nandi, S.; et al. The Effect of the COVID-19 Pandemic on Electively Scheduled Hip and Knee Arthroplasty Patients in the United States. *J. Arthroplast.* **2020**, *35*, S49–S55. [CrossRef] [PubMed]
2. Lanham, N.S.; Bockelman, K.J.; McCriskin, B.J. Telemedicine and Orthopaedic Surgery: The COVID-19 Pandemic and Our New Normal. *JBJS Rev.* **2020**, *8*, e2000083. [CrossRef] [PubMed]
3. Chen, J.S.; Buchalter, D.B.; Sicat, C.S.; Aggarwal, V.K.; Hepinstall, M.S.; Lajam, C.M.; Schwarzkopf, R.S.; Slover, J.D. Telemedicine during the COVID-19 pandemic: Adult reconstructive surgery perspective. *Bone Jt. J.* **2021**, *103*, 196–204. [CrossRef] [PubMed]
4. Menendez, M.E.; Jawa, A.; Haas, D.A.; Warner, J.J.P.; Codman Shoulder, S. Orthopedic surgery post COVID-19: An opportunity for innovation and transformation. *J. Shoulder Elb. Surg.* **2020**, *29*, 1083–1086. [CrossRef] [PubMed]
5. Day, J.S.; Lau, E.; Ong, K.L.; Williams, G.R.; Ramsey, M.L.; Kurtz, S.M. Prevalence and projections of total shoulder and elbow arthroplasty in the United States to 2015. *J. Shoulder Elb. Surg./Am. Shoulder Elb. Surg.* **2010**, *19*, 1115–1120. [CrossRef] [PubMed]
6. Kim, S.H.; Wise, B.L.; Zhang, Y.; Szabo, R.M. Increasing incidence of shoulder arthroplasty in the United States. *J. Bone Jt. Surgery. Am. Vol.* **2011**, *93*, 2249–2254. [CrossRef] [PubMed]
7. Kurtz, S.M.; Lau, E.; Ong, K.; Zhao, K.; Kelly, M.; Bozic, K.J. Future young patient demand for primary and revision joint replacement: National projections from 2010 to 2030. *Clin. Orthop. Relat. Res.* **2009**, *467*, 2606–2612. [CrossRef]
8. Moverman, M.A.; Puzzitiello, R.N.; Pagani, N.R.; Barnes, C.L.; Jawa, A.; Menendez, M.E. Public Perceptions of Resuming Elective Surgery During the COVID-19 Pandemic. *J. Arthroplast.* **2021**, *36*, 397–402.e392. [CrossRef]
9. Meneghini, R.M. Resource Reallocation during the COVID-19 Pandemic in a Suburban Hospital System: Implications for Outpatient Hip and Knee Arthroplasty. *J. Arthroplast.* **2020**, *35*, S15–S18. [CrossRef] [PubMed]
10. Stambough, J.B.; Deen, J.T.; Walton, S.L.; Kerr, J.M.; Zarski, M.J.; Yates, A.J., Jr.; Andrawis, J.P. Arthroplasty During COVID-19: Surveillance of AAHKS Members in the First Year of the Pandemic. *Arthroplast. Today* **2021**, *7*, 209–215. [CrossRef] [PubMed]
11. Menendez, M.E.; Lawler, S.M.; Carducci, M.P.; Ring, D.; Mahendraraj, K.A.; Jawa, A. Delayed hospital discharge after total shoulder arthroplasty: Why, and who is at risk? *JSES Open Access* **2019**, *3*, 130–135. [CrossRef] [PubMed]
12. Duchman, K.R.; Anthony, C.A.; Westermann, R.W.; Pugely, A.J.; Gao, Y.; Hettrich, C.M. Total Shoulder Arthroplasty: Is Less Time in the Hospital Better? *Iowa Orthop. J.* **2017**, *37*, 109–116. [PubMed]
13. Brolin, T.J.; Throckmorton, T.W. Outpatient Shoulder Arthroplasty. *Orthop. Clin. N. Am.* **2018**, *49*, 73–79. [CrossRef] [PubMed]

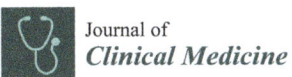 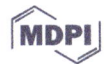

Brief Report

Current Concepts in Humeral Component Design for Anatomic and Reverse Shoulder Arthroplasty

Joaquin Sanchez-Sotelo

Division of Shoulder, Elbow Surgery Mayo Clinic Rochester, Rochester, MN 55905, USA; sanchezsotelo.joaquin@mayo.edu

Abstract: The history of humeral component design has evolved from prostheses with relatively long stems and limited anatomic head options to a contemporary platform with short stems and stemless implants with shared instrumentation and the ability to provide optimal shoulder reconstruction for both anatomic and reverse configurations. Contemporary humeral components aim to preserve the bone, but they are potentially subject to malalignment. Modern components are expected to favorably load the humerus and minimize adverse bone reactions. Although there will likely continue to be further refinements in humeral component design, the next frontiers in primary shoulder arthroplasty will revolve around designing an optimal plan, including adequate soft tissue tension and providing computer-assisted tools for the accurate execution of the preoperative plan in the operating room.

Keywords: shoulder; arthroplasty; anatomic arthroplasty; reverse arthroplasty

---

Citation: Sanchez-Sotelo, J. Current Concepts in Humeral Component Design for Anatomic and Reverse Shoulder Arthroplasty. *J. Clin. Med.* **2021**, *10*, 5151. https://doi.org/10.3390/jcm10215151

Academic Editor: Markus Scheibel

Received: 7 September 2021
Accepted: 18 October 2021
Published: 2 November 2021

Publisher's Note: MDPI stays neutral with regard to jurisdictional claims in published maps and institutional affiliations.

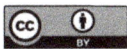

Copyright: © 2021 by the author. Licensee MDPI, Basel, Switzerland. This article is an open access article distributed under the terms and conditions of the Creative Commons Attribution (CC BY) license (https://creativecommons.org/licenses/by/4.0/).

The design of the humeral component in shoulder arthroplasty has evolved tremendously over the last two decades. When discussing the general principles of shoulder replacement, glenoid reconstruction is reviewed frequently. Interestingly, the humeral side of the joint is discussed less often. The purpose of this review article is to provide an update on the principles driving contemporary humeral component design.

1. Brief Historical Perspective

The history of humeral component design has evolved over a few important milestones that have had a major impact on where we are today.

1.1. From Monoblock and Cemented to Modular Cementless

Neer is considered by some to be the father of modern shoulder surgery in North America [1]. The original Neer prosthesis was a smooth monoblock hemiarthroplasty with a narrow stem and three sizes. Because the stem was narrow and designed for a cemented application, it could be "floated" in the canal in whichever location was best to position the prosthetic humeral head anatomically [2]. Although early on the original Neer prosthesis was implanted without cement, in the absence of surface treatment, cementless implantation led to a high rate of radiographic loosening [3]. The development of technology to treat the stem with ingrowth-friendly surfaces led to the successful survival of cementless humeral components [4]. At the same time, modular anatomic humeral heads were introduced to allow a humeral head size selection independent of the stem size selection [5]. Currently, most surgeons agree on trying to avoid the use of cement for humeral component fixation at the time of primary arthroplasty; If component revision becomes necessary, cement removal could substantially increase the difficulties associated with the revision procedure.

1.2. A More Sophisticated Understanding of Humeral Geometry

Traditional cementless ingrowth stems with standard modular heads were noted as not allowing for the anatomic restoration of the proximal humerus geometry in many shoulders: the fit of the stem in the humeral canal dictated where the head would "land".

This prompted studies on the variability of proximal humerus morphology [6] and on the design of implants with various features to adjust the position of the prosthetic head relative to the stem in terms of inclination, eccentricity, and offset [7].

1.3. Reverse Arthroplasty

Grammont revolutionized the field of shoulder arthroplasty with the development of the reverse prosthesis concept: a more constrained implant of reverse geometry that would increase the moment arm of the deltoid to compensate for the rotator cuff insufficiency [8]. Despite becoming an incredibly successful implant in terms of the restoration of active elevation and the long-term survivorship, [9] the limitations of the traditional Grammont-style prosthesis included poor restoration of the internal and external rotation as well as excessive impingement of the humeral polyethylene with the medial scapular pillar, leading to polyethylene wear, bone loss (notching), and eventually loosening [10]. Frankle modified the reverse principles to optimize the impingement-free range of motion and the tension of the axial rotator cuff with the design of a reverse prosthesis with a less truncated sphere and a more vertical polyethylene (135-degree opening angle) [11,12]. Contemporary designs follow the modifications of reverse introduced by Frankle.

1.4. Shorter Stems, Resurfacing, and Stemless

The length of most of the traditional stems was arbitrarily set to occupy the upper third to half of the humerus. Standard-length stems have demonstrated outstanding performance and survivorship [13]. However, avoiding relatively long stems is attractive for several reasons, including easier revision, easier implantation of an ipsilateral total elbow arthroplasty, and maybe easier management of periprosthetic fractures. Resurfacing arthroplasty represented a first attempt to avoid stem use, [14] but resurfacing components have fallen out of favor since incomplete head removal made glenoid access more difficult, and the prosthetic head sizes with various degrees of offset and eccentricity could not be used. As such, the design has evolved into the use of short-stem and stemless prostheses. The length of most of the short stems has been chosen arbitrarily, with few exceptions. For anatomic arthroplasty, stemmed and stemless prostheses seem to provide equivalent results, provided satisfactory implantation is achieved at the time of surgery [15,16].

1.5. Malalignment and Adverse Bone Reactions

One benefit of longer stems is that a tight stem fit into the endosteal canal facilitates adequate alignment. Ultrashort stems introduce two potential problems: poor alignment and adverse bone reactions.

Stems that do not engage the cylindrical portion of the endosteal canal can easily be misaligned. Excessive valgus or varus will lead to a poor humeral head position in anatomic arthroplasty. Similarly, poor alignment can lead to a reverse polyethylene that is excessively horizontal with an increased risk of notching, or to a more vertical polyethylene that may facilitate dislocation. Certain short stems have been designed with just enough length to avoid malalignment [17]. Stemless prostheses are also at risk for malalignment (Figure 1). As such, care must be taken to optimize the humeral head cut to minimize the chances of malalignment with ultrashort stem and stemless prostheses.

Certain ultrashort stems need larger diameters to achieve primary stability in the absence of diaphyseal contact. This concept has been captured with the fill–fit ratio popularized by Walch et al. [18]. Severe stress shielding with resorption of the greater tuberosity, and in extreme cases in areas of complete cortical defect, has been reported with the implantation of larger sizes of certain stems, and malalignment may accentuate these adverse bone reactions through point contact of the stem on the cortical bone, further shielding the proximal bone from stress (Figure 2). Thus, it is important to design implants that do not shield the metaphysis from stress.

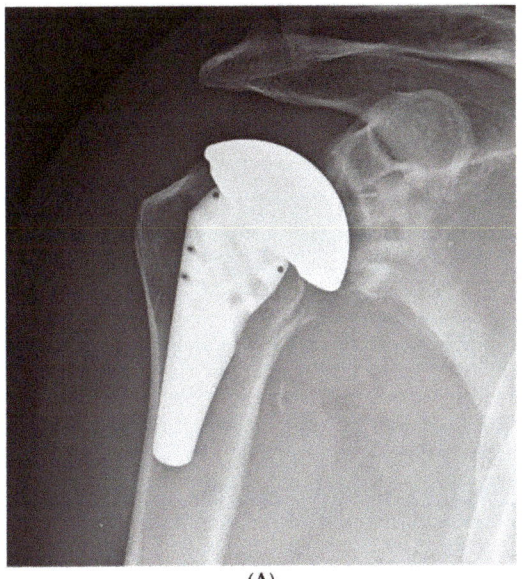 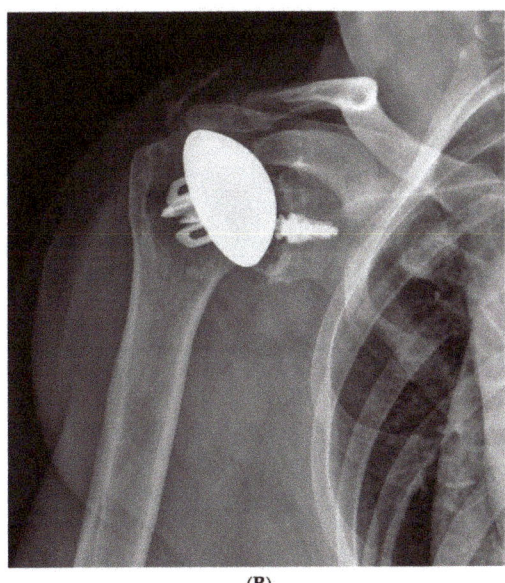

Figure 1. Ultrashort stems (**A**) and stemless prostheses (**B**) are at increased risk for malalignment.

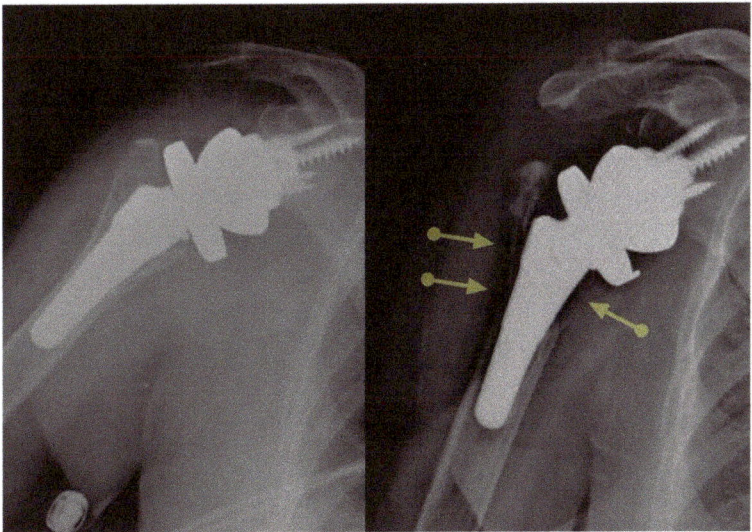

Figure 2. Certain ultrashort stems are associated with substantial stress shielding.

1.6. Preoperative Planning Software and Surgical Execution

The development and widespread use of preoperative planning software has revolutionized the field of shoulder arthroplasty. I trained at a time when plain radiographs were the only imaging study obtained before shoulder arthroplasty. Today, the vast majority of shoulder arthroplasty surgeons rely on computer tomography to understand each shoulder to be replaced and to plan the surgery accordingly. Furthermore, preoperative planning software has advanced the field to a whole other level: three-dimensional renderings, automated measurements, and virtual implant overlays allow for accurate planning of the implant positioning to optimize orientation, seating, contact, motion free of impingement, and other variables [19–21]. Such software can then be used for artificial intelligence predictive algorithms, manufacturing patient-specific guides, and using computer-assisted surgery with navigation or robotics.

In the field of reverse shoulder arthroplasty, preoperative planning software reveals that using a larger glenoid with a larger lateral offset and an inferior overhang is the most successful strategy to optimize the range of motion free of impingement, especially when combined with a more vertical (typically 135 degree) polyethylene opening angle [22].

1.7. Same-Day Surgery and Ambulatory Surgery Centers

In the United States, there is a growing interest in same-day discharge after shoulder arthroplasty, as well as in performing these procedures in ambulatory surgery centers. This is driven by two main forces: the potential for certain financial gain and the need to decrease hospitalizations, especially considering the current COVID-19 pandemic [23]. Ambulatory surgery centers have less capacity to process large inventories and instrument trays. As such, there is the need for streamlined instrumentation and shared instruments between stem and stemless designs. Patient-matched implants and preoperative planning software may further help decrease inventory.

1.8. Proximal Humerus Bone Density

Understanding the bone mineral density of the proximal humerus is paramount to optimizing the primary stability of modern humeral components. In the osteoarthritic shoulder, the strongest bone is at the periphery and is closer to the superior aspect of the humeral head. As such, fixation is theoretically optimized by achieving a prosthetic fit to the periphery of the metaphysis and with a slightly higher humeral head cut [24]. However, one downside of performing a higher humeral head cut is the more difficult access to the glenoid.

1.9. Implications for Humeral Component Design

The brief historical review summarized above provides the grounds for design features that are perceived as desirable when considering contemporary humeral component design (Table 1).

Table 1. Desirable features for contemporary humeral component design.

- Platform: same component for anatomic and reverse arthroplasty
- Multiple anatomic head options for accurate restoration of humeral geometry
- Reverse configuration must accommodate large glenospheres with lateral offset and inferior overhang
- Proximal coating and proximal loading
- Peripheral metaphyseal fixation
- Short-stem and stemless offerings
- Streamlined instrumentation shared for stem and stemless
- Accurate execution of implant placement
    - Preoperative planning software
    - Cutting guides
    - Patient-specific guides
    - Navigation
    - Robotics

2. Implant Configurations: What Are Our Targets on the Humeral Side Currently?

2.1. Anatomic Shoulder Arthroplasty

When performing an anatomic shoulder arthroplasty, the main goal on the humeral side is to restore the overall geometry of the proximal humerus. Considering the variability of the human shoulder (in terms of size, retroversion, and other parameters), as well as the need to adapt to the final position of the humeral stem or stemless nucleus, it is necessary to design systems with multiple head sizes and thicknesses as well as with a mechanism to offset the humeral head with respect to the final position of the humeral stem/nucleus (Figure 3). In most shoulders, the restoration of the premorbid anatomy provides the best outcome. However, in certain shoulders, the humeral head version, diameter, thickness, and/or eccentricity may need to be adapted to the condition of the soft tissues. For example, in a shoulder with substantial posterior subluxation and chronic stretching of the posterior rotator cuff and capsule, it may be necessary to implant a humeral head that is thicker than the premorbid native head to properly tension the soft tissue envelope posteriorly.

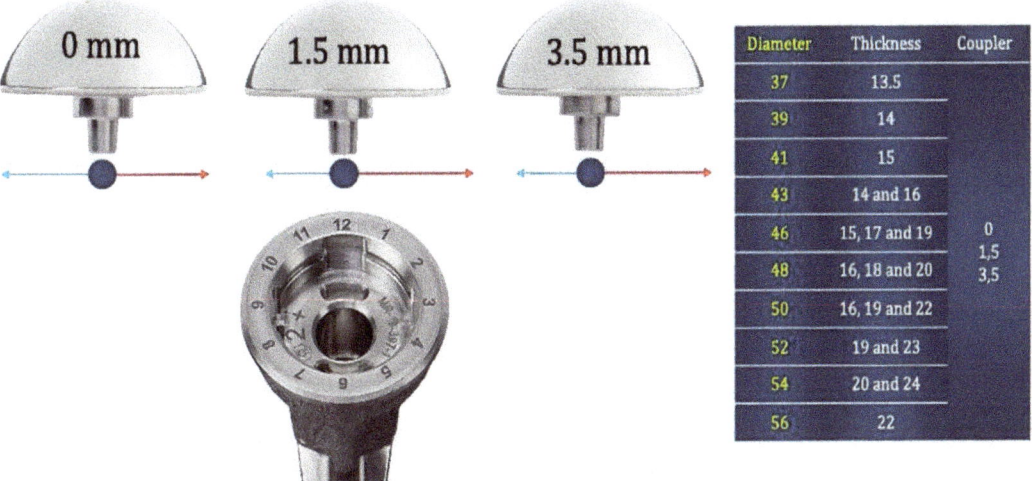

Figure 3. Options for replacement of the humeral head with one system for anatomic shoulder arthroplasty.

2.2. Reverse Shoulder Arthroplasty

Understanding the nuances associated with the design and implantation of the humeral component in reverse shoulder arthroplasty is not possible without considering the glenoid side [22]. Currently, most would agree that reverse shoulder arthroplasty requires a fine balance between (1) maximizing impingement-free range of motion and (2) optimizing soft tissue tension and muscle function around the shoulder.

Avoiding any impingement between the medial aspect of the polyethylene and the body of the scapula and scapular pillar essentially requires displacing the proximal humerus laterally and posteroinferiorly. This is best achieved by implanting a larger glenosphere with a posteroinferior overhang in reference to the glenoid vault combined with a larger lateral offset of the glenoid component. Larger lateral offsets may be achieved with thicker glenospheres, structural bone grating between the native glenoid and the baseplate (bio-RSA), or thicker (augmented) baseplates (Figure 4). The benefit of bio-RSA and augmented baseplates over thicker glenospheres is that both bone graft and metal augments provide adequate correction of angular deformities (inclination and retroversion) without reaming excessively, which can lead to impingement as well.

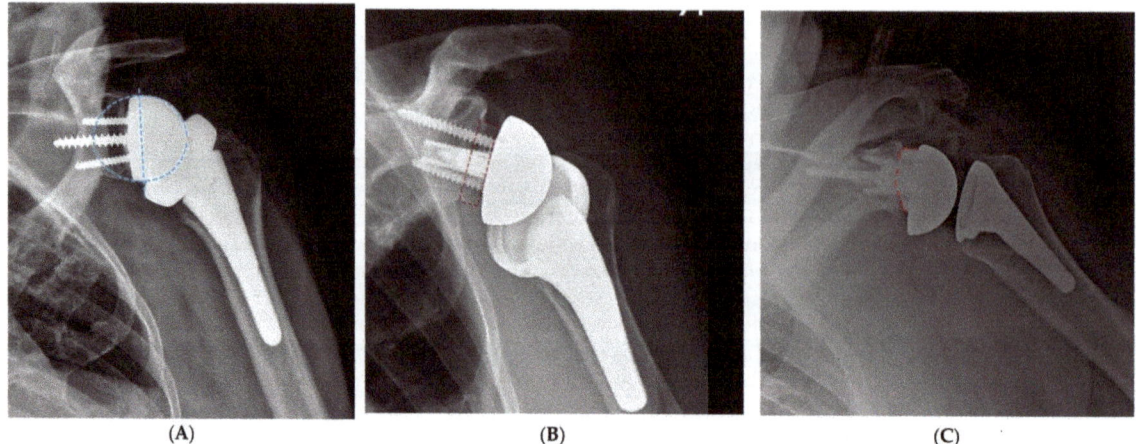

Figure 4. (**A**), Impingement-free range of motion is optimized with implantation of larger glenospheres with a lateral offset and an inferior overhang. Glenoid lateralization may be achieved with thicker glenospheres (**B**), the use of a bone graft under the baseplate (BIO-RSA), or the use of augmented baseplates (**C**).

Provided the surgeon commits to implantation of large glenospheres with an inferior overhang and a lateral offset using any of the three methods above, the humeral component must allow for a minimal thickness above the cut surface in order to avoid excessive soft tissue tension secondary to lateralization, distalization, or both. A relatively easy way to design humeral components that allow for anatomic and reverse compatibility is to design humeral bearings that rest on the cut surface of the humerus, so-called onlay systems. The downside of onlay systems for those surgeons who maximize impingement-free motion on the glenoid side is that the soft tissue tension may be excessive. This can be compensated for by lowering the humeral cut, which may be acceptable in the cuff-deficient shoulder but not in the cuff-intact osteoarthritic shoulder, where a lower cut would damage the rotator cuff. As such, if the surgeon chooses to maximize impingement-free range of motion through glenoid implantation, the thinnest humeral bearing construct should place the pivot point at or below the humeral cut. When the pivot point (the deepest portion of the polyethylene) is below the humeral cut, implants are classified as inlays.

However, *the onlay vs. inlay controversy should probably be abandoned* for two reasons. Firstly, there is a high level of variability regarding how much lateralization and distalization are provided by the many implants in the market [25]. Classifying them as onlays or inlays is an oversimplification. What matters is where the humerus "lands" for a specific glenoid reconstruction, depending on the humeral implant selected and where it is implanted. This will affect the length and the moment arm of the deltoid and rotator cuffs [26]. Secondly, surgeons may implant inlay components in an onlay fashion or the other way around. For example, the original prosthesis designed by Dr. Frankle was an inlay design; however, its proximal portion was relatively large and could not be fully inset in the humeral metaphysis of many patients, thus resulting in an onlay application of an inlay design (Figure 5). By the same token, if thicker polyethylene bearings or a metal spacer are added to an inlay prosthesis to guarantee adequate stability, the pivot point is at an onlay level despite the implant being designed as an inlay. Consequently, even though implants that allow placement of the pivot point at or below the cut surface of the humerus are necessary to optimize soft tissue tension across the whole spectrum of shoulder replacements, in many shoulders, these inlay components will behave as onlay ones because thicker polyethylenes may be needed to avoid dislocation, especially in the cuff-deficient shoulder. The ideal degree of humeral lateralization probably varies from individual to individual depending on the underlying diagnosis and other characteristics.

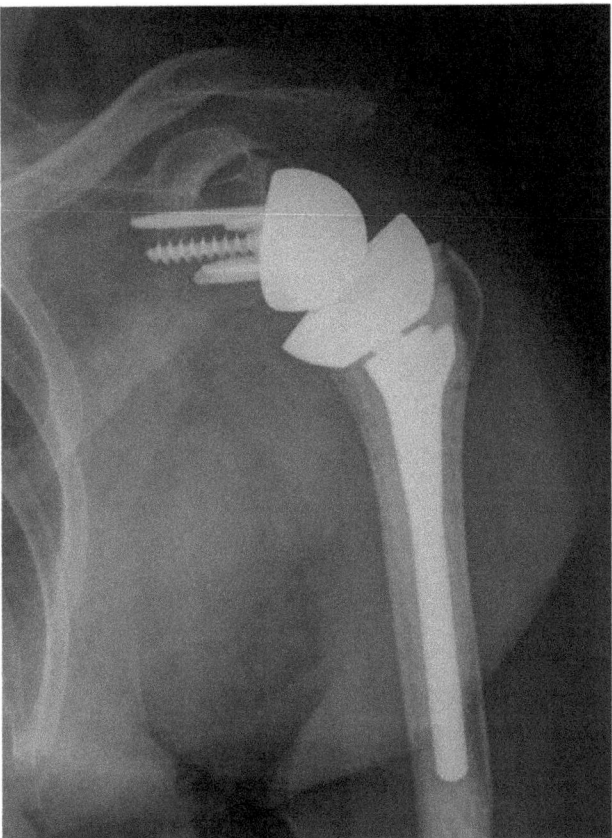

Figure 5. This implant was designed as an inlay, but its large size resulted in an onlay application most of the time.

3. From Design to Implantation: Pearls and Pitfalls Learned with Use of a Contemporary Humeral Component

Hopefully, a review of the history of implant component design and an understanding of what are considered contemporary targets today will help drive the surgical techniques for implantation of contemporary humeral components (Figure 6).

3.1. Anatomic Arthroplasty

3.1.1. Preoperative Planning

Our preference is to plan the humeral head osteotomy at 2–3 mm proximal to the transition between the rotator cuff attachment and the humeral head. Some surgeons prefer performing the osteotomy at fixed angles, typically 135 degrees of inclination and 30 degrees of retroversion. Others prefer to make the cut at the exact location of the anatomic humeral neck. In such a case, it is possible that the stem will end up oriented inside the canal in varus or valgus, and the implications of malalignment in anatomic arthroplasty are less substantial, provided the humeral head is reconstructed anatomically.

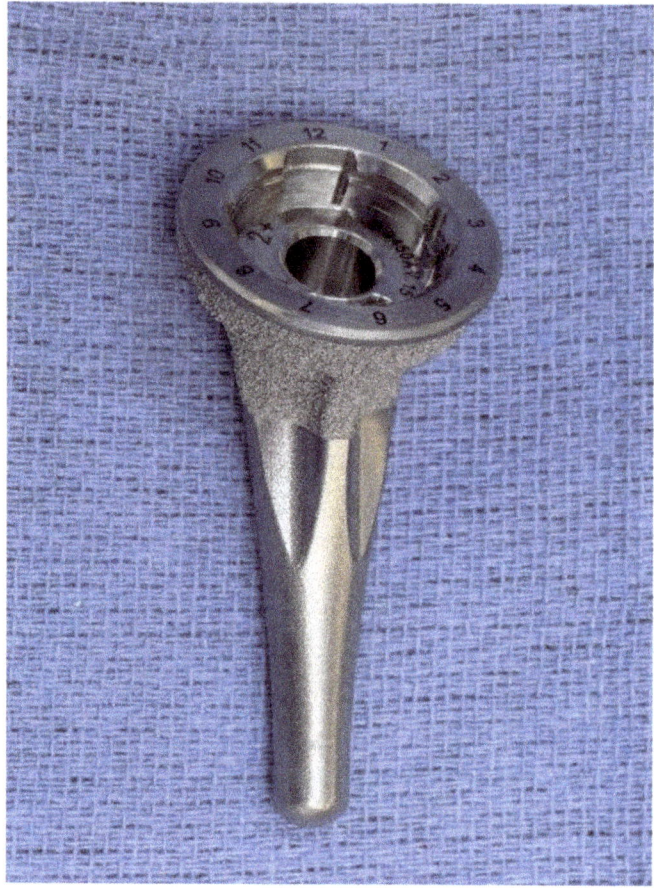

Figure 6. Contemporary platform of a short-stem humeral component designed for proximal fixation and loading.

3.1.2. Humeral Osteotomy

Many surgeons are used to performing the humeral head osteotomy with so-called freehand techniques. However, for those implants with a fixed neck–shaft angle, it may be advantageous to use an extramedullary or an intramedullary guide. Our preference is to use an intramedullary guide, and the selection of the entry point of the guide is paramount to avoid a varus or valgus cut. A C–guide may then be used to select the ideal cut height (Figure 7).

3.1.3. Sizing

The preparation of the metaphysis for modern components that rely on peripheral fixation typically aims to place the component "bowl" so that it will leave 2–4 mm of cancellous bone between the component and the cortical rim of the metaphysis (Figure 8). A wider distance may be advantageous in patients with a stronger bone that does not require maximizing peripheral fixation. The guide pin for the reaming of the metaphysis may be centered using a trial humeral head or sizing discs.

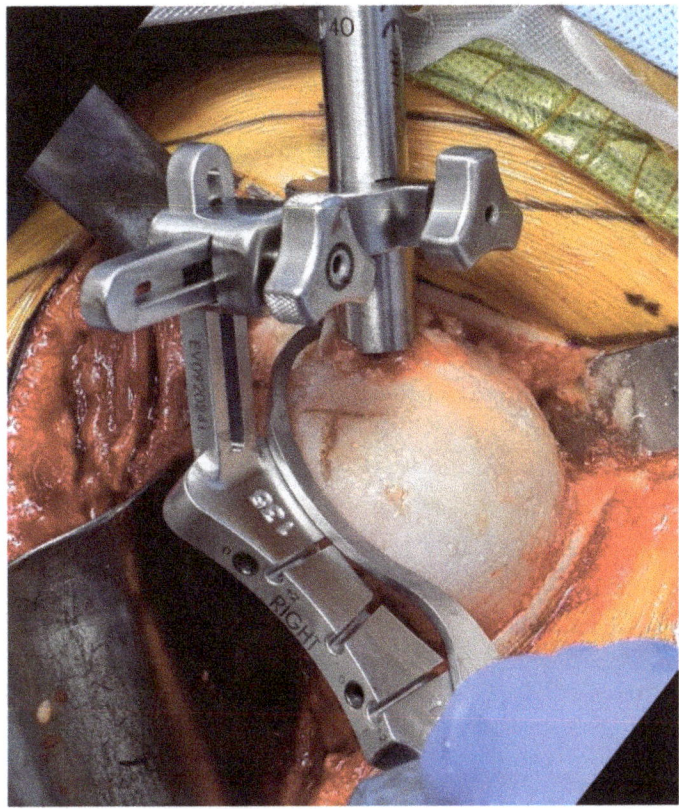

Figure 7. Use of an extramedullary cutting guide may facilitate predictable osteotomy of the humerus in a specific degree of inclination.

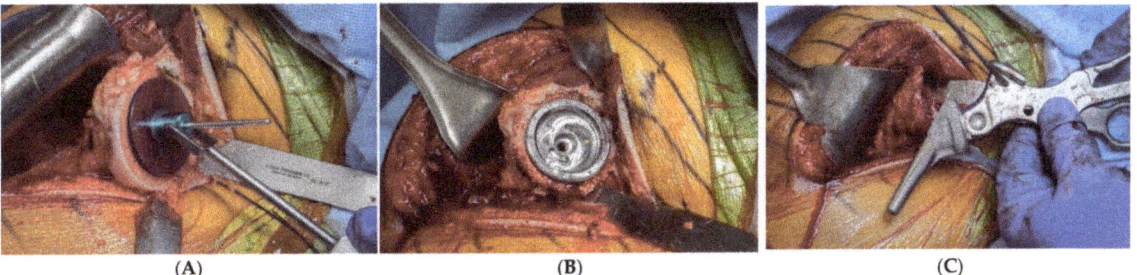

Figure 8. Primary component stability may be optimized by the implant fit at the periphery of the proximal humerus, within 2–4 mm of the cortical rim. (**A**), Sizing disk; (**B**), Trial; (**C**), Humeral component.

3.1.4. Humeral Preparation and Implantation

Since short and stemless humeral components do not provide selfaligning features, surgeons must be extremely careful at the time of compactor preparation and component implantation to replicate the desired alignment based on the preoperative planning and the osteotomy performed. The most common pitfall is to place the component in an excessive varus. As such, an effort must be made to use the compactor/inserter handle when pushing into the varus.

3.1.5. Humeral Head Selection

The resected humeral head provides a great reference for the selection of the correct diameter and also for the thickness. The geometry of the humeral head can be perfectly replicated by selecting the right combination of diameter, thickness, and eccentricity. In shoulders with a severe preoperative soft tissue imbalance, changes in the humeral head thickness or in diameter may be needed. As mentioned previously, arthritic shoulders with a severe posterior subluxation may require the use of a thicker humeral head to properly tension the posterior capsule and cuff. In shoulders with avascular necrosis, it may be wise to downsize the humeral head since there is a higher risk of stiffness. Intraoperative testing may be used to confirm an adequate soft tissue balance in anatomic shoulder arthroplasty (Table 2).

Table 2. Intraoperative assessment of the soft tissue balance in anatomic shoulder arthroplasty.

- Passive posterior translation of the humeral head in reference to the glenoid component of approximately 50% with spontaneous relocation (arm at 30 degrees of external rotation)
- Subscapularis can be repaired without excessive tension
- Satisfactory passive elevation, external rotation, and internal rotation
- The humeral head "spins" on the glenoid component surface in rotation without excessive translation

3.2. Reverse Arthroplasty

As mentioned before, humeral and glenoid planning are intimately related in reverse arthroplasty. The configuration and placement of the glenoid component have a major impact on the range of motion free of impingement. Humeral planning is then completed to select the correct size and alignment of the humeral component. My preference is to select a polyethylene opening angle of 135 degrees. The combined configuration of the glenoid and humeral components will lead to specific arcs of motion free of impingement. It will also lead to a specific position of the humerus in space in reference to the scapula, which will impact soft tissue tension. Currently, there is no consensus regarding the ideal position of the humerus in reference to the scapula in reverse arthroplasty, but most aim to replicate the anatomic position of the greater tuberosity from lateral to medial.

An accurate humeral cut and a correct implantation of the humeral component at the time of surgery are important to replicate the polyethylene opening angle desired for a given shoulder. The same considerations described for anatomic shoulder arthroplasty regarding humeral osteotomy and sizing, as well as humeral preparation and implantation, apply to most platform stems. However, reverse arthroplasty is more constrained than anatomic arthroplasty, and achieving primary stability of the humeral component is maybe more important. As such, we have a low threshold to implant the so-called "plus sizes", which are slightly oversized in reference to the standard sizes to provide a tighter fit.

Regarding the bearing selection, the thinnest polyethylene will result in a pivot point at the level of the humeral cut. Thicker bearings with or without the addition of a metal tray will move the pivot point proximal and medial with reference to the geometric center of the proximal humerus, and as such will increase humeral lateralization and distalization. The ideal bearing thickness is typically selected based on intraoperative trialing, and currently there are no good objective parameters to guide the bearing selection. Bearings with improved wear performance, such as vitamin E polyethylene, are definitively attractive.

4. Future Directions

The evolution of humeral component design has been quite remarkable. Contemporary implants provide the opportunity for bone preservation, platform convertibility, the anatomic reconstruction of the proximal humerus when anatomic arthroplasty is performed, and optimal arcs of motion free of impingement with adequate soft tissue tension when reverse arthroplasty is performed. However, the jury is still out regarding the potential for component malalignment and bone adaptation to these newer components over time. The preoperative planning software is very refined, but the execution of the plan is still evolving. Various navigation and robotic systems are being developed and will likely translate into a more accurate execution of the preoperative plans.

Funding: This research received no external funding.

Institutional Review Board Statement: Not applicable.

Informed Consent Statement: Not applicable.

Conflicts of Interest: The author declares no conflict of interest.

References

1. Neer, C.S., II; Watson, K.C.; Stanton, F.J. Recent experience in total shoulder replacement. *J. Bone Joint Surg. Am.* **1982**, *64*, 319–337. [CrossRef]
2. Sanchez-Sotelo, J.; O'Driscoll, S.W.; Torchia, M.E.; Cofield, R.H.; Rowland, C.M. Radiographic assessment of cemented humeral components in shoulder arthroplasty. *J. Shoulder Elb. Surg.* **2001**, *10*, 526–531.
3. Sanchez-Sotelo, J.; Wright, T.W.; O'Driscoll, S.W.; Cofield, R.H.; Rowland, C.M. Radiographic assessment of uncemented humeral components in total shoulder arthroplasty. *J. Arthroplast.* **2001**, *16*, 180–187. [CrossRef] [PubMed]
4. Cil, A.; Veillette, C.J.; Sanchez-Sotelo, J.; Sperling, J.W.; Schleck, C.D.; Cofield, R.H. Survivorship of the humeral component in shoulder arthroplasty. *J. Shoulder Elb. Surg.* **2010**, *19*, 143–150.
5. Mileti, J.; Sperling, J.W.; Cofield, R.H.; Harrington, J.R.; Hoskin, T.L. Monoblock and modular total shoulder arthroplasty for osteoarthritis. *J. Bone Joint Surg. Br.* **2005**, *87*, 496–500. [CrossRef] [PubMed]
6. Boileau, P.; Walch, G. The three-dimensional geometry of the proximal humerus. Implications for surgical technique and prosthetic design. *J. Bone Joint Surg. Br.* **1997**, *79*, 857–865.
7. Walch, G.; Boileau, P. Prosthetic adaptability: A new concept for shoulder arthroplasty. *J. Shoulder Elb. Surg.* **1999**, *8*, 443–451. [CrossRef]
8. Baulot, E.; Sirveaux, F.; Boileau, P. Grammont's idea: The story of Paul Grammont's functional surgery concept and the development of the reverse principle. *Clin. Orthop. Relat. Res.* **2011**, *469*, 2425–2431. [CrossRef]
9. Bacle, G.; Nové-Josserand, L.; Garaud, P.; Walch, G. Long-Term Outcomes of Reverse Total Shoulder Arthroplasty: A Follow-up of a Previous Study. *J. Bone Joint Surg. Am.* **2017**, *99*, 454–461.
10. Spiry, C.; Berhouet, J.; Agout, C.; Bacle, G.; Favard, L. Long-term impact of scapular notching after reverse shoulder arthroplasty. *Int. Orthop.* **2021**, *45*, 1559–1566.
11. Cuff, D.J.; Pupello, D.R.; Santoni, B.G.; Clark, R.E.; Frankle, M.A. Reverse Shoulder Arthroplasty for the Treatment of Rotator Cuff Deficiency: A Concise Follow-Up, at a Minimum of 10 Years, of Previous Reports. *J. Bone Joint Surg. Am.* **2017**, *99*, 1895–1899.
12. Kennon, J.C.; Songy, C.; Bartels, D.; Statz, J.; Cofield, R.H.; Sperling, J.W.; Sanchez-Sotelo, J. Primary reverse shoulder arthroplasty: How did medialized and glenoid-based lateralized style prostheses compare at 10 years? *J. Shoulder Elb. Surg.* **2020**, *29*, S23–S31.
13. Nguyen, N.T.V.; Martinez-Catalan, N.; Songy, C.E.; Sanchez-Sotelo, J. Radiological humeral adaptative changes five years after anatomical total shoulder arthroplasty using a standard-length cementless hydroxyapatite-coated humeral component. *Bone Joint J.* **2021**, *103*, 958–963. [CrossRef]
14. Thomas, S.R.; Sforza, G.; Levy, O.; Copeland, S.A. Geometrical analysis of Copeland surface replacement shoulder arthroplasty in relation to normal anatomy. *J. Shoulder Elb. Surg.* **2005**, *14*, 186–192.
15. Willems, J.I.P.; Hoffmann, J.; Sierevelt, I.N.; van den Bekerom, M.P.J.; Alta, T.D.W.; van Noort, A. Results of stemless shoulder arthroplasty: A systematic review and meta-analysis. *EFORT Open Rev.* **2021**, *6*, 35–49.
16. Märtens, N.; Heinze, M.; Awiszus, F.; Bertrand, J.; Lohmann, C.H.; Berth, A. Long-term survival and failure analysis of anatomical stemmed and stemless shoulder arthroplasties. *Bone Joint J.* **2021**, *103*, 1292–1300.
17. Cagle, P.J.; Patel, A.V.; Zastrow, R.W.; Esper, R.; Greiwe, R.M.; Sanchez-Sotelo, J. Radiographic alignment of short stem humeral components in shoulder arthroplasty: A multicenter study. *Semin. Arthroplast. JSES* **2020**, *30*, 195–199.
18. Raiss, P.; Schnetzke, M.; Wittmann, T.; Kilian, C.M.; Edwards, T.B.; Denard, P.J.; Neyton, L.; Godenèche, A.; Walch, G. Postoperative radiographic findings of an uncemented convertible short stem for anatomic and reverse shoulder arthroplasty. *J. Shoulder Elb. Surg.* **2019**, *28*, 715–723.
19. Gauci, M.O.; Athwal, G.S.; Sanchez-Sotelo, J.; Chaoui, J.; Urvoy, M.; Boileau, P.; Walch, G. Identification of threshold pathoanatomic metrics in primary glenohumeral osteoarthritis. *J. Shoulder Elb. Surg.* **2021**, *30*, 2270–2282. [CrossRef]
20. Gauci, M.O.; Deransart, P.; Chaoui, J.; Urvoy, M.; Athwal, G.S.; Sanchez-Sotelo, J.; Boileau, P.; Walch, G. Three-dimensional geometry of the normal shoulder: A software analysis. *J. Shoulder Elb. Surg.* **2020**, *29*, e468–e477.
21. Raiss, P.; Walch, G.; Wittmann, T.; Athwal, G.S. Is preoperative planning effective for intraoperative glenoid implant size and type selection during anatomic and reverse shoulder arthroplasty? *J. Shoulder Elb. Surg.* **2020**, *29*, 2123–2127.
22. Sanchez-Sotelo, J.; Athwal, G.S. How to Optimize Reverse Shoulder Arthroplasty for Irreparable Cuff Tears. *Curr. Rev. Musculoskelet. Med.* **2020**, *13*, 553–560. [CrossRef] [PubMed]

23. Vajapey, S.P.; Contreras, E.S.; Neviaser, A.S.; Bishop, J.Y.; Cvetanovich, G.L. Outpatient Total Shoulder Arthroplasty: A Systematic Review Evaluating Outcomes and Cost-Effectiveness. *JBJS Rev.* **2021**, *9*, e20. [CrossRef]
24. Reeves, J.M.; Athwal, G.S.; Johnson, J.A. An assessment of proximal humerus density with reference to stemless implants. *J. Shoulder Elb. Surg.* **2018**, *27*, 641–649. [CrossRef]
25. Werthel, J.D.; Walch, G.; Vegehan, E.; Deransart, P.; Sanchez-Sotelo, J.; Valenti, P. Lateralization in reverse shoulder arthroplasty: A descriptive analysis of different implants in current practice. *Int. Orthop.* **2019**, *43*, 2349–2360. [PubMed]
26. Burnier, M.; Hooke, A.; Gil, J.; Sanchez-Sotelo, J.; Elhassan, B. Biomechanical Analysis of the Subscapularis, Infraspinatus and Teres Minor Length and Moment Arm after Reverse Shoulder Arthroplasty: A Cadaveric Study. *Semin. Arthroplast. JSES* **2021**. [CrossRef]

Journal of Clinical Medicine

Article

Can Lateralization of Reverse Shoulder Arthroplasty Improve Active External Rotation in Patients with Preoperative Fatty Infiltration of the Infraspinatus and Teres Minor?

Marko Nabergoj [1,2], Shinzo Onishi [3], Alexandre Lädermann [4,5,6,*], Houssam Kalache [7], Rihard Trebše [1,2], Hugo Bothorel [8] and Philippe Collin [9]

1. Valdoltra Orthopaedic Hospital, 6280 Ankaran, Slovenia; mmarkoj@gmail.com (M.N.); rihard.trebse@ob-valdoltra.si (R.T.)
2. Faculty of Medicine, University of Ljubljana, Vrazov trg 2, 1000 Ljubljana, Slovenia
3. Department of Orthopaedic Surgery, Faculty of Medicine, University of Tsukuba, Tsukuba 305-8575, Japan; onishishinzo@gmail.com
4. Division of Orthopaedics and Trauma Surgery, La Tour Hospital, 1217 Meyrin, Switzerland
5. Faculty of Medicine, University of Geneva, 1211 Geneva, Switzerland
6. Division of Orthopaedics and Trauma Surgery, Department of Surgery, Geneva University Hospitals, 1205 Geneva, Switzerland
7. Hôpital Saint-Camille, 2 Rue des Pères Camilliens, 94360 Bry-sur-Marne, France; kalache.houssam@gmail.com
8. Research Department, La Tour Hospital, 1217 Meyrin, Switzerland; hugo.bothorel@latour.ch
9. Clinique Victor Hugo 5 Bis Rue du Dôme, 75116 Paris, France; docphcollin@gmail.com
* Correspondence: alexandre.laedermann@gmail.com; Tel.: +41-22-719-75-55

Abstract: (1) Background: Postoperative recovery of external rotation after reverse shoulder arthroplasty (RSA) has been reported despite nonfunctional external rotator muscles. Thus, this study aimed to clinically determine the ideal prosthetic design allowing external rotation recovery in such a cohort. (2) Methods: A monocentric comparative study was retrospectively performed on patients who had primary RSA between June 2013 and February 2018 with a significant preoperative fatty infiltration of the infraspinatus and teres minor. Two groups were formed with patients with a lateral humerus/lateral glenoid 145° onlay RSA—the onlay group (OG), and a medial humerus/lateral glenoid 155° inlay RSA—the inlay group (IG). Patients were matched 1:1 by age, gender, indication, preoperative range of motion (ROM), and Constant score. The ROM and Constant scores were assessed preoperatively and at a minimum follow-up of two years. (3) Results: Forty-seven patients have been included (23 in OG and 24 in IG). Postoperative external rotation increased significantly in the OG only ($p = 0.049$), and its postoperative value was significantly greater than that of the IG by 11.1° ($p = 0.028$). (4) Conclusion: The use of a lateralized humeral stem with a low neck-shaft angle resulted in significantly improved external rotation compared to a medialized humeral 155° stem, even in cases of severe fatty infiltration of the infraspinatus and teres minor. Humeral lateralization and a low neck-shaft angle should be favored when planning an RSA in a patient without a functional posterior rotator cuff.

Keywords: prosthesis; design; range of motion; degeneration; PROMs; results; complication

1. Introduction

The treatment of rotator cuff tears was revolutionized with the introduction of RSA, which provides significant improvements in functional and clinical outcomes for many different shoulder pathologies [1]. Studies reporting on long-term outcomes of Grammont-style designs have reported consistent limited restoration of external rotation [2]. This could be explained by the slackening of the remaining rotator cuff or various impingements, since the original Grammont-type RSA design has a medialized center of rotation compared to the native glenohumeral joint [3]. Several biomechanical [4,5] and clinical studies [6] have observed an increase in lateralization which led to improved rotational movements. Thus, the implant design was evolved so that the center of rotation was lateralized compared to the Grammont-type RSA, though remaining medialized compared to the native shoulder joint [2].

Lateralization can be achieved on the glenoid side, the humeral side, or both. It can be promoted by using an additional metal or bone stock on the glenoid side [4], or by using a neck-shaft angle of 135° or 145° as well as a curved or onlay stem on the humeral side [7]. Comparative clinical studies between lateralized and medialized humeral components have been previously reported [8]. However, there are no published studies in the literature that have specifically analyzed the clinical results of primary RSA using a medialized or lateralized humeral component in patients with a nonfunctional posterior rotator cuff.

The purpose of this study was thus to compare ROM and clinical outcomes between different RSA humeral designs in patients with preoperative grade 3 to 4 fatty infiltration of the posterior rotator cuff. The hypothesis was that lateralized RSA using an onlay 145° stem would be associated with an improved external rotation compared to medialized RSA using an inlay 155° stem.

2. Materials and Methods

2.1. Patient Selection

Between June 2013 and February 2018, 651 RSAs (primary RSA, revision of RSA, and conversion from anatomical shoulder prothesis to RSA) performed by the senior author (P.C.) were considered potentially eligible for inclusion in this retrospective, comparative study using a prospectively collected database. Inclusion criteria consisted of (1) patients who underwent implantation of a primary RSA for rotator cuff arthropathy due to massive rotator cuff tear type E (supraspinatus, infraspinatus, and teres minor) [9], (2) a preoperative grade 3 or 4 fatty infiltration of infraspinatus and teres minor based on the Goutallier classification [10] characterized using non-contrast computer tomography (CT) scans, (3) positive external rotation LAG sign of more than 40° [11], and (4) a minimum follow-up of two years. The exclusion criteria were: incomplete documentation, revision cases, other indication for surgery, and a shorter follow-up.

The included patients were categorized into two groups based on the type of prostheses they received: lateralized RSA (Onlay Group, OG): onlay 145° curved, short stem (lateralized humerus and glenoid); or medialized RSA (Inlay Group, IG): inlay 155° straight standard stem (medialized humerus/lateralized glenoid. Patients were matched in the largest possible ratio (1:1) by age, gender, indication, preoperative range of motion, and Constant score [12].

The study protocol was approved by the hospital ethics committee (CERC-VS-2018-06-1), and all patients gave informed written consent.

2.2. Surgical Technique and Implant Design

Patients were operated on under the combination of general anesthesia and interscalene block, and exclusively by a standard deltopectoral approach. An onlay curved short stem with a neck shaft angle of 145° was used in the OG (Ascend Flex, Wright Medical, Memphis, TN, USA), and an inlay straight standard stem with a neck shaft angle of 155° was implanted in the IG (Aequalis II; Wright Medical, Memphis, TN, USA). The stems were impacted with a retroversion of 20°. A bony cylindrical autograft of 7 mm thick was harvested from the native humeral head and systematically used on the glenoid side. The glenoid implant was composed of a 25 mm long peg to safely fix the graft beneath the baseplate, two compression screws, and two locking screws. An angle of 10° of inferior tilt was targeted. A glenosphere with a 36 mm diameter was used [13,14]. Table 1 summarizes the differences in lateralization between the two RSA designs that were implanted in our study.

Table 1. Lateralization (Expressed in MM) of Different Components Used in Our Study.

Manufacturer	Implant	Gleno-Humeral Construct	Humeral Offset	Glenoid Offset	Global Offset	Glenoid Contribution	Humeral Contribution
Wright	Ascend Flex 145°	LGLH	14.2	17.3	31.5	42%	58%
Wright	Aequalis II 155°	LGMH	8	14.6	22.6	57%	43%

LG—lateralized glenoid, MH—medialized humerus, LH—lateralized humerus, °—degrees

2.3. Postoperative Rehabilitation Protocol

Postoperatively, the arm was placed in a sling for four weeks. Our physiotherapy protocol after RSA was based on three goals. The goal during the first four weeks was to recover the passive anterior forward flexion and external rotation according to a previously validated protocol [3]. After four weeks, the goal was to recover ROM, based on the deltoid reactivation and strengthening in "zero position" according to Saha [15]. The third goal was to recover functional shoulder movements for the daily activities, using neuromuscular techniques to pass from active elevation to functional movements. Strengthening was not recommended.

2.4. Study Variables

The main outcomes of interest were the improvements in active external rotation, and in clinical scores in relation to the prosthetic designs. The following patient characteristics were assessed: age, sex, length of follow-up, and ROM.

2.5. Clinical Evaluation

All patients were clinically evaluated preoperatively and at the final follow-up. A goniometer was used to assess anterior forward flexion and external rotation for the active ROM assessment. The external rotation was measured with the arm by the side of the body, whereas the internal rotation was measured by the highest vertebral spinous process reached by the patient's extended thumb. Internal rotation was scored by the following discrete assignment: $0° = 0$, buttocks = 1, sacrum = 2, L5 = 3, L4 = 4, L3 = 5, L2 = 6, L1 = 7, Th12 = 8, Th11 = 9, Th10 = 10, Th9 = 11, Th8 = 12, Th7 = 13, Th6 = 14. The assessment included the Constant score [12].

2.6. Statistical Analysis

The Shapiro–Wilk test was used to check the normality of distributions. Descriptive statistics were presented in terms of means, standard deviations (SD), medians, and ranges. The significance of pre- vs. postoperative differences within each group was determined using the Wilcoxon signed-rank test for non-normally distributed data and using the paired Student t-test for normally distributed data. The significance of differences between groups was determined using the Mann–Whitney U test (Wilcoxon rank-sum test) for non-normally distributed quantitative data, the Student unpaired t-test for normally distributed data, and the Fisher exact test for categorical data. Statistical analyses were performed using R version 3.6.2 (R Foundation for Statistical Computing, Vienna, Austria). p values < 0.05 were considered statistically significant.

3. Results

Forty-seven patients participated in a matched analysis (23 in OG and 24 in IG). Cohorts were comparable in terms of age, gender, surgical indication, preoperative ROM, and Constant score (Table 2).

Table 2. Comparison Analysis of Pre- and Postoperative Data between Onlay and Inlay Groups.

	Onlay Group (OG, n = 23 Patients)			Inlay Group (IG, n = 24 Patients)			p-Value
	N (%)			N (%)			
	Mean ± SD	Median	(Range)	Mean ± SD	Median	(Range)	
Male sex	9 (39.1%)			9 (37.5%)			1.000
Age at index operation (yrs)	74.6 ± 7.6	77.0	(59.0–87.0)	75.0 ± 5.4	75.0	(65.0–87.0)	0.848
Follow-up (months)	27.3 ± 2.9	28.0	(24.0–31.0)	52.0 ± 14.6	48.5	(24.0–89.0)	<0.001
Anterior forward flexion							
preoperative	92.4 ± 40.3	90.0	(15.0–160.0)	87.9 ± 43.9	80.0	(10.0–165.0)	0.416
postoperative	128.9 ± 26.8	140.0	(70.0–160.0)	140.4 ± 33.1	150.0	(35.0–180.0)	0.032
improvement	36.5 ± 41.8	30.0	(−20.0–145.0)	52.5 ± 41.1	65.0	(−15.0–120.0)	0.112
p-value *	<0.001			<0.001			
Internal rotation (°)							
preoperative	4.2 ± 3.3	4.0	(1.0–12.5)	5.1 ± 4.3	4.0	(1.0–13.0)	0.728
postoperative	4.7 ± 2.8	4.0	(1.0–8.0)	3.5 ± 2.7	4.0	(1.0–13.0)	0.109
improvement	0.4 ± 3.7	0.0	(−4.5–7.0)	−1.6 ± 5.1	0.0	(−11.0–6.0)	0.341
p-value *	0.726			0.247			
External rotation (°)							
preoperative	4.6 ± 8.9	0.0	(0.0–30.0)	0.8 ± 4.1	0.0	(−10.0–10.0)	0.133
postoperative	12.0 ± 15.8	0.0	(0.0–45.0)	1.9 ± 3.8	0.0	(0.0–10.0)	0.028
improvement	7.4 ± 16.2	0.0	(−30.0–40.0)	1.0 ± 5.1	0.0	(−10.0–10.0)	0.191
p-value *	0.049			0.416			
Constant score							
preoperative	33.4 ± 15.5	28.0	(13.0–69.0)	33.3 ± 14.6	32.5	(5.0–65.0)	0.790
postoperative	67.5 ± 14.3	71.0	(35.0–93.0)	67.7 ± 14.1	72.0	(31.0–87.0)	0.898
improvement	34.1 ± 20.4	34.0	(−20.0–80.0)	34.4 ± 19.2	34.5	(3.0–76.0)	0.882
p-value *	<0.001			<0.001			

* Between pre- and post-operative measurements. Underlined p-values indicate those below 0.05. °—degrees.

The postoperative results are summarized in Table 2. Patients in the IG had a significantly greater follow-up compared to the OG (52.0 ± 14.6 vs. 27.3 ± 2.9 months; $p < 0.001$). Anterior forward flexion improved significantly in both groups but was significantly greater postoperatively in the IG compared to the OG (140.4 ± 33.1 vs. 128.9 ± 26.8; $p = 0.032$). External rotation improved significantly only in the OG (preop: 4.6° ± 8.9° vs. postop: 12.0° ± 15.8°; $p = 0.049$) and was also significantly greater postoperatively in the OG compared to the IG (12.0 ± 15.8 vs. 1.9 ± 3.8; $p = 0.028$). In the OG, external rotation improved in 9 cases (10° to 40°), remained comparable in 11 cases, and worsened in 3 cases (5° to 30°). In the IG, external rotation improved in 5 cases (5° to 10°), remained comparable in 17 cases, and worsened in 2 cases (10°). Postoperative internal rotation did not increase in any members of the two groups and was not significantly different between the groups. The Constant score improved significantly in both groups.

4. Discussion

The results of this study confirmed our hypothesis; prosthetic designs play a significant role in postoperative active ROM, despite nonfunctional rotator cuffs. Even if functional scores were similar between the two groups, IG had better postoperative anterior forward flexion, and OG a better postoperative active external rotation, even if the infraspinatus and teres minor presented severe fatty infiltration.

We observed a statistically significant increase in external rotation by 7.4° in the OG with lateralized humerus compared to IG with medialized humerus. This result might be related to (1) an increased humeral lateralization, either due to the use of an onlay design or due to the use of a more varus neck-shaft angle stem (145° vs. 155°) [14,16], (2) a tenodesis effect and a retensioning of the remnant posterior cuff (Figure 1), (3) a better recruitment of the posterior deltoid (Figure 1), and (4) less scapular notching [17].

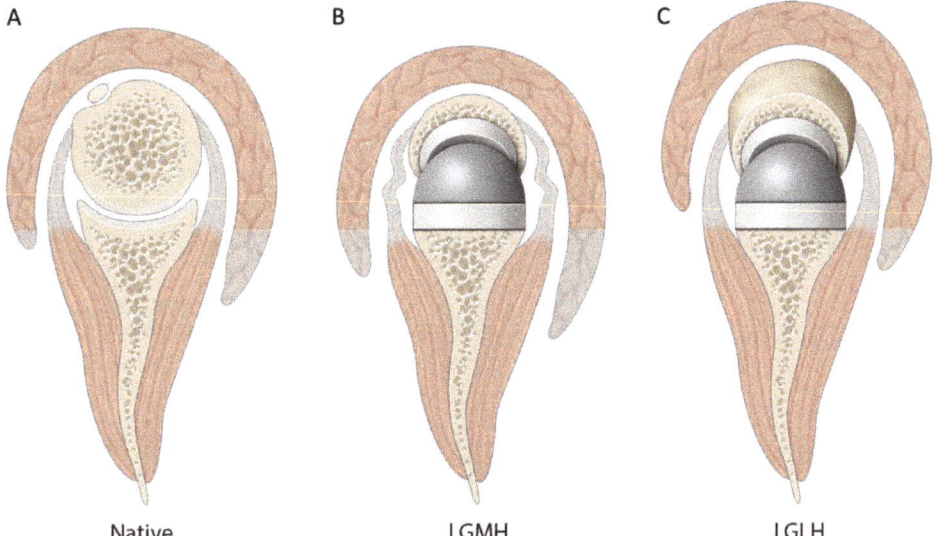

Figure 1. Factors influencing postoperative external rotation. (**A**) Native shoulder. The center of rotation is in the humeral head, and the level of deltoid arm does not allow deltoid recruitment. (**B**) A combination of lateral glenoid/medial humerus RSA. As in native shoulders, the bony lateralization of the center of rotation decreases recruitment of the deltoid for rotation. Additionally, due to the medialized center of rotation compared to the native shoulder, the rotator cuff is slackened and thus less efficient in rotatory motion. (**C**) A combination of lateral glenoid/lateral humerus RSA. Additional lateralization on the humeral side allows important deltoid recruitment and a tenodesis effect and a retensioning of the remnant posterior cuff.

Increased lateralization on the humeral side might have important biomechanical consequences and affect clinical outcomes. This is theorized to increase the tension of the rotator cuff muscles, so that their rotational capacities improve [14,18,19]. Lädermann et al. have shown that the greatest lengthening of the infraspinatus is achieved when a combination of bone increased offset RSA with a 145° onlay stem is used [14]. Several biomechanical studies showed improvement of rotator cuff (especially infraspinatus and teres minor) and posterior deltoid moment arms in lateralized humeral designs [20,21]. The increase in lateralization could potentially improve the length–tension relationship of the posterior remnant of the rotator cuff and thus increase its efficiency. However, the increase of external rotation, we found, may be mainly due to a so-called "tenodesis effect" of the remnant posterior cuff, which could prevent some loss of active external rotation.

Humeral lateralization improves deltoid muscle efficiency. The increase of external rotation could perhaps be explained through the "wrapping effect" of the posterior deltoid when a prosthetic design of lateralized humerus is used [22]. By lateralizing the center of rotation, a major part of the posterior deltoid fibers is preserved for rotational motion, which allows for a possible increase in active external rotation [20,23,24]. The moment arm for the posterior part of the deltoid is approximately 20% of that for the infraspinatus and teres minor [20,23]. Collin et al. showed that patients with an absence of posterosuperior rotator cuff (type E rotator cuff tear) still have an external rotation of 20° at 90° of abduction, potentially generated by the posterior deltoid [9].

A low neck-shaft angle, limiting inferior friction-type impingement, and consequently, scapular notching, could also explain the difference in external rotation between the two groups of the present study [17,25–27]. Only one clinical study, performed by Merolla et al., compared the same groups as ours using an OG and IG RSA design with a minimum follow-up of 2 years [28]. Both implants showed similar postoperative ROM between the low (OG) and high (IG) neck-shaft angles, although the former was associated with significantly greater delta scores of external rotation and lower rates of scapular notching [28]. Lateralization seems to play a significant role in scapular notching [29].

Simovitch et al. reported on the minimal clinically important difference (MCID) for different shoulder outcome metrics and ROM after shoulder arthroplasty. They noted that the MCID in terms of active forward anterior forward flexion is $12° \pm 4°$ and for active external rotation is $3° \pm 2°$ [30]. With that knowledge in mind, we can explain why we were not able to find any statistical difference between the clinical outcomes of the OG and the IG. We noticed a significant improvement of movement in one plane in each group. In OG, it was external rotation, whereas in IG, it was abduction, which in the end negated each other; consequently, we could not find a substantial difference between the clinical outcomes of the two analyzed groups.

All previously mentioned findings are crucial when planning RSA in a patient with a loss of active external rotation. Effectively, it has traditionally been implied for this condition that a latissimus dorsi transfer +/− teres major tendon transfer(s) be undertaken [31,32]. Our study demonstrated that an adequate prosthetic design could be sufficient to restore active external rotation, confirming other reports [33]. Consequently, due to the additional difficulty, increased operative time, associated loss of internal rotation [34], and increased neurological complication rate [35], primary transfers do no longer seem justified, as a simple change in prosthetic design could achieve similar results.

Strengths and Limitations

This study compared two groups of patients that were operated on by the same surgeon, using the same surgical technique, with the same glenoid configuration. Furthermore, the control group was matched according to age, gender, indication, preoperative ROM, and Constant score. This is the first report to specifically analyze the effect of the lateralized humeral stem in primary lateralized glenoid RSA in patients with preoperative third- or fourth-grade fatty infiltration of the infraspinatus and teres minor. We acknowledge, however, several limitations. First, the retrospective design of this study; however, observation and recollection biases were reduced by prospective collection of the data. Second, this is not a randomized study, which might create a sample bias. Third, we did not perform an a priori sample size calculation. Due to a limited number of patients, we did not divide patients within the OG between those who had a satisfying postoperative external rotation and those who did not, preventing analysis of the main predictive factor for this outcome. Lastly, patients in the IG had a significantly longer follow-up compared to those in the OG. As external rotation improves with time [36], the difference in range of motion could have been even more important with a similar follow-up.

5. Conclusions

The use of lateralized RSA with a low neck-shaft angle humeral stem results in significantly improved external rotation compared to medialized RSA with a 155° humeral stem, even in cases of severe fatty infiltration of the infraspinatus and the teres minor. Humeral lateralization and a low neck-shaft angle should be favored when planning an RSA in patients without a functional posterior rotator cuff. On the other hand, the medialized humerus with a 155° inlay stem contributed to a greater anterior forward flexion than the other configuration. However, the change in ROM amongst groups did not affect the postoperative clinical outcome.

Author Contributions: Conceptualization: A.L. and P.C.; methodology: H.B.; formal analysis: H.B.; investigation: S.O., H.K. and M.N.; resources: P.C.; data curation: S.O. and H.B.; writing: M.N., R.T. and A.L.; original draft preparation: M.N., S.O. and H.K.; writing—review and editing: P.C., A.L. and R.T.; project administration: P.C. All authors have read and agreed to the published version of the manuscript.

Funding: This research was founded by a grant from FORE (Foundation for Research and Teaching in Orthopaedics, Sports Medicine, Trauma and Imaging in the Musculoskeletal System): grant number 2021-1.

Institutional Review Board Statement: The study was conducted according to the guidelines of the Declaration of Helsinki, and approved by the Institutional Review Board (or Ethics Committee) of Recherche Clinique Vivalto Santé (protocol code CERC-VS-2018-06-1, date of approval: 29 June 2018).

Informed Consent Statement: Informed consent was obtained from all subjects involved in the study.

Data Availability Statement: All the available data have been presented in this study. Details regarding where data supporting reported results can be requested at the following e-mail address: hugo.bothorel@latour.ch.

Conflicts of Interest: Alexandre Lädermann reports grants and personal fees from Arthrex, grants and personal fees from Medacta, grants and personal fees from Stryker, outside the submitted work. He is the founder of the FORE, of BeeMed, and Med4cast. Philippe Collin reports that he is a paid consultant for Stryker and Arthrex and receives royalties from Stryker. Rihard Trebše reports personal fees from Zimmer Biomet, personal fees from Medacta, personal fees from De Puy. Other authors declare no conflict of interest.

References

1. Shah, S.S.; Roche, A.M.; Sullivan, S.W.; Gaal, B.T.; Dalton, S.; Sharma, A.; King, J.J.; Grawe, B.M.; Namdari, S.; Lawler, M.; et al. The Modern Reverse Shoulder Arthroplasty & an Updated Systematic Review for Each Complication: Part II. *JSES Int.* **2021**, *5*, 121–137. [PubMed]
2. Parry, S.; Stachler, S.; Mahylis, J. Lateralization in reverse shoulder arthroplasty: A review. *J. Orthop.* **2020**, *22*, 64–67. [CrossRef] [PubMed]
3. Collin, P.; Liu, X.; Denard, P.J.; Gain, S.; Nowak, A.; Ladermann, A. Standard versus bony increased-offset reverse shoulder arthroplasty: A retrospective comparative cohort study. *J. Shoulder Elb. Surg.* **2018**, *27*, 59–64. [CrossRef] [PubMed]
4. Gutiérrez, S.; Comiskey Iv, C.A.; Luo, Z.P.; Pupello, D.R.; Frankle, M.A. Range of impingement-free abduction and adduction deficit after reverse shoulder arthroplasty. Hierarchy of surgical and implant-design-related factors. *J. Bone Jt. Surg. Am.* **2008**, *90*, 2606–2615. [CrossRef] [PubMed]
5. Werner, B.S.; Chaoui, J.; Walch, G. The influence of humeral neck shaft angle and glenoid lateralization on range of motion in reverse shoulder arthroplasty. *J. Shoulder Elb. Surg.* **2017**, *26*, 1726–1731. [CrossRef] [PubMed]
6. Frankle, M.; Siegal, S.; Pupello, D.; Saleem, A.; Mighell, M.; Vasey, M. The Reverse Shoulder Prosthesis for glenohumeral arthritis associated with severe rotator cuff deficiency. A minimum two-year follow-up study of sixty patients. *J. Bone Jt. Surg. Am.* **2005**, *87*, 1697–1705. [CrossRef]
7. Werthel, J.D.; Walch, G.; Vegehan, E.; Deransart, P.; Sanchez-Sotelo, J.; Valenti, P. Lateralization in reverse shoulder arthroplasty: A descriptive analysis of different implants in current practice. *Int. Orthop.* **2019**, *43*, 2349–2360. [CrossRef]
8. Polisetty, T.S.; Baessler, A.M.; Levy, J.C.; Badman, B.L. Onlay versus inlay reverse total shoulder arthroplasty: A retrospective comparison of radiographic and clinical outcomes. *Semin. Arthroplast.* **2021**, *31*, 202–208. [CrossRef]
9. Collin, P.; Matsumura, N.; Ladermann, A.; Denard, P.J.; Walch, G. Relationship between massive chronic rotator cuff tear pattern and loss of active shoulder range of motion. *J. Shoulder Elb. Surg.* **2014**, *23*, 1195–1202. [CrossRef]
10. Goutallier, D.B.I.P.D. Assessment of the trophicity of the muscles of the ruptured rotator cuff by CT scan. *Surg. Shoulder St Louis MO Mosby Year Book 1* **1990**, *304*, 1–13.
11. Collin, P.; Treseder, T.; Denard, P.J.; Neyton, L.; Walch, G.; Ladermann, A. What is the Best Clinical Test for Assessment of the Teres Minor in Massive Rotator Cuff Tears? *Clin. Orthop. Relat. Res.* **2015**, *473*, 2959–2966. [CrossRef] [PubMed]
12. Constant, C.R.; Murley, A.H. A clinical method of functional assessment of the shoulder. *Clin. Orthop. Relat Res.* **1987**, *214*, 160–164. [CrossRef]
13. Boileau, P.; Moineau, G.; Roussanne, Y.; O'Shea, K. Bony increased-offset reversed shoulder arthroplasty: Minimizing scapular impingement while maximizing glenoid fixation. *Clin. Orthop. Relat. Res.* **2011**, *469*, 2558–2567. [CrossRef]
14. Lädermann, A.; Denard, P.J.; Collin, P.; Zbinden, O.; Chiu, J.C.H.; Boileau, P.; Olivier, F.; Walch, G. Effect of humeral stem and glenosphere designs on range of motion and muscle length in reverse shoulder arthroplasty. *Int. Orthop.* **2020**, *44*, 519–530. [CrossRef] [PubMed]
15. Saha, A.K. Zero position of the gleno-humeral joint: Its recognition and clinical importance: Hunterian Lecture delivered at the Royal College of Surgeons of England on 10th July 1957. *Ann. R. Coll. Surg. Engl.* **1958**, *22*, 223.
16. Lädermann, A.; Denard, P.J.; Boileau, P.; Farron, A. Effect of humeral stem design on humeral position and range of motion in reverse shoulder arthroplasty. *Int. Orthop.* **2015**, *39*, 2205–2213. [CrossRef] [PubMed]
17. Lädermann, A.; Gueorguiev, B.; Charbonnier, C.; Stimec, B.V.; Fasel, J.H.D.D.; Zderic, I.; Hagen, J.; Walch, G. Scapular notching on kinematic simulated range of motion after reverse shoulder arthroplasty is not the result of impingement in adduction. *Medicine* **2015**, *94*, e1615. [CrossRef]

18. Greiner, S.; Schmidt, C.; König, C.; Perka, C.; Herrmann, S. Lateralized reverse shoulder arthroplasty maintains rotational function of the remaining rotator cuff shoulder. *Clin. Orthop. Rel. Res.* **2013**, *471*, 940–946. [CrossRef]
19. Herrmann, S.; König, C.; Heller, M.; Perka, C.; Greiner, S. Reverse shoulder arthroplasty leads to significant biomechanical changes in the remaining rotator cuff. *J. Orthop. Surg. Res.* **2011**, *6*, 42. [CrossRef] [PubMed]
20. Hamilton, M.A.; Roche, C.P.; Diep, P.; Flurin, P.H.; Routman, H.D. Effect of prosthesis design on muscle length and moment arms in reverse total shoulder arthroplasty. *Bull. NYU Hosp. Jt. Dis.* **2013**, *71* (Suppl. 2), S31–S35.
21. Chan, K.; Langohr, G.D.G.; Mahaffy, M.; Johnson, J.A.; Athwal, G.S. Does Humeral Component Lateralization in Reverse Shoulder Arthroplasty Affect Rotator Cuff Torque? Evaluation in a Cadaver Model. *Clin. Orthop. Relat. Res.* **2017**, *475*, 2564–2571. [CrossRef]
22. Gruson, K.I. CORR Insights((R)): Does Humeral Component Lateralization in Reverse Shoulder Arthroplasty Affect Rotator Cuff Torque? Evaluation in a Cadaver Model. *Clin. Orthop. Relat. Res.* **2017**, *475*, 2572–2574. [CrossRef]
23. Hamilton, M.A.; Diep, P.; Roche, C.; Flurin, P.H.; Wright, T.W.; Zuckerman, J.D.; Routman, H. Effect of reverse shoulder design philosophy on muscle moment arms. *J. Orthop. Res.* **2015**, *33*, 605–613. [CrossRef]
24. Valenti, P.; Sauzieres, P.; Katz, D.; Kalouche, I.; Kilinc, A.S. Do less medialized reverse shoulder prostheses increase motion and reduce notching? *Clin. Orthop. Relat. Res.* **2011**, *469*, 2550–2557. [CrossRef]
25. Gutiérrez, S.; Walker, M.; Willis, M.; Pupello, D.R.; Frankle, M.A. Effects of tilt and glenosphere eccentricity on baseplate/bone interface forces in a computational model, validated by a mechanical model, of reverse shoulder arthroplasty. *J. Shoulder Elb. Surg.* **2011**, *20*, 732–739. [CrossRef] [PubMed]
26. Lévigne, C.; Boileau, P.; Favard, L.; Garaud, P.; Molé, D.; Sirveaux, F.; Walch, G. Scapular notching in reverse shoulder arthroplasty. *J. Shoulder Elb. Surg.* **2008**, *17*, 925–935. [CrossRef] [PubMed]
27. Li, X.; Dines, J.S.; Waren, R.F.; Craig, E.V.; Dines, D.M. Inferior glenosphere placement reduces scapular notching in reverse total shoulder arthroplasty. *Orthopedics* **2015**, *38*, e88–e93. [CrossRef] [PubMed]
28. Merolla, G.; Walch, G.; Ascione, F.; Paladini, P.; Fabbri, E.; Padolino, A.; Porcellini, G. Grammont humeral design versus onlay curved-stem reverse shoulder arthroplasty: Comparison of clinical and radiographic outcomes with minimum 2-year follow-up. *J. Shoulder Elb. Surg.* **2018**, *27*, 701–710. [CrossRef] [PubMed]
29. Shah, S.S.; Gaal, B.T.; Roche, A.M.; Namdari, S.; Grawe, B.M.; Lawler, M.; Dalton, S.; King, J.J.; Helmkamp, J.; Garrigues, G.E.; et al. The modern reverse shoulder arthroplasty and an updated systematic review for each complication: Part I. *JSES Int.* **2020**, *4*, 929–943. [CrossRef]
30. Simovitch, R.; Flurin, P.H.; Wright, T.; Zuckerman, J.D.; Roche, C.P. Quantifying success after total shoulder arthroplasty: The minimal clinically important difference. *J. Shoulder Elb. Surg.* **2018**, *27*, 298–305. [CrossRef]
31. Boileau, P.; Rumian, A.P.; Zumstein, M.A. Reversed shoulder arthroplasty with modified L'Episcopo for combined loss of active elevation and external rotation. *J. Shoulder Elb. Surg.* **2010**, *19* (Suppl. 2), 20–30. [CrossRef] [PubMed]
32. Puskas, G.J.; Catanzaro, S.; Gerber, C. Clinical outcome of reverse total shoulder arthroplasty combined with latissimus dorsi transfer for the treatment of chronic combined pseudoparesis of elevation and external rotation of the shoulder. *J. Shoulder Elb. Surg.* **2014**, *23*, 49–57. [CrossRef]
33. Young, B.L.; Connor, P.M.; Schiffern, S.C.; Roberts, K.M.; Hamid, N. Reverse shoulder arthroplasty with and without latissimus and teres major transfer for patients with combined loss of elevation and external rotation: A prospective, randomized investigation. *J. Shoulder Elb. Surg.* **2020**, *29*, 874–881. [CrossRef]
34. Flury, M.; Kwisda, S.; Kolling, C.; Audigé, L. Latissimus dorsi muscle transfer reduces external rotation deficit at the cost of internal rotation in reverse shoulder arthroplasty patients: A cohort study. *J. Shoulder Elb. Surg.* **2019**, *28*, 56–64. [CrossRef]
35. Sheth, M.; Ko, J.K.; Namdari, S. Reverse Shoulder Arthroplasty and Latissimus Dorsi Tendon Transfer. *Am. J. Orthop.* **2017**, *46*, e287–e292. [PubMed]
36. Collin, P.; Matsukawa, T.; Denard, P.J.; Gain, S.; Lädermann, A. Pre-operative factors influence the recovery of range of motion following reverse shoulder arthroplasty. *Int. Orthop.* **2017**, *41*, 2135–2142. [CrossRef] [PubMed]

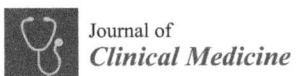

Article

Negligible Correlation between Radiographic Measurements and Clinical Outcomes in Patients Following Primary Reverse Total Shoulder Arthroplasty

Daniel P. Berthold [1,2,*], Daichi Morikawa [1,3], Lukas N. Muench [1,2], Joshua B. Baldino [1], Mark P. Cote [1], R. Alexander Creighton [4], Patrick J. Denard [5], Reuben Gobezie [6], Evan Lederman [7], Anthony A. Romeo [8], Knut Beitzel [2,9] and Augustus D. Mazzocca [1]

1. Department of Orthopaedic Surgery, University of Connecticut, Farmington, CT 06030, USA; idarimo@hotmail.com (D.M.); lukas.muench@mri.tum.de (L.N.M.); baldino@uchc.edu (J.B.B.); mcote@uchc.edu (M.P.C.); mazzocca@uchc.edu (A.D.M.)
2. Department of Orthopaedic Sports Medicine, Technical University of Munich, 81675 Munich, Germany; beitzelknut@tum.de
3. Department of Orthopaedic Surgery, Juntendo University, Tokio 113-8421, Japan
4. UNC Orthopaedics, University of North Carolina at Chapel Hill, Chapel Hill, NC 27599, USA; alex_creighton@med.unc.edu
5. Southern Oregon Orthopedics, Medford, OR 97504, USA; pjdenard@gmail.com
6. The Cleveland Shoulder Institute, Beachwood, OH 44194, USA; clevlandshoulder@gmail.com
7. Department of Orthopaedic Sports Medicine, University of Arizona College of Medicine, Tucson, AZ 85006, USA; elederman1@icloud.com
8. Dupage Medical Group, Elmhurst, IL 60126, USA; romeoortho@gmail.com
9. Arthroscopy and Orthopedic Sportsmedicine, ATOS Orthoparc Clinic, 50858 Cologne, Germany
* Correspondence: daniel.berthold@tum.de; Tel.: +49-89-4140-7842

Abstract: Previous attempts to measure lateralization, distalization or inclination after reverse total shoulder arthroplasty (rTSA) and to correlate them with clinical outcomes have been made in the past years. However, this is considered to be too demanding and challenging for daily clinical practice. Additionally, the reported findings were obtained from heterogeneous rTSA cohorts using 145° and 155° designs and are limited in external validity. The purpose of this study was to investigate the prognostic preoperative and postoperative radiographic factors affecting clinical outcomes in patients following rTSA using a 135° prosthesis design. In a multi-center design, patients undergoing primary rTSA using a 135° design were included. Radiographic analysis included center of rotation (COR), acromiohumeral distance (AHD), lateral humeral offset (LHO), distalization shoulder angle (DSA), lateralization shoulder angle (LSA), critical shoulder angle (CSA), and glenoid and baseplate inclination. Radiographic measurements were correlated to clinical and functional outcomes, including the American Shoulder and Elbow Surgeons (ASES), Simple Shoulder Test (STT), Single Assessment Numeric Evaluation (SANE), and Visual Analogue Scale (VAS) score, active forward elevation (AFE), external rotation (AER), and abduction (AABD), at a minimum 2-year follow-up. There was a significant correlation between both DSA ($r = 0.299$; $p = 0.020$) and LSA ($r = -0.276$; $p = 0.033$) and the degree of AFE at final follow-up. However, no correlation between DSA ($r = 0.133$; $p = 0.317$) and LSA ($r = -0.096$; $p = 0.471$) and AER was observed. Postoperative AHD demonstrated a significant correlation with final AFE ($r = 0.398$; $p = 0.002$) and SST ($r = 0.293$; $p = 0.025$). Further, postoperative LHO showed a significant correlation with ASES ($r = -0.281$; $p = 0.030$) and LSA showed a significant correlation with ASES ($r = -0.327$; $p = 0.011$), SANE ($r = -0.308$; $p = 0.012$), SST ($r = -0.410$; $p = 0.001$), and VAS ($r = 0.272$; $p = 0.034$) at terminal follow-up. All other correlations were found to be non-significant ($p > 0.05$, respectively). Negligible correlations between pre- and postoperative radiographic measurements and clinical outcomes following primary rTSA using a 135° prosthesis design were demonstrated; however, these observations are of limited predictive value for outcomes following rTSA. Subsequently, there remains a debate regarding the ideal placement of the components during rTSA to most sufficiently restore active ROM while minimizing complications such as component loosening and scapular notching. Additionally, as the data from this study show,

Citation: Berthold, D.P.; Morikawa, D.; Muench, L.N.; Baldino, J.B.; Cote, M.P.; Creighton, R.A.; Denard, P.J.; Gobezie, R.; Lederman, E.; Romeo, A.A.; et al. Negligible Correlation between Radiographic Measurements and Clinical Outcomes in Patients Following Primary Reverse Total Shoulder Arthroplasty. *J. Clin. Med.* **2021**, *10*, 809. https://doi.org/10.3390/jcm10040809

Academic Editor: Markus Scheibel
Received: 25 January 2021
Accepted: 11 February 2021
Published: 17 February 2021

Publisher's Note: MDPI stays neutral with regard to jurisdictional claims in published maps and institutional affiliations.

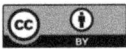

Copyright: © 2021 by the authors. Licensee MDPI, Basel, Switzerland. This article is an open access article distributed under the terms and conditions of the Creative Commons Attribution (CC BY) license (https://creativecommons.org/licenses/by/4.0/).

there is still a considerable lack of data in assessing radiographic prosthesis positioning in correlation to clinical outcomes. As such, the importance of radiographic measurements and their correlation with clinical and functional outcomes following rTSA may be limited.

Keywords: reverse total shoulder arthroplasty; DSA; LSA; lateralization; distalization; radiographic analysis

1. Introduction

In the past years, the prevalence and clinical use of reverse total shoulder arthroplasty (rTSA) in the USA has dramatically increased by 40.8%, with 30,850 procedures being performed in 2013 compared to 21,916 in 2011 [1]. First designed by Paul Grammont in 1985 for the treatment of arthritic shoulders with severe cuff insufficiency [2,3], the rationale of rTSA was to medialize the center of rotation, and to distalize the humerus relative to the acromion, resulting in increased deltoid muscle tension in an attempt to facilitate active forward elevation (AFE) [4]. The initial design with a humeral inclination of 155° showed promising long-term functional outcomes, however it failed to restore active external rotation (AER) and led to significant scapular notching, which has been reported to occur in 74% to 88% of cases [2,3,5–8].

Thus, recent studies have focused on significant design modifications to improve active range of motion (ROM) by increasing lateralization on the glenoid side, implementing a more anatomic humeral inclination of 135°, and decreasing distalization of the humeral shaft [5,6,9–12]. As a result, Boileau et al. demonstrated that lateralization of the glenoid improved postoperative AER, and subsequently decreased the risk of scapular notching [5]. However, the increased use of rTSAs still elicits high rates of postoperative complications, occurring in 39% to 59% of cases [13,14]. However, of interest, Mahendraraj et al. recently showed that the distalization shoulder angle (DSA) and lateralization shoulder angle (LSA) may be reproducible measures, but seem to have only marginal correlation with postoperative clinical outcomes. As such, further investigations into the prognostic utility of minimally cumbersome rTSA measurement methodologies are warranted [15].

As intraoperative implant positioning has been shown to influence complication rates, attempts have been made to correlate pre- and postoperative radiographic measurements to clinical and functional outcomes [16,17]. However, these measurements and their correlation to outcomes in patients following rTSA are controversial among shoulder surgeons, while current evidence on the importance of these measurements is still lacking. Previous attempts to measure distalization of the humerus as well as medialization of the center of rotation have been considered to be too demanding for daily clinical practice [18,19], which has led Boutsiadis et al. to introduce more reproducible measurements and to evaluate their impact on postoperative clinical outcomes [20]. The authors showed that a lateralization shoulder angle (LSA) of 75° to 95° was correlated wirh increased AER, whereas a distalization shoulder angle (DSA) of 40° to 65° was correlated with increased AFE. However, the reported findings were obtained from a heterogeneous rTSA cohort using 145° and 155° designs and were limited in external validity and due to small sample sizes. Further, Jeon et al. found insufficient AFE in patients with increased postoperative lateral humeral offset (LHO) [21]. However, this was only observed when rTSAs were performed using medialized implants, to increase the force on the anterior deltoid (in patients with severe cuff tear arthropathy). As such, data on patients undergoing rTSA using a 135° prosthesis design remain limited.

The purpose of this study was to determine prognostic radiographic factors affecting clinical and functional outcomes in patients undergoing primary rTSA using a design with a humeral inclination of 135°. The authors hypothesized that there would be no significant correlation between radiographic measurements and clinical and functional outcomes following primary rTSA.

2. Methods

2.1. Study Design

A retrospective multi-center review was conducted on rTSA cases performed by 5 independent surgeons from 5 separate institutions between June 2013 and January 2018. Institutional review board permission was obtained prior to initiation of the study (IRB 17-202-2). Patients who underwent primary rTSA using an implant with a 135° humeral inclination for the treatment of cuff tear arthropathy or primary glenohumeral arthritis with a minimum follow-up of 2 years were included in the study. Patients were excluded if they underwent rTSA using a 155° prothesis design, were revision cases, had concomitant fractures of the humeral head or glenoid requiring surgery, or had neurovascular injuries.

2.2. Outcome Measures

American Shoulder and Elbow Surgeons (ASES), Simple Shoulder Test (SST), Single Assessment Numeric Evaluation (SANE) and Visual Analogue Scale (VAS) scores were collected preoperatively and at final follow-up [22,23]. Furthermore, range of motion, consisting of active forward elevation (AFE), active abduction (AABD) and active external rotation (AER), were recorded preoperatively and at final follow-up.

2.3. Surgical Procedure

All surgical procedures were performed utilizing a uniform implant design (Univers Reverse; Arthrex Inc., Naples, FL, USA). A deltopectoral approach was used in all cases. Subscapularis repair was based on surgeon preference. On the glenoid side, this system provides a 36, 39, or 42 mm glenosphere with neutral, 4 mm lateralized, or 2.5 mm inferior eccentric options. Inclination angle, glenosphere size and offset were based on intraoperative deltoid tension, implant stability, and notching according to surgeon's preference. On the humeral side, the prosthesis has a modular cup which allows the surgeon to implant the component with either 135° or 155° of inclination. All humeral components were implanted by press-fitting. No patients required bone grafting.

2.4. Radiographic Evaluation

All patients had standard preoperative and postoperative radiographs (true anteriorposterior, y view and axillary view). Radiographic assessment was performed by two independent viewers blinded to patient outcomes. Radiographic measurements were performed on standard anteroposterior (AP) view performed at the most recent preoperative and last postoperative visit. Preoperative measurements included center of rotation (COR), critical shoulder angle (CSA) acromiohumeral distance (AHD), lateral humeral offset (LHO), and glenoid inclination (GI). Postoperative measurements included AHD, LHO, baseplate inclination (BI), distalization shoulder angle (DSA), and lateralization shoulder angle (LSA) [20,21,24–26].

AHD was measured by calculating the perpendicular distance between the most lateral portion of the undersurface of the acromion and a line parallel to the superior border of the greater tuberosity [21] (Figure 1). LHO was measured by determining the distance from the AHD line to the most lateral projection of the greater tuberosity [21] (Figure 2). LSA was measured by drawing a line from the superior glenoid tubercle to the most lateral border of the acromion and a second line from the most lateral border of the acromion to the most lateral border of the greater tuberosity. The angle between these two lines formed the LSA [20] (Figure 3a). DSA was measured by drawing a line between the most lateral border of the acromion and the superior glenoid tubercle and drawing a second line to connect the superior glenoid tubercle with the most superior border of the greater tuberosity. The angle between these two lines formed the DSA [20] (Figure 3b). Glenoid and baseplate were determined as the angle between the floor of the supraspinatus fossa and the glenoid fossa [25] (Figure 4). COR was measured by determining the best fit circle flush to the articular surface, identifying the center of the circle in the humeral head, and then measuring the distance of the perpendicular line between the center of the humeral head and the midpoint of the line connecting the superior and inferior glenoid tubercles [24] (Figure 5b). CSA was measured by a line from the superior pole to the inferior pole of the glenoid and a line from the inferior pole to the lateral edge of the acromion [26] (Figure 5a). In addition, scapular notching was graded according to the Nerot–Sirveaux classification and severity of preoperative cuff tear arthropathy was evaluated according to the Hamada classification [27,28].

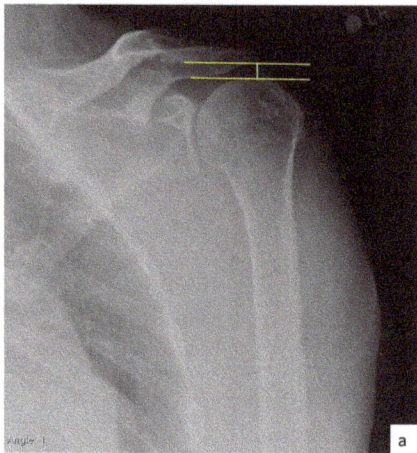 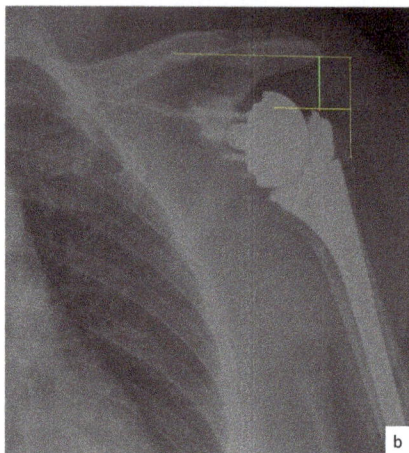

Figure 1. (**a**) Preoperative acromiohumeral distance (AHD; green line); (**b**) postoperative acromiohumeral distance (AHD; green line).

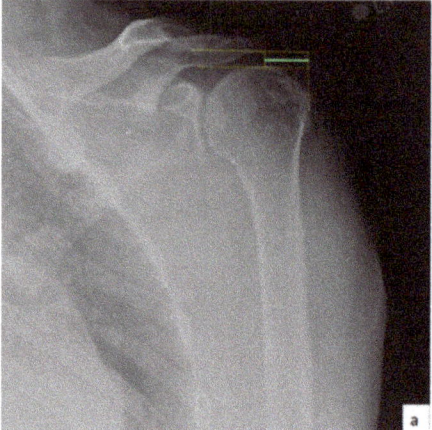 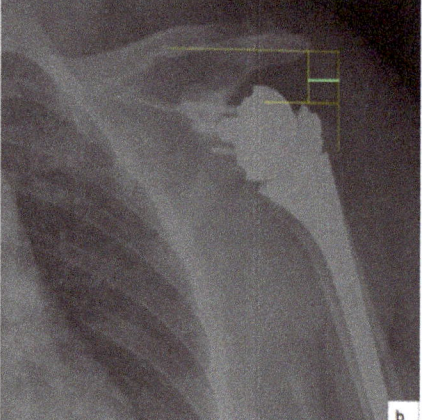

Figure 2. (**a**) Preoperative lateral humeral offset (LHO; green line); (**b**) postoperative lateral humeral offset (LHO; green line).

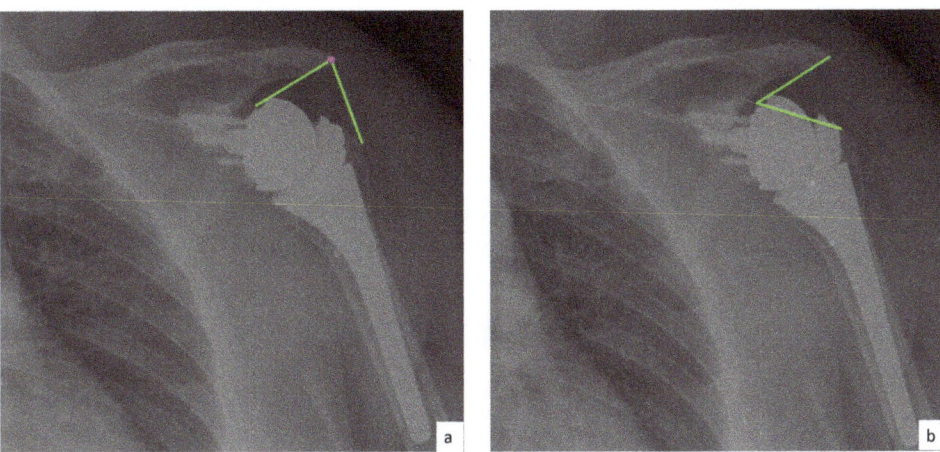

Figure 3. (**a**) Lateralization shoulder angle (LSA); (**b**) distalization shoulder angle (DSA).

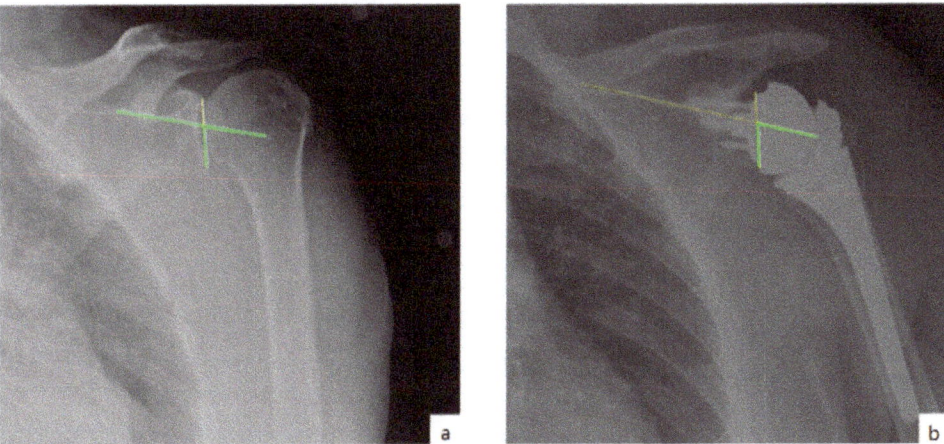

Figure 4. (**a**) Glenoid inclination (green angle); (**b**) baseplate inclination (green line).

2.5. Statistical Analysis

Descriptive statistics including mean and standard deviation for continuous variables and frequency and proportion for categorical variables were calculated to characterize the study groups. The relationships between clinical outcome measures and radiographic measurements were examined graphically with scatterplots and with Pearson correlation coefficients (rho). The effect of DSA and LSA on postoperative forward elevation was examined using a mixed effects linear model to account for patients nesting within surgeon's practices. An interclass correlation coefficient (ICC) was calculated to determine reproducibility of the radiographic measurements. A p-value < 0.05 was considered statistically significant. All analyses were performed with Stata statistical software (StataCorp. 2017. Stata Statistical Software: Release 15. College Station, TX: StataCorp LLC).

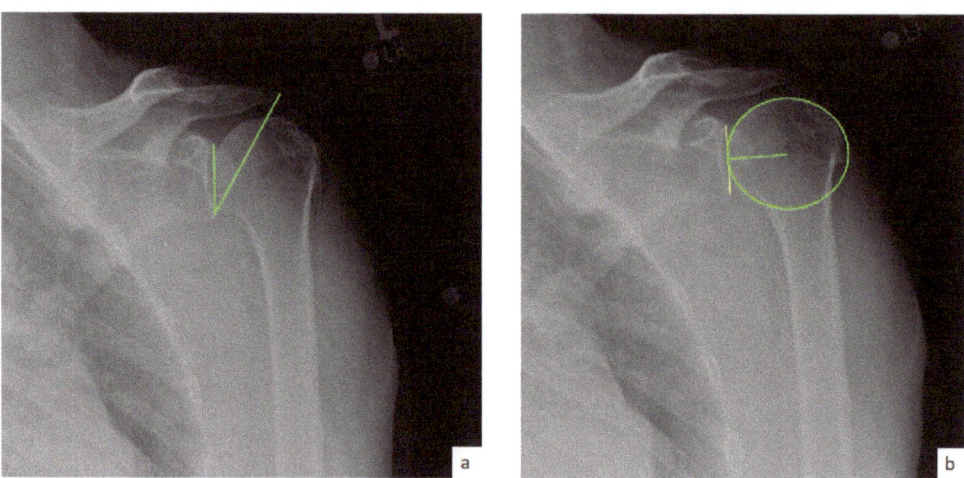

Figure 5. (**a**) Critical shoulder angle (CSA; green angle); (**b**) center of rotation (COI; green line).

3. Results

3.1. Subjects

Ninety-four rTSAs meeting the study criteria were performed during the study period. Of those, 61 were available at final follow-up (Figure 6). The mean age of patients was 69.2 ± 8.2 years (range: 53–88) with a mean follow-up of 3.1 ± 0.7 years (range: 2.0–4.2) years. Most patients were female (55.7%). Patient demographics are demonstrated in Table 1.

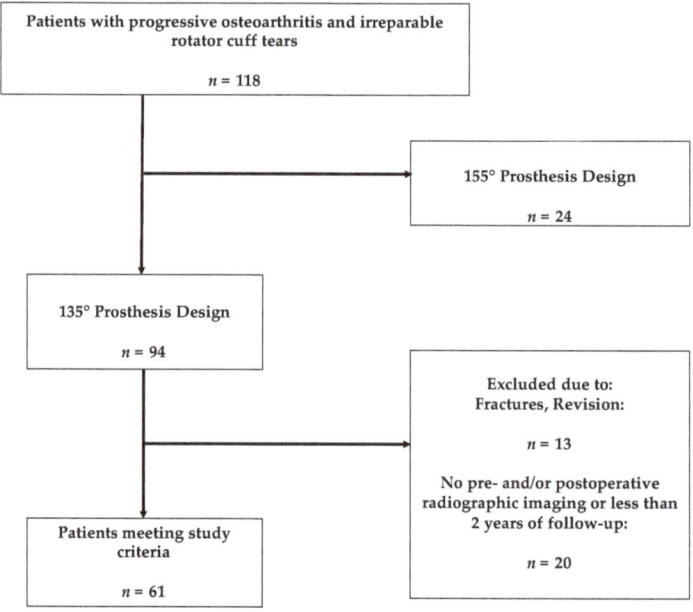

Figure 6. Flowchart displaying inclusion criteria.

Table 1. Patient demographics ($N = 61$).

	n	%
Sex		
Male	27	44.3
Female	34	55.7
Mean age ± SD (years)	69.2 ± 8.2	
Mean follow-up ± SD (years)	3.1 ± 0.7	
Dominant Arm Involved	32	52.0
Right Shoulders	33	54.0
BMI	29.9 ± 7.0	

3.2. Clinical Outcome

Overall, there was significant improvement in all clinical outcome measures from pre- to postoperative. SST improved from $2.5 \pm 1.8_{pre}$ to $8.0 \pm 2.6_{post}$, SANE improved from $28.9 \pm 22.7_{pre}$ to $80.7 \pm 20.1_{post}$, VAS improved from $6.0 \pm 2.2_{pre}$ to $1.4 \pm 2.3_{post}$, ASES improved from $37 \pm 14.5_{pre}$ to $78.1 \pm 21.6_{post}$. At final follow-up, there was no significant difference in SST, SANE, VAS, and ASES when comparing patient populations of the different institutions.

In addition, there was significant improvement in ROM from pre-to postoperative. AFE improved from $92 \pm 36°_{pre}$ to $131 \pm 27°_{post}$, AABD improved from $69 \pm 35°_{pre}$ to $109 \pm 38°_{post}$, AER improved from $29 \pm 18°_{pre}$ to $42 \pm 19°_{post}$ at final follow-up ($p < 0.01$, respectively). When comparing ROM of patients at the different institutions, no significant difference was found for AFE, AABD, or AER.

3.3. Inter-Rater Reliability of Radiographic Analysis

Inter-rater reliability was calculated for COR, Pre-CSA, Pre-AHD, Post-AHD, DSA, Pre-LHO, Post-LHO, LSA, glenoid inclination, baseplate inclination, Hamada and Notching grades. Reliability was found to be good for most of the radiographic measurements. However, Pre-AHD (ICC = 0.37; CI: 0.18–0.55) showed only poor reliability. Moderate to good ICC was found for COR (ICC = 0.68; CI: 0.51–0.8), DSA (ICC = 0.66; CI: 0.32–0.82) and glenoid inclination (ICC = 0.66; CI: 0.47–0.79). Mean values of radiographic measurements with corresponding inter-rater reliability are demonstrated in Table 2.

Table 2. Inter-rater reliability for all radiographic measurements and mean values for radiographic analysis.

	Mean ± SD	ICC	ICC 95% CI	Reliability
COR	20.9 ± 3.9 mm	0.68	[0.51, 0.8]	Moderate-Good
Pre CSA	35.2 ± 4.5 deg	0.9	[0.9, 0.94]	Good
Pre AHD	5.1 ± 3.2 mm	0.37	[0.18, 0.55]	Poor
Post AHD	26.3 ± 9.5 mm	0.88	[0.82, 0.93]	Good
DSA	38.6 ± 9.6 deg	0.66	[0.32, 0.82]	Moderate-Good
Pre LHO	9.9 ± 5.7 mm	0.86	[0.79, 0.91]	Good
Post LHO	9.5 ± 6 mm	0.84	[0.75, 0.89]	Good
LSA	89.2 ± 11.9 deg	0.84	[0.73, 0.9]	Good
Glenoid inclination	81.2 ± 6.8 deg	0.66	[0.47, 0.79]	Moderate-Good
Baseplate inclination	83.2 ± 6.4 deg	0.79	[0.69, 0.86]	Good

Abbreviation: COR = center of rotation; Pre CSA = preoperative critical shoulder angle; Pre AHD = preoperative acromiohumeral distance; Post AHD = postoperative acromiohumeral distance; DSA = distalization shoulder angle; Pre LHO = preoperative lateral humeral offset; Post LHO = postoperative lateral humeral; LSA = lateralization shoulder angle.

3.4. Correlation between Preoperative Radiographic Measurements and Clinical Outcomes

Pre-AHD was found to have a significant correlation with final AER ($p = 0.016$; $r = 0.314$). Additionally, Pre-LHO showed a significant correlation with final ASES ($p = 0.032$; $r = -0.277$). COR, CSA, and glenoid inclination had no significant influence on clinical outcomes at terminal follow-up ($p > 0.05$, respectively) (Appendix A Table A1).

3.5. Correlation between Lateralization and Clinical Outcomes

Post-LHO was found to significantly correlate with final ASES ($p = 0.03$; $r = -0.281$). Further, there was a significant correlation of LSA with final SST ($p = 0.001$; $r = -0.41$), final pain score ($p = 0.034$; $r = 0.272$), final SANE ($p = 0.018$, $r = -0.308$), and final ASES ($p = 0.011$; $r = -0.327$). Further, there was a significant correlation between LSA and final AFE ($p = 0.033$; $r = -0.276$). Correlations of LSA with final AER ($p = 0.471$; $r = -0.096$) and AABD ($p = 0.824$; r = 0.030) were found to be non-significant (Appendix A Table A1).

3.6. Correlation between Distalization and Clinical Outcomes

Post-AHD had a significant correlation with final SST ($p = 0.025$; $r = 0.293$). On the contrary, DSA showed no significant correlation to any clinical outcome measures. Post-AHD demonstrated a significant correlation to final AER ($p = 0.002$; $r = 0.398$). In addition, DSA significantly influenced final AFE ($p = 0.02$; $r = 0.299$). No significant correlations were found between DSA and final AER ($p = 0.317$; $r = 0.133$) and AABD ($p = 0.283$; $r = 0.145$).

3.7. Prediction of Active ROM

The highest degree in AFE was observed in patients presenting with a postoperative DSA between 40° and 60°. Patients with an AFE < 100° (n = 5) were further shown to have a DSA smaller than 40° (Figure 7). When looking at the LSA, patients with an AFE < 100° (n = 4) had an LSA greater than 95°. The highest degree in AFE was observed in patients having an LSA between 75° to 95° (Figure 8). However, there was no statistically significant correlation between distalization ($p = 0.317$) and lateralization ($p = 0.471$) to AER at final follow-up.

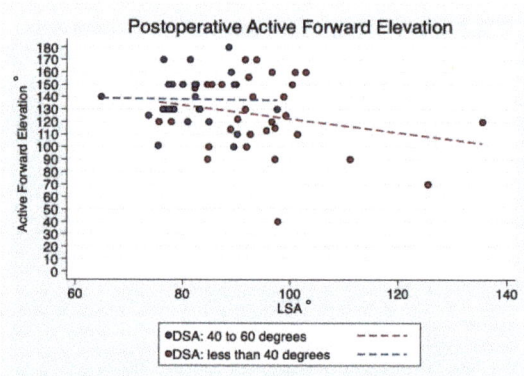

Figure 7. Scatterplot showing the linear correlation between DSA and LSA for final AFE. Good final AFE could be seen for DSA between 40 and 60° and LSA between 80 and 100°; Abbreviations: DSA = distalization shoulder angle; LSA = lateralization shoulder angle; AFE = active forward elevation.

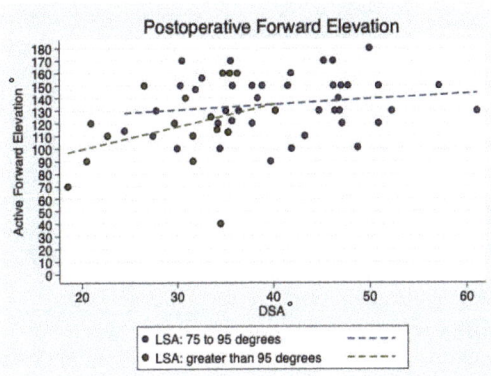

Figure 8. Scatterplot showing the linear correlation between LSA and DSA for final AFE. Good final AFE could be seen for DSA between 40 and 60° and LSA between 80 and 100°. Abbreviations: DSA = distalization shoulder angle; LSA = lateralization shoulder angle; AFE = active forward elevation.

4. Discussion

The most important finding of this study was that there was only a negligible correlation between radiographic measurements and clinical and functional outcomes following primary rTSA using a design with a humeral inclination of 135°. Even though statistically significant correlations between postoperative outcomes scores and radiographic measurements were found, these observations are of limited predictive value for outcomes following rTSA. The data gathered from this multi-center study indicate that the importance of radiographic measurements and their correlation with outcomes following rTSA may be limited.

In the postoperative setting, lateralization in rTSA can be expressed by different radiographic variables, including LHO, LSA, and COR. In their retrospective study, Jeon et al. demonstrated that an increased postoperative LHO was found to be a significant risk factor for poor restoration of postoperative AFE, when using an implant designed to be medialized [21]. In contrast, the data from this study showed that in a cohort using a lateralized implant, no significant relationship between preoperative and postoperative LHO and AFE could be demonstrated. However, in this study, post-LHO was found to significantly influence final ASES score, which may be of limited predictive value, as this finding did not allow for drawing a definite conclusion.

Increasing the lateralization of the COR in rTSA using a medialized implant design has been shown to result in greater active ROM [9]. As only few studies have focused on measuring COR in lateralized implants [18,29], the authors from this study could not find a significant relationship between COR, clinical outcomes, and final active ROM when using a lateralized rTSA design. Similar to a previous study by Boutsiadis et al. [20], who reported that patients achieved the highest degree in postoperative AFE and AABD with a DSA between 40° and 65° and the highest degree in AER when having a LSA of 75° to 95°, the findings of this study demonstrated a significant correlation between LSA and AFE as well as DSA and AFE. Additionally, the highest degree in AER was noted in patients having LSA values between 75° and 95°; however, a direct correlation of LSA and DSA with final AER and AABD could not be confirmed [20]. This may be explained by existing differences in implant designs being used, as all included patients uniformly underwent rTSA using a lateralized design with a humeral inclination of 135°. In contrast, Boutsiadis et al. included patients with two different implant designs (145° and 155° humeral inclination) [20].

Additionally, a positive correlation between LSA and DSA could be shown, which is consistent with the current literature [20]. In a lateralized rTSA design, a lower LSA, which corresponds to a more medialized implant, is associated with a larger DSA, indicating a greater distance between the acromion and humerus. To this, the findings from this study suggest that a LSA greater than 100° correlates with a DSA of less than 40°, thus reducing final AFE. Considering the current literature, lateralization of rTSA has been shown to increase postoperative AFE and AER by restoring the anatomic COR, while optimizing recruitment of the muscle fibers [6,30,31]. However, LSA was noted to be between 75° and 95° for optimal implant lateralization, with excessive lateralization resulting in less active ROM.

Increasing distalization, in order to improve tension on the deltoid muscle, has been shown to play an important role in rTSA [4]. In a computer-based model using different humeral offset and stem designs, Lädermann et al. demonstrated a strong positive linear relationship between AHD and AFE and AABD [6]. Furthermore, the authors showed that AHD decreased by 6 mm when switching from a 155° inlay design to a 135° onlay design. Even though it was shown that a higher AHD, expressed as arm lengthening, was related to a higher degree in AFE [6], the exact amount of arm lengthening remains inconclusive [6,18,32,33].

First introduced by Moor et al. [26], the CSA has been reported to be a reproducible radiographic index. As a larger CSA has been found to be associated with degenerative rotator cuff tears, there is still limited knowledge regarding its influence on rTSA [34]. Even though Roberson et al. [34] reported improved AFE in patients with a lower CSA, no significant relationship between CSA and clinical outcomes scores or final active ROM was found in this study.

Taking these findings into account, there remains a debate regarding the ideal placement of the components during rTSA to most sufficiently restore active ROM while minimizing complications such as component loosening and scapular notching. Additionally, as this study further verified, there is still a considerable lack of data in assessing radiographic prosthesis positioning in correlation with clinical outcomes. This may lead shoulder surgeons to overestimate current data and the importance of radiographic measurements and their correlation with outcomes following rTSA.

There are several limitations to the study. First, the study cohort was not randomized. Second, although outcomes were collected prospectively, data were reviewed retrospectively, which could create selection bias. Third, all radiographic measurements are highly dependent on patient orientation during radiographic imaging, as angles and distances are influenced by the position of the scapula as well as rotation of the humerus. However, this reflects daily clinical practice, as radiographic imaging, even if standardized, can show significant variances. Fourth, the multi-center design of this study including five surgeons from different sites leads to differences in implant positioning and intraoperative and postoperative outcomes. However, for the purpose of this study, the authors intended to demonstrate that even with high experience and expertise in this field, the observations and findings from this study and its subsequent comparison to the current literature should be interpreted with careful attention.

5. Conclusions

Negligible correlations between pre- and postoperative radiographic measurements and clinical outcomes following primary rTSA using a 135° prosthesis design were demonstrated. However, these observations are of limited predictive value for outcomes following rTSA. Subsequently, there remains a debate regarding the ideal placement of the components during rTSA to most sufficiently restore active ROM while minimizing complications such as component loosening and scapular notching. Additionally, as the data from this study showed, there is still a considerable lack of data in assessing radiographic prosthesis positioning in correlation to clinical outcomes. As such, the importance of radiographic measurements and their correlation with clinical and functional outcomes following rTSA may be limited.

Author Contributions: D.P.B. and L.N.M. wrote the manuscript. D.M. contributed to study design and data conception. M.P.C. contributed to the statistical analysis. J.B.B. helped with data conception. R.A.C. helped with interpretation of data and radiographic measurements. A.D.M., A.A.R., P.J.D., R.G., E.L. helped with data conception and analysis. K.B. served as important reviewer and helped with data interpretation. All authors have read and agreed to the published version of the manuscript.

Funding: The University of Connecticut Health Center/UConn Musculoskeletal Institute has received direct funding and material support from Arthrex Inc. (Naples, Fl). The company had no influence on study design, data collection, or interpretation of the results or the final manuscript.

Institutional Review Board Statement: Ethical approval was obtained via Human Research Determination Form to the institutional review board (IRB) of the University of Connecticut (IRB 17-202-2).

Informed Consent Statement: Informed consent was obtained from all subjects involved in the study.

Data Availability Statement: The data presented in this study are available on request from the corresponding author. The data are not publicly available due to ethical reasons.

Conflicts of Interest: Authors B.D.P., M.D., M.L.M. and B.J.B., C.A.R. declare that they have no conflict of interest. A.D.M. reports research grants from Arthrex Inc., is a consultant for Arthrex Inc. and receives royalties from Arthrex Inc. D.P.J. is a consultant for Arthrex Inc. and receives royalties from Arthrex Inc. L.E. is a consultant for Arthrex Inc. and receives royalties from Arthrex Inc. C.M.P. receives personal fees from Arthroscopy Association of North America (AANA). Gobezie R is a consultant for Arthrex Inc. and receives royalties from Arthrex Inc. R.A.R. receives material or orther financial support from AANA; is a board or committee member of Amercian Shoulder and Elbow Surgeons; Receives financial and material support from Arthrex Inc. ansd receives royalties from Arthrex Inc; receives other financial or material support from Mayor League Baseball; is an Editorial or governing board for Orthopedics and a board or committee member for Orthopedics Today; receives research support from Paragen Technologies and holds stock or stock options for Paragen Technologies; Is an editorial or governing board for SAGE; receives royalties and material support by Saunders/Mosby-Elsevier; receives royalties or material support for SLACK incorporated and is a editorial or governing board for SLACK incorporated; is an editorial or governing board for Wolters Kluwer Health. K Beitzel is a consultant for Arthrex Inc. and receives royalties from Arthrex Inc.

Appendix A

Table A1. Table showing correlation between radiographic analysis and final clinical outcome scores.

		ASES	SANE	SST	VAS	FE	ABD	ER
COR	r	−0.079	0.080	0.006	0.154	0.170	−0.176	−0.011
	p−value	0.547	0.545	0.966	0.235	0.194	0.190	0.937
Pre CSA	r	−0.035	0.056	−0.056	0.051	−0.211	−0.212	−0.187
	p−value	0.794	0.672	0.677	0.697	0.105	0.113	0.156
Pre AHD	r	0.085	0.142	0.124	−0.059	−0.051	−0.015	0.314
	p−value	0.518	0.284	0.349	0.652	0.697	0.910	**0.016**
Pre LHO	r	−0.277	−0.243	−0.251	0.177	−0.048	−0.037	0.035
	p−value	**0.032**	0.064	0.055	0.173	0.716	0.783	0.790
Post−AHD	r	0.150	0.179	0.293	−0.135	0.398	0.111	0.233
	p−value	0.253	0.174	**0.025**	0.299	**0.002**	0.411	0.075
Post LHO	r	−0.281	−0.215	−0.197	0.193	0.086	0.045	−0.003
	p−value	**0.030**	0.102	0.135	0.136	0.513	0.739	0.985
DSA	r	0.169	0.099	0.234	−0.145	0.299	0.145	0.133
	p−value	0.198	0.456	0.075	0.266	**0.020**	0.283	0.317
LSA	r	−0.327	−0.308	−0.410	0.272	−0.276	0.030	−0.096
	p−value	**0.011**	**0.012**	**0.001**	**0.034**	**0.033**	0.824	0.471

Table A1. Cont.

		ASES	SANE	SST	VAS	FE	ABD	ER
Inclination Glenoind.	r	−0.066	−0.156	−0.095	0.132	0.072	0.176	0.104
	p−value	0.614	0.238	0.473	0.310	0.583	0.191	0.435
Inclination Baseplate	r	−0.121	0.038	−0.102	0.123	0.122	0.106	0.050
	p−value	0.356	0.776	0.442	0.347	0.353	0.433	0.710
Hamada	r	−0.009	0.067	−0.031	0.013	0.156	−0.141	−0.289
	p−value	0.947	0.613	0.817	0.919	0.233	0.297	0.026
Notching	r	−0.030	−0.165	0.042	0.151	−0.246	−0.133	−0.214
	p−value	0.818	0.213	0.754	0.244	0.058	0.325	0.104

Significant values ($p < 0.05$) are highlighted. Abbreviation: COR = center of rotation; Pre CSA = preoperative critical shoulder angle; Pre AHD = preoperative acromiohumeral distance; Post AHD = postoperative acromiohumeral distance; DSA = distalization shoulder angle; Pre LHO = preoperative lateral humeral offset; Post LHO = postoperative lateral humeral; LSA = lateralization shoulder angle; FE = postoperative forward elevation; ABD = postoperative abduction; ER = postoperative external rotation; ASES = Postoperative American Shoulder and Elbow Surgeons; SST = Postoperative Simple Shoulder Test; VAS = Postoperative Visual Analogue Scale; SANE = Postoperative Single Assessment Numeric Evaluation.

References

1. Routman, H.D.; Flurin, P.H.; Wright, T.W.; Zuckerman, J.D.; Hamilton, M.A.; Roche, C.P. Reverse Shoulder Arthroplasty Prosthesis Design Classification System. *Bull. NYU Hosp. Jt. Dis.* **2015**, *73*, S5–S14.
2. Grammont, P. Etude et réalisation d'une nouvelle prothèse d'épaule. *Rheumatologie* **1987**, *39*, 27–38.
3. Grammont, P.M.; Baulot, E. Delta shoulder prosthesis for rotator cuff rupture. *Orthopedics* **1993**, *16*, 65–68. [CrossRef]
4. Boileau, P.; Watkinson, D.J.; Hatzidakis, A.M.; Balg, F. Grammont reverse prosthesis: Design, rationale, and biomechanics. *J. Shoulder Elbow Surg.* **2005**, *14*, 147s–161s. [CrossRef] [PubMed]
5. Boileau, P.; Moineau, G.; Roussanne, Y.; O'Shea, K. Bony increased-offset reversed shoulder arthroplasty: Minimizing scapular impingement while maximizing glenoid fixation. *Clin. Orthop. Relat. Res.* **2011**, *469*, 2558–2567. [CrossRef]
6. Ladermann, A.; Denard, P.J.; Boileau, P. Effect of humeral stem design on humeral position and range of motion in reverse shoulder arthroplasty. *Int. Orthop.* **2015**, *39*, 2205–2213. [CrossRef]
7. Bacle, G.; Nove-Josserand, L.; Garaud, P.; Walch, G. Long-Term Outcomes of Reverse Total Shoulder Arthroplasty: A Follow-up of a Previous Study. *J. Bone Jt. Surg. Am.* **2017**, *99*, 454–461. [CrossRef]
8. Mizuno, N.; Denard, P.J.; Raiss, P.; Walch, G. The clinical and radiographical results of reverse total shoulder arthroplasty with eccentric glenosphere. *Int. Orthop.* **2012**, *36*, 1647–1653. [CrossRef] [PubMed]
9. Gutierrez, S.; Levy, J.C.; Frankle, M.A. Evaluation of abduction range of motion and avoidance of inferior scapular impingement in a reverse shoulder model. *J. Shoulder Elbow Surg.* **2008**, *17*, 608–615. [CrossRef]
10. Berliner, J.L.; Regalado-Magdos, A.; Ma, C.B.; Feeley, B.T. Biomechanics of reverse total shoulder arthroplasty. *J. Shoulder Elbow Surg.* **2015**, *24*, 150–160. [CrossRef] [PubMed]
11. Frankle, M.; Levy, J.C.; Pupello, D. The reverse shoulder prosthesis for glenohumeral arthritis associated with severe rotator cuff deficiency. a minimum two-year follow-up study of sixty patients surgical technique. *J. Bone Jt. Surg. Am.* **2006**, *88*, 178–190. [CrossRef]
12. Katz, D.; Valenti, P.; Kany, J.; Elkholti, K.; Werthel, J.D. Does lateralisation of the centre of rotation in reverse shoulder arthroplasty avoid scapular notching? Clinical and radiological review of one hundred and forty cases with forty five months of follow-up. *Int. Orthop.* **2016**, *40*, 99–108. [CrossRef]
13. Ernstbrunner, L.; Suter, A.; Catanzaro, S.; Rahm, S.; Gerber, C. Reverse Total Shoulder Arthroplasty for Massive, Irreparable Rotator Cuff Tears Before the Age of 60 Years: Long-Term Results. *J. Bone Jt. Surg. Am.* **2017**, *99*, 1721–1729. [CrossRef] [PubMed]
14. Gerber, C.; Canonica, S.; Catanzaro, S.; Ernstbrunner, L. Longitudinal observational study of reverse total shoulder arthroplasty for irreparable rotator cuff dysfunction: Results after 15 years. *J. Shoulder Elbow Surg.* **2018**, *27*, 838. [CrossRef]
15. Mahendraraj, K.A.; Colliton, E.; Muniz, A.; Menendez, M.E.; Jawa, A. Assessing the validity of the distalization and lateralization shoulder angles following reverse total shoulder arthroplasty. *Semin. Arthroplast. JSES* **2020**. [CrossRef]
16. Li, X.; Knutson, Z.; Choi, D. Effects of glenosphere positioning on impingement-free internal and external rotation after reverse total shoulder arthroplasty. *J. Shoulder Elbow Surg.* **2013**, *22*, 807–813. [CrossRef]
17. Berhouet, J.; Garaud, P.; Favard, L. Evaluation of the role of glenosphere design and humeral component retroversion in avoiding scapular notching during reverse shoulder arthroplasty. *J. Shoulder Elbow Surg.* **2014**, *23*, 151–158. [CrossRef] [PubMed]
18. Jobin, C.M.; Brown, G.D.; Bahu, M.J. Reverse total shoulder arthroplasty for cuff tear arthropathy: The clinical effect of deltoid lengthening and center of rotation medialization. *J. Shoulder Elbow Surg.* **2012**, *21*, 1269–1277. [CrossRef] [PubMed]
19. Marcoin, A.; Ferrier, A.; Blasco, L.; De Boissieu, P.; Nerot, C.; Ohl, X. Reproducibility of a new method for measuring lowering and medialisation of the humerus after reverse shoulder arthroplasty. *Int. Orthop.* **2018**, *42*, 141–147. [CrossRef]
20. Boutsiadis, A.; Lenoir, H.; Denard, P.J. The lateralization and distalization shoulder angles are important determinants of clinical outcomes in reverse shoulder arthroplasty. *J. Shoulder Elbow Surg.* **2018**, *27*, 1226–1234. [CrossRef]

21. Jeon, Y.S.; Rhee, Y.G. Factors associated with poor active anterior elevation after reverse total shoulder arthroplasty. *J. Shoulder Elbow Surg.* **2018**, *27*, 786–793. [CrossRef]
22. Richards, R.R.; An, K.N.; Bigliani, L.U. A standardized method for the assessment of shoulder function. *J. Shoulder Elbow Surg.* **1994**, *3*, 347–352. [CrossRef]
23. Lippitt, S. A practical tool for evaluating shoulder function. The Simple Shoulder Test. *Shoulder A Balance Mobil. Stab.* **1993**, 501–518.
24. Rhee, S.M.; Lee, J.D.; Park, Y.B.; Yoo, J.C.; Oh, J.H. Prognostic Radiological Factors Affecting Clinical Outcomes of Reverse Shoulder Arthroplasty in the Korean Population. *Clin. Orthop. Surg.* **2019**, *11*, 112–119. [CrossRef] [PubMed]
25. Maurer, A.; Fucentese, S.F.; Pfirrmann, C.W. Assessment of glenoid inclination on routine clinical radiographs and computed tomography examinations of the shoulder. *J. Shoulder Elbow Surg.* **2012**, *21*, 1096–1103. [CrossRef]
26. Moor, B.K.; Bouaicha, S.; Rothenfluh, D.A.; Sukthankar, A.; Gerber, C. Is there an association between the individual anatomy of the scapula and the development of rotator cuff tears or osteoarthritis of the glenohumeral joint?: A radiological study of the critical shoulder angle. *Bone Jt. J.* **2013**, *95*, 935–941. [CrossRef]
27. Sirveaux, F.; Favard, L.; Oudet, D.; Huquet, D.; Walch, G.; Mole, D. Grammont inverted total shoulder arthroplasty in the treatment of glenohumeral osteoarthritis with massive rupture of the cuff: Results of a multicentre study of 80 shoulders. *J. Bone Jt. Surg. Br. Vol.* **2004**, *86*, 388–395. [CrossRef]
28. Hamada, K.; Yamanaka, K.; Uchiyama, Y.; Mikasa, T.; Mikasa, M. A radiographic classification of massive rotator cuff tear arthritis. *Clin. Orthop. Relat. Res.* **2011**, *469*, 2452–2460. [CrossRef] [PubMed]
29. Sabesan, V.J.; Lombardo, D.; Josserand, D. The effect of deltoid lengthening on functional outcome for reverse shoulder arthroplasty. *Musculoskelet. Surg.* **2016**, *100*, 127–132. [CrossRef]
30. Werner, B.S.; Chaoui, J.; Walch, G. The influence of humeral neck shaft angle and glenoid lateralization on range of motion in reverse shoulder arthroplasty. *J. Shoulder Elbow Surg.* **2017**, *26*, 1726–1731. [CrossRef]
31. Greiner, S.; Schmidt, C.; Konig, C.; Perka, C.; Herrmann, S. Lateralized reverse shoulder arthroplasty maintains rotational function of the remaining rotator cuff. *Clin. Orthop. Relat. Res.* **2013**, *471*, 940–946. [CrossRef]
32. Gutierrez, S.; Comiskey, C.A.; Luo, Z.P.; Pupello, D.R.; Frankle, M.A. Range of impingement-free abduction and adduction deficit after reverse shoulder arthroplasty. Hierarchy of surgical and implant-design-related factors. *J. Bone Jt. Surg. Am.* **2008**, *90*, 2606–2615. [CrossRef] [PubMed]
33. Schwartz, D.G.; Cottrell, B.J.; Teusink, M.J. Factors that predict postoperative motion in patients treated with reverse shoulder arthroplasty. *J. Shoulder Elbow Surg.* **2014**, *23*, 1289–1295. [CrossRef]
34. Roberson, T.A.; Shanley, E.; Abildgaard, J.T. The influence of radiographic markers of biomechanical variables on outcomes in reverse shoulder arthroplasty. *JSES Open Access* **2019**, *3*, 59–64. [CrossRef]

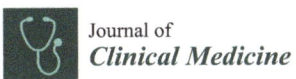

Article

Clinical and Radiologic Outcomes after Anatomical Total Shoulder Replacement Using a Modular Metal-Backed Glenoid after a Mean Follow-Up of 5.7 Years

Emil Noschajew [1], Felix Rittenschober [1], Harald Kindermann [2] and Reinhold Ortmaier [1,*]

1. Department of Orthopedic Surgery, Ordensklinikum Barmherzige Schwestern Linz, Vinzenzgruppe Center of Orthopedic Excellence, Teaching Hospital of the Paracelsus Medical University, 5020 Salzburg, Austria
2. Department of Marketing and Electronic Business, University of Applied Sciences Upper Austria, Campus 4400 Steyr, 4600 Wels, Austria
* Correspondence: reinhold.ortmaier@ordensklinikum.at

Abstract: Background: Glenoid wear is a common complication of anatomical total shoulder arthroplasty (aTSA) with a metal-backed glenoid (MBG), and the clinical and radiological results of historical implants are poor. The aim of this work was to evaluate the clinical and radiological results of 25 participants as well as the longevity after implantation of an anatomic shoulder prosthesis with a recent, modular cementless flat metal-backed glenoid component after a mean follow-up of 5.7 years. Methods: Clinically, the Simple Shoulder Test (SST), UCLA Activity Score (UCLA), and Constant Murley Score (CMS) were evaluated. Radiographically, the radiolucent lines (RLs), humeral head migration (HHM), and lateral glenohumeral offset (LGHO) were assessed. Survival was calculated with Kaplan–Meier curves and life-table analysis. Results: The mean CMS at follow-up was 46.2 points (range: 14–77; SD: 19.5). In terms of the SST score, the average value was 6.5 points (range: 1–10; SD: 3.5). The UCLA activity score showed a mean value of 5.9 points (range: 1–9; SD: 2.1). There were 17 revisions after a mean follow-up of 68.2 months (range: 1.8–119.6; SD: 27.9). HHM occurred in every patient, with a mean measurement of 6.4 mm (range: 0.5–13.4; SD: 3.9; $p < 0.0001$). The mean LGHO between the initial postoperative and follow-up images was 2.6 mm (range: 0–4.0; SD: 1.5; $p < 0.0001$). RLs were found in 22 patients (88%) around the glenoid and in 21 patients (84%) around the humeral head prosthesis. Conclusion: The clinical and radiographic outcomes after metal-backed glenoids were poor at 2.2 to 8.4 years of follow-up. We determined devastating survival in the majority of cases (68%), with mostly inlay wear (71%) as the main reason that led to revision surgery. The use of metalback genoids cannot be recommended based on the data of this study.

Keywords: clinical outcome; metal back glenoid; midterm results; prosthesis; radiologic outcome; shoulder

1. Introduction

Over the past decades, the total number of implanted TSAs has increased significantly, and this trend continues [1,2]. Despite a huge overhand of reverse total shoulder implants (RSA), the main indication for aTSA is indicated in patients with primary osteoarthritis (OA) with an intact rotator cuff (RTC) and no severe glenoid retroversion, biconcavity, or bone defect and younger age [3]. In this patient group, aTSA was still the implant of choice.

Longevity and low complication rates are crucial for patients, especially younger individuals. For aTSA survival, the glenoid component represents the weak link [4–6]. There are two types of glenoid components: cemented all-polyethylene glenoids (PEGs) and MBGs.

The usual pick for aTSA is the cemented all-PEG. However, high rates of glenoid component loosening and wear are reported in cemented all-PEGs [6]. The first attempts to improve the stability of glenoid components have led to the development of metal-backed

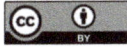

implants. As a rule, MBG components consist of the "metal back" itself and a polyethylene (PE) component that articulates with the humeral head component. This creates a further contact surface between two different materials with possible complications, e.g., dissociation of the two parts or abrasion of the components. Additionally, these glenoids can increase the width of the two components or reduce the PE content and may stress shield the underlying bone due to primary stable fixation [7]. The results of historical metalback glenoids in the literature are rather poor, and based on a systematic review of Papadonikolakis and Matsen carried out in 2014, it was determined that MBGs are not advisable as they have higher failure rates [6]. Following the success of reverse prostheses, the development of modular MBG implants is currently attracting renewed interest. These implants have the potential to be used for both anatomical and reverse shoulder endoprostheses. Revision surgery should theoretically be less complicated as the glenoid baseplate does not require removal [8]. The purpose is thus to lower glenoid component loosening rates and raise the possibility of revising the implant via RSA due to the modularity of most implants. Despite concerning reports of high complication rates of MBGs in aTSA, newer designs promise to lower the complication rate and yield better results with the possibility of converting the prosthesis very easily to a reverse implant if necessary [8]. In this study, we evaluated the clinical and radiological results, as well as the survival rate of the aTSA with a modular cementless flat MBG.

2. Materials and Methods

2.1. Study Population

All subjects gave their informed consent for inclusion before participating in the study. The study was conducted in accordance with the Declaration of Helsinki, and the protocol was approved by the local Ethics Committee of the state of Upper Austria (Study number 1167/2020). The case number consisted of 25 patients (15 women) who underwent shoulder arthroplasty in the period from 01/2009 to 07/2020. Included in the study were all patients who received an aTSA with a flat MBG in the specified period. The indication for implantation was an intact RTC without severe fatty infiltration (Fuchs grade ≤ 2) as well as radiographically determined omarthrosis, which was accompanied by severe pain in the shoulder joint and restricted movement of the affected arm and glenoid morphology according to Walch A1, 2 and B1 [9,10]. The exclusion criteria for performing aTSA included a full-thickness RTC tear and/or fatty infiltration of the RTC (Fuchs grade > 2), glenoid morphology according to Walch B2, B3, C, and D.

The minimum follow-up time from prosthesis implantation to the last reevaluation was 24 months, with a mean follow-up time of 68.6 months (range: 25.9–100.7). All patients were required to have pre- and postoperative radiographic images of the operated shoulder. Exclusion criteria for participating in the study were neurologic abnormalities or inability to fulfill the study requirements.

2.2. Data Collection and Assessment

Clinically, the postoperative Constant Murley Score (CMS), UCLA-Score, and the Simple Shoulder Test (SST) were assessed at the final follow-up. Radiologically, every patient had preoperative X-rays in two planes (anterior-posterior (AP) and axillary or y-view) and MRI or CT. CT and MRI were used for the classification of the preoperative glenoid morphology, according to Walch et al. [10], and RTC degeneration, according to Fuchs et al. [9]. Immediately postoperatively and at final follow-up, all patients received at least an X-ray in two planes (AP and axillary or y-view).

The postoperative X-ray images were calibrated over the known head size of the implanted humeral head. Radiolucent lines (RLs) around the humeral and glenoid components were assessed from the postoperative X-rays. Postoperative X-rays were also used to evaluate the center of rotation (COR). Postoperative radiographs were needed to measure the humeral head migration (HHM) and lateral glenohumeral offset (LGHO). HHM was measured via the smallest distance between the COR and the dense cortical bone marking the underside of the acromion. The difference between immediately postoperative AP X-rays and AP X-rays at final follow-up was calculated. The COR was determined as described by Alolabi et al. [11]. The debridement of the PE was measured using the LGHO as a difference (millimeter) of LGHO from immediately postoperative AP X-rays and LGHO from AP X-rays at final follow-up, which was determined by the distance from the medial edge of the baseplate to the most lateral point of the greater tuberosity (Figure 1).

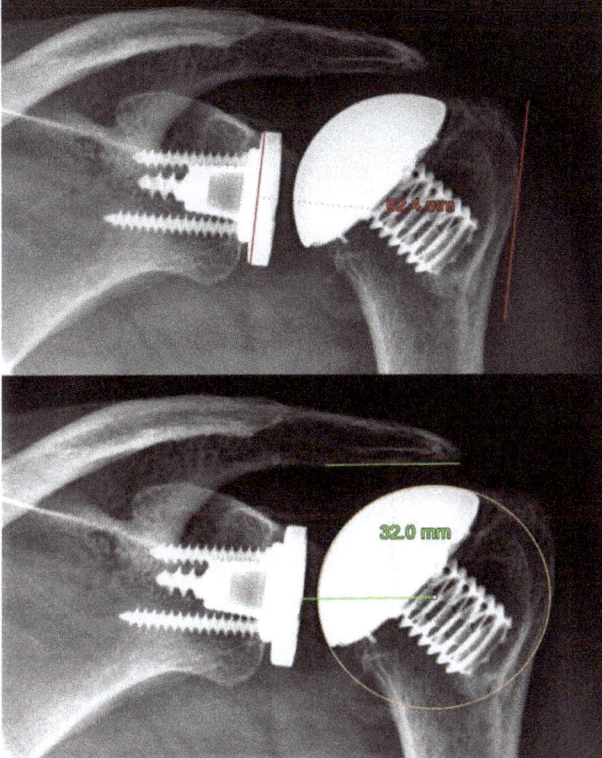

Figure 1. Postoperative radiographs of a left shoulder demonstrate the measurement method of the lateral glenohumeral offset (above X-ray image) and the humeral head migration (below X-ray image).

To evaluate RLs around the glenoid, the Lazarus scoring system, originally described for pegged glenoid components, was applied [12]. To evaluate the RLs around the humeral component in our study, the AP radiographs were assessed, and the axillary view was taken by dividing the implant-bone interface into three different sections.

Similarly, the radiolucent lines around the humeral component were assessed using eight distinct zones. For the humeral components, the analysis was based on the classification by Molé et al. [13] (Figure 2).

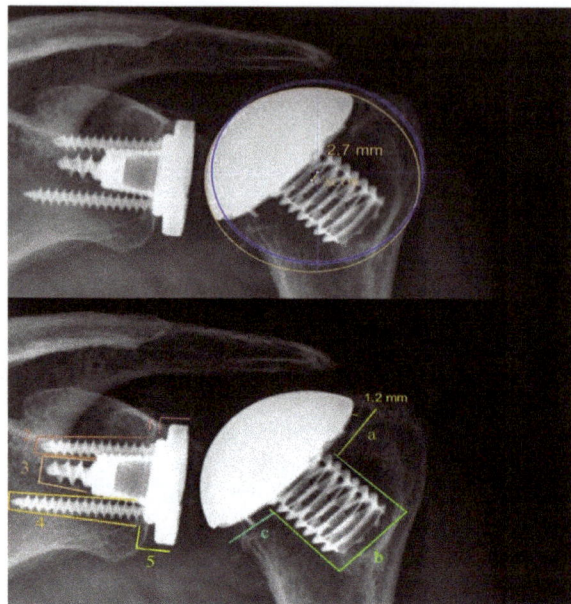

Figure 2. Postoperative radiographs of the left shoulder. The above X-ray image shows the anatomical circle (blue) and the implant-matched circle (orange), according to Alolabi et al. [11]. The distance between the two centers was measured (ΔCOR). In the X-ray image below, an assessment of radiolucent lines (RLs) for the glenoid and humeral components is shown. Glenoid RLs were quantified in 5 zones (1–5) considering their thickness, while the humeral RLs were quantified in 3 different zones (a, b, and c). The Radiograph shows radiolucency in zone a.

2.3. Statistical Analysis

For statistical analysis, a comparison was made between the values originally collected postoperatively and those collected at the follow-up examination. If the Shapiro–Wilk test did not obtain a normal distribution, the Wilcoxon test for paired samples was used instead. We also used descriptive statistics for data evaluation. The data were evaluated and compared using Origin Pro® 9.0 (OriginLab Corp, Northampton, MA, USA) and SPSS® 26.0 software (IBM Corp, Armonk, NY, USA). OriginLab® was used to create a Kaplan–Meier plot for the endpoints defined as revision for conversion to RSA and revision for any reason. Furthermore, common statistical methods, such as the mean values, medians, effect sizes, ranges, and standard deviations (SDs), were used in this study.

3. Results

None of the patients were lost to the follow-up. The average age of the patients at the time of surgery was 64.8 years (SD: 11.0) and, on the day of the examination, 70.9 (SD: 8.7) years. Most of the subjects received the prosthesis on their left shoulder, comprising 13 patients (52%). Among them, 12 patients were right-handed. A total of 12 patients had prostheses implanted on the non-dominant side. In all patients, an Eclipse™ humeral prosthesis combined with a Universal Glenoid™ baseplate from Arthrex® was implanted. The Univers 3D Metal Back is made of the Material Ti6Al4V. The Eclipse™ Humeral Head is made of the material CoCr, and the inlay is made of PE. The company of the tools, Arthrex Inc., is based in Naples, FL (34108-1945), USA. Details of the implants used in every patient were documented, and acceptable combinations between the size of the baseplate and humeral head in which the radii fit together properly were chosen for every patient. Table 1 shows patients' demographics, implant details, preoperative glenoid morphology, RTC degeneration, and postoperative deviation from the native center of rotation.

Table 1. Patient demographics and implants.

Case	Age at Implantation	Gender	Indication	Prosthesis Side r: Right l: Left	Baseplate Size	Inlay Size	Humeral Head Size	Preoperative CT/MRI	Walch Classification of the Glenoid	Fuchs Classification of Rotator Cuff	ΔCOR in mm
1	74	f	OA	r	m	m	45	MRI	A1	SC: 1, SS: 1, IS: 1, TM: 2	2.7
2	58	f	OA	l	s	s	39	MRI	A2	SC: 1, SS: 2, IS: 2, TM: 1	1.5
3	73	m	OA	r	l	l	47	MRI	A2	SC: 1, SS: 2, IS: 1, TM: 1	4.0
4	78	f	OA	l	m	m	43	MRI	A2	SC: 1, SS: 2, IS: 1, TM: 1	1.8
5	67	m	OA	r	l	l	47	MRI	A2	SC: 1, SS: 2, IS: 1, TM: 1	1.5
6	59	f	OA	r	s	s	41	MRI	A2	SC: 1, SS: 1, IS: 1, TM: 1	2.8
7	70	f	pOA	r	m	m	47	MRI	A1	SC: 1, SS: 1, IS: 1, TM: 1	2.6
8	74	f	OA	r	l	l	49	MRI	A2	SC: 2, SS: 2, IS: 2, TM: 1	1.2
9	76	f	OA	l	m	m	43	MRI	A1	SC: 1, SS: 2, IS: 2, TM: 1	4.1
10	49	m	OA	r	m	m	43	MRI	A2	SC: 1, SS: 1, IS: 1, TM: 1	0.8
11	45	f	OA	r	m	m	43	CT	A1	SC: 1, SS: 1, IS: 1, TM: 1	1.6
12	68	f	OA	l	m	m	43	MRI	A1	SC: 1, SS: 1, IS: 1, TM: 1	1.7
13	56	m	OA	r	m	m	45	CT	A1	SC: 1, SS: 1, IS: 1, TM: 1	1.1
14	68	m	OA	l	m	m	43	MRI	A2	SC: 1, SS: 1, IS: 1, TM: 2	0.9
15	65	f	OA	l	s	s	41	MRI	A1	SC: 1, SS: 1, IS: 1, TM: 1	0.8
16	60	f	OA	r	m	m	41	MRI	A2	SC: 1, SS: 1, IS: 1, TM: 1	1.2
17	62	m	OA	l	s	s	41	MRI	A1	SC: 1, SS: 1, IS: 1, TM: 1	2.5
18	59	f	OA	l	s	s	43	MRI	A1	SC: 1, SS: 1, IS: 1, TM: 1	1.5
19	56	m	OA	l	m	m	47	CT	A1	SC: 1, SS: 1, IS: 1, TM: 1	1.6
20	63	m	OA	l	s	s	41	MRI	A1	SC: 1, SS: 1, IS: 1, TM: 1	2.2
21	61	f	OA	l	s	s	39	MRI	A1	SC: 1, SS: 1, IS: 1, TM: 1	1.0
22	80	f	pOA	r	m	m	47	MRI	A2	SC: 1, SS: 1, IS: 1, TM: 1	1.5
23	72	m	OA	l	l	l	43	MRI	A2	SC: 1, SS: 1, IS: 1, TM: 1	2.3
24	49	f	OA	l	m	m	43	MRI	A2	SC: 1, SS: 2, IS: 1, TM: 1	1.5
25	76	m	OA	r	l	l	43	MRI	A1	SC: 1, SS: 1, IS: 1, TM: 1	1.8

Abbreviations: SC: M. subscapularis, SS: M. supraspinatus, IS: M. infraspinatus, TM: M. teres minor, OA: osteoarthritis, pOA: posttraumatic OA.

3.1. Clinical Outcome

The total score of CMS on the implanted arm at follow-up was, on average, 46.2 points (range: 14–77; SD: 19.5) in 25 patients. Of those patients, the average total score on the unaffected arm was 75.4 points (range: 22–100; SD: 18.4). On the assessment day, the average score on the affected arm in the strength area was 3.8 points (SD: 3.7). The patients rated the subjective pain classification using the VAS ranging from 0 to 15, with an average of 9.7 (SD: 3.7) out of 15 points. Only one participant (4%) achieved complete freedom from pain. The mean score for everyday activities was 12.8 (range: 3–20; SD: 5.3). At the follow-up examination, the mean score in the mobility range was 19.9 (range: 4–38; SD: 9.9). The results of the SST in the surveys had a mean score of 6.5 (range: 1–10; SD: 3.5), with a median of 8. The UCLA score was, on average, 5.9 (range: 1–9; SD: 2.1), with the median lying at 5 points.

3.2. Radiologic Outcome

In 22 patients (88%), RLs around the glenoid component were found. In 21 (84%) patients, the humeral component showed RLs. The overall mean Lazarus grade for the glenoid component was 2.1 points (range: 0–4; SD: 1.1; $p < 0.001$; effect size: 2.0). There were only two patients with an RL thicker than 2 mm. In detail, there were three patients with a Lazarus grade of 0 (12%), three patients with a grade of 1 (12%), eight patients with a grade of 2 (32%), ten patients with a grade of 3 (40%), one patient with a grade of 4 (4%) and none with a grade of 5. The overall mean points given by the classification according to Molé et al. [13] were 3.4 (range: 0–7; SD: 2.17; $p < 0.001$; effect size: 1.6). Most patients had a score of 3, followed by a score of 0 and 6, each with the same number of frequencies. No patient had a score of 1, and only one had a score of 7.

Upward migration of the humeral head was observed in all of the patients. The mean difference between the HHM value of the initial postoperative radiograph and the latest follow-up was 6.4 mm (range: 0.5–13.4; SD: 3.9; $p < 0.001$; effect size: 1.6). In 7 study participants, the humeral head migrated more than 10 mm. On the other hand, only two patients had an HHM of less than 1 mm.

In 23 out of 25 cases, polyethylene wear was detected after a mean follow-up of 62.3 months. For LGHO, the mean difference between the first postoperative radiograph and the last follow-up was 2.6 mm (range: 0–4.0; SD: 1.5; $p < 0.001$; effect size: 1.7). In most patients (9), the inlay wore between 2 and 4 mm. On the other hand, only four patients had an LGHO difference of 1 to 2 mm.

3.3. Complications and Revisions

Seventeen patients (8 women) were revised, mostly because of polyethylene wear. In patients undergoing revision surgery for any reason, the mean age at implantation of the anatomic prosthesis was 63.3 years (range: 45–80; SD: 10.5), and at revision, the average age was 68.8 years (range: 51–84; SD: 9.6). Among our study group, the probability of prosthesis survival was 32% (17 revisions) after a mean follow-up of 68.2 months (range: 1.8–119.6; SD: 27.9). In 12 cases (71%), PE wear was the most prevalent reason for revision surgery. Three patients had RTC injuries, and one patient had glenoid loosening as the cause of the revision. Only one patient developed a wound infection after surgery, resulting in the need for revision. Figure 3 shows the overall implant survival curve of our study. There, after around 75 months, the median has been reached. Afterward, the revision cases occurred more frequently in less amount of time. Censored were all patients on their last follow-up time who did not undergo revision surgery. In the graph, it can be seen that the first revision occurred quite early, after 1.8 months. The last revision occurred after 119.6 months. The graph shows that the first half of the revisions took 3/4 of the total time span. In contrast, most of the revisions were done after the midpoint of the timeline.

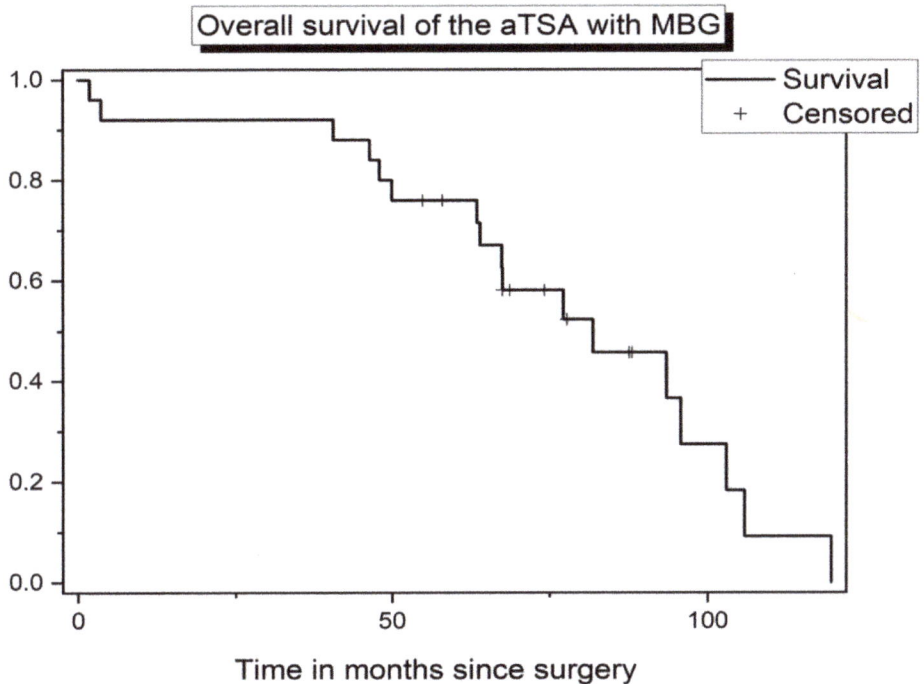

Figure 3. Kaplan–Meier plot depicting survival of the aTSA with MBG from implant revision for any reason among the study population.

Altogether, thirteen patients, seven of whom were female, were converted to RSA. Out of the 13 revision cases, there were different reasons for conversion to an RSA. With 85% (11 cases), the most common indication for revision was polyethylene wear. The remaining 2 cases had secondary RTC tears as reasons. In all of them, an explantation of the Eclipse™ implant and switch to Arthrex Reverse TSA was performed. The mean time to revision for conversion to RSA was 80.7 months (range: 40.5–152.6; SD: 30.9), whereas the mean age of the patients at revision was 71.2 years (range: 61–84; SD: 7.9). Figure 4 shows the Kaplan–Meier survival curve from conversion to RSA. The survival rate free of revision for conversion to RSA was 48% at 80.7 months. After approximately 85 months, half of the patients got conversion surgery to RSA. The median of revisions came in later than in the first Kaplan–Meier curve. The first conversion to RSA happened after 40.5 months and the last much later at 152.6 months, as seen in the Kaplan–Meier curve (Figure 4).

The time interval between the first and last revision is described in Figure 4 as considerably higher. Figure 5 shows a radiograph taken right before a revision for conversion to RSA, highlighting both PE wear and humeral implant loosening with varus-tilting.

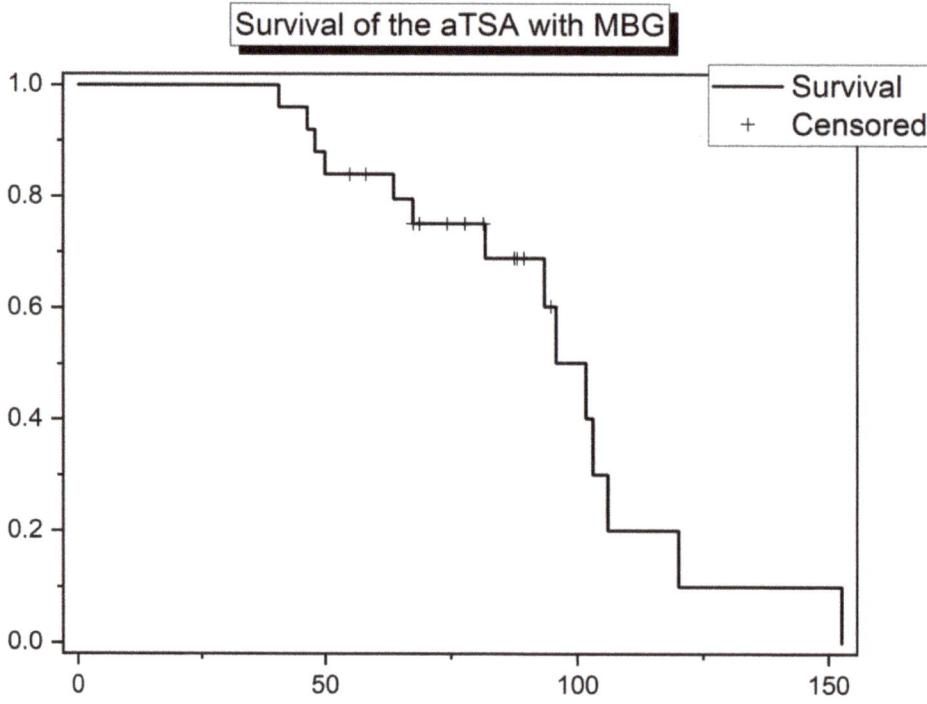

Figure 4. Kaplan–Meier plot depicting survival of the aTSA with MBG from implant revision for conversion to RSA among the study population.

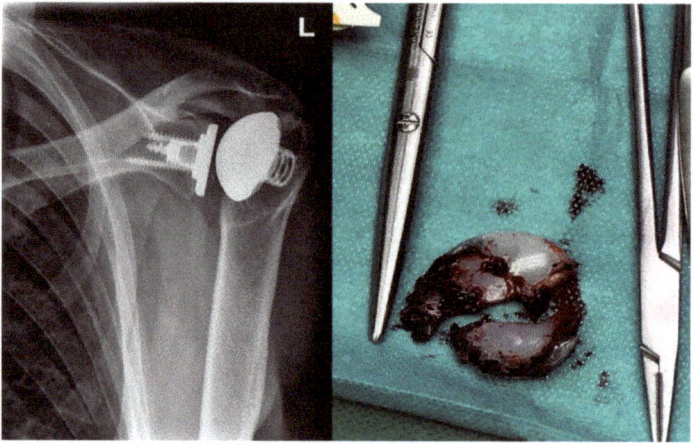

Figure 5. The image on the left side shows an X-ray taken shortly before a revision operation for conversion to RSA, demonstrating inlay abrasion with a tilt of the humeral head towards the metalback as a direct sign of inlay abrasion and loosening of the humeral component with varus-tilt due to osteolysis and PE wear. The image on the right side presents an intraoperative situs of the inlay after removal.

4. Discussion

Anatomical shoulder arthroplasty is an effective method for treating degenerative joint diseases if the bone substance is enough and the RTC is intact [14]. Nevertheless, compared to knee or hip replacements, TSAs have a relatively short lifespan, averaging ten years [15]. Therefore, each component of the shoulder prosthesis should be well chosen, aiming for the longest possible survival. Any part of the prosthesis can lead to revision surgery if it is not harmonized with the other components or is flawed.

At a mean follow-up of 68.2 months (range: 1.8–119.6; SD: 27.9), complete revision in our study cohort was required in 17 patients (68%), and 71% of shoulders undergoing revision (12 of 17) had PE wear as the main reason. These results were similar to findings from a study by Gauci et al. [16], in which a total of 26 out of 69 shoulders were revised, including 16 out of 26 shoulders in the MBG group. After a follow-up period of 12 years, the survival of the implants was 24% (SD: 0.10) for the metal-backed components. PE wear with metal-on-metal contact, RTC deficiency, and instability accounted for revision in the MBG group [16]. Gauci et al. [16] had a similar patient number, indications for revision, and survival rates. However, their follow-up period was longer than ours, so their findings may indicate what we have to deal with in the future, namely, a decrease in the survival of the implants. Over time, the chances of degenerative changes in the bone and deterioration of the inlay increase due to extended use of the shoulder joint after implantation of the prosthesis.

Another study conducted by Boileau et al. [17], also showed with 46% a very poor survival rate in 165 TSAs with 2 to 16 years of follow-up and a mean age of 68 years. These patients were diagnosed with primary OA and then treated with aTSA using an uncemented MBG component. The outcome for the survival rate free of revision was 46% at 12 years, with the endpoint for the survival curve defined as either complete or partial revision. Of the study population, 61 patients, or 37%, had undergone revision surgery after a mean follow-up of 8.5 years, 49 of whom had evidence of PE inlay wear [17]. It is worth mentioning that in our study, a similar rate of revisions was caused by PE wear. For the survival rates in our study, the longevity of the prostheses until revision surgery was reported. The mean follow-up was greater than ours, and our study's indication for aTSA with MBG was also mainly OA. The revisions of the patients in our study came in earlier. However, this study has a higher patient coverage.

To date, with 570 metal-backed TSAs, the most extensive series show low survival rates with MBG implants in aTSA with 95 revisions from a total of 121 accounting for metal-backed prostheses after 15 years [18]. This shows that prostheses with MBGs lead to increasing revision rates over time, rendering MBGs inadvisable for long-term use. A systematic literature search was conducted by Papadonikolakis and Matsen [19] regarding papers stating radiographic leakage, loosening, or revision of the glenoid component in aTSAs that had been carried out in patients of all ages and with any diagnosis. They found that when comparing 1571 MBG and 3035 full-PEG implants, the revision rate was more than three times higher for MBG components (14%) than for full-PE components (3.8%), according to the authors' findings. As many as 77% of revisions of full-PE components were due to loosening, whereas 62% of revisions of MBG components occurred due to other causes, such as PE wear, metal wear, component dissociation or fracture, screw fracture, and RTC tear [20]. Our age distribution correlates with similar results of specific studies published by Gauci et al. [16] and Taunton et al. [21]. Age could also play a considerable part in the results since older patients may have a lower functional demand than younger patients or tend to have higher rates of RTC deficiency, which correlates with patient age [22]. It has been argued that, in comparison to older patients, young patients have higher functional demands and higher expectations of enhanced capacity for social interaction, participation in sports, and exercise [23].

The mean age of our patients was 70.9 years. Similar mean patient age of 68 years was found in the study by Taunton et al. [21]. It was also found that at an average follow-up of 9.5 years, the five-year survival rate in this study was 79.9%, and the 10-year survival rate was 51.9%, leading the authors to express significant concern about the utilization of metal-backed, uncemented glenoid components [21,24].

In our study, the objective and subjective clinical results were poor. The clinical outcomes of our study were, in general, worse than those in similar studies on the topic of aTSA with MBG, especially for CMS. The flat profile design of our MBG and the screws with a small diameter that we used could contribute to the worse outcome, as not all studies compared had a flat MBG or utilized screws with a small diameter. Altogether, with the ADL score, which was on average 12.8 (64%), the most important domains for patients' quality of life were not as poor as might be expected. This could be mainly due to the advanced age of the patients and the relatively inactive life they lead. Almost all study participants were retirees who did not require high mobility. A similar negative result was found in a study by Clement et al. [25]. Therein, 49 shoulders with metal-backed glenoids of 39 patients had an average CMS of 33.5 after a minimum follow-up of 132 months. However, no patient was able to abduct their arm to 90 degrees pre- or postoperatively [25]. A study by Fucentese et al. [26] that examined the clinical and radiographic outcomes associated with the use of an uncemented soft-metal-backed glenoid component found a CMS of 65.9 in 22 patients after a mean follow-up of 50 months [26]. The study from Gauci et al. [16] had a CMS of 64, similar to the one from Fucentese et al. [26], which was found in 7 shoulders with MBG from 23 MBG prostheses, of which 16 were lost to follow-up, at a mean follow-up of 10.3 years [16]. In 2017, Kany et al. [27] noted a mean CMS of 56.6 and a mean SST of 6.7 points in their study of 14 TSAs with MBG [27]. This implies a poor outcome in MBG prostheses, which was also apparent in our case. Another study by Kany et al. [28] found a mean CMS score of 60 in a total of 26 cases, 16 of whom had TSA with MBG and a mean SST score of 8 [28]. The study by Kany et al. [28] had a similar patient outcome but a moderately better CMS and SST score than ours.

The radiological results are in concordance with the clinical results of our study. These radiographic results reaffirm the poor clinical scores. The radiological results correlate with the clinical results.

In our study, there was a huge difference in RLs from the first postoperative radiographic control to the follow-up. At follow-up, 22 patients (88%) had one or more RLs on the glenoid, and 21 patients (84%) had RLs on the humeral components, whereas none were found at the first postoperative admission. In contrast, the study by Boileau et al. [29] showed RLs in only 5 of a total of 20 shoulders with an MBG after a mean follow-up of 38.4 months [29]. For the humeral component, Gallacher et al. [14] analyzed a total of 100 shoulders from 86 patients with a mean follow-up of 35.4 months (range 24–76 months). The study found that 12% had incomplete RLs, and 4% had complete RLs [14]. Magosch et al. [30] conducted a study of 48 TSA-implanted patients with MBG who were clinically and radiologically followed up with a mean of 49 months. They found in total 4 cases of incomplete RLs, two cases with under 1 mm of thickness, and 2 cases with RLs < 2 mm. As in our study, they did not find glenoid component loosening in their cases. However, we had more cases with RLs using the same prosthesis type as Magosch et al. [30]. In summary, 8 cases from their study required revision [30,31]. Unlike other studies, ours had a large number of RLs. The high amount of PE wear could be responsible for this. However, none of the MBGs at the follow-up were loose despite RLs and rarefication due to PE wear. Furthermore, in the literature, it has been reported that the prevalence of RLs in TSA ranges from 22% to 95%, and they occur in both types of glenoids, whether they are cemented or uncemented. However, evaluation of radiolucency from radiographs is prone to error, with standardization of patient position being difficult due to scapulothoracic mobility and individual anatomic differences. The lack of a standardized scoring system makes the comparison of findings challenging [32]. RLs rates were shown to be highly variable throughout studies, complicating comparisons of related factors.

HHM was detected on the AP radiographs in all patients within our study. Clinically, proximal humerus migration is important because it implicates a disturbance of normal glenohumeral kinematics from which advanced RTC disease is often a sign [33]. There was a mean difference between the HHM of the first postoperative radiograph and the last follow-up of 6.4 mm (range: 0.5–13.4; SD: 3.9; effect size: 1.6). This indicates a serious disturbance of normal glenohumeral kinematics. Montoya et al. [34] observed HHM in 8 of 53 patients after a mean follow-up of 64 months [34]. A comparison of HHM between our study and other findings in the literature reveals that HHM is more common in our study, but for the most part, the level of upward migration is rather moderate.

Regarding the LGHO, we see a similar pattern. Among 25 patients, 23 developed PE wear. In some patients, the MBG also showed signs of wear to some extent. The LGHO in our study had a mean difference between the first postoperative imaging and the follow-up of 2.6 mm (range: 0–4.0; SD: 1.5; effect size: 1.7). All patients who underwent revision had radiographic signs of wear of the glenoid component as well as superior HHM at follow-up. It has been shown by biomechanical and clinical studies that MBG implants used in aTSA have adverse effects on both the PE and the underlying glenoid bone [20]. In the future, finite element computational analysis (in silico) will allow implant designs to be tested and improved in advance. This could help reduce PE wear and therefore support the longevity of shoulder prostheses with an MBG [35,36].

Long-term studies of MBG implants and their LGHO measurements on radiographs are lacking, making comparative studies scarce. Nevertheless, this is an important issue that can be used to dispute the beneficial effect of MBG components in aTSA, as almost all individuals in the study population received HHM, RLs, and LGHO. Analysis of the results for clinical scores showed a similar trend as described above for radiological outcomes.

In summary, the propagated advantage of the new modular MBG components concerning prosthesis survivability cannot be confirmed in our study. The clinical results are consistent with the radiological results, which are also unacceptably poor.

The study conducted had some limitations. The number of patients was relatively low at 25. We did not include a control group for comparison purposes. A comparison group would be desirable, especially in view of the unusually high complication and revision rate. The results of the present study are also compared against old MBGs with known technical problems and a significantly longer follow-up.

Due to the fact that angles and lengths are impacted by the location of the scapula and the humerus rotation, all radiographic measures are strongly reliant on the patient's orientation during radiographic imaging. Radiographic imaging, even when standardized, can reveal massive differences. However, no patients were lost to follow-up. In addition, the same implant was used throughout the entire study population, with the same surgical technique being performed by two experienced shoulder surgeons.

5. Conclusions

In conclusion, considering all previously mentioned aspects, aTSAs with MBG provide poor clinical and radiological outcomes. Concerns from previous studies were fulfilled in that anatomic shoulder prostheses with an MBG present rapid inlay wear and have a low survival rate, reaching 32% in our study at 68.2 months. In the future, further long-term follow-up studies on modern MBGs need to be carried out, with more participants and the inclusion of a control group.

Author Contributions: Conceptualization, E.N. and R.O.; methodology, R.O.; software, E.N.; validation, R.O., E.N. and F.R.; formal analysis, H.K.; investigation, E.N.; resources, F.R.; data curation, E.N.; writing—original draft preparation, E.N.; writing—review and editing, E.N.; visualization, E.N.; supervision, R.O.; project administration, R.O.; funding acquisition, R.O. All authors have read and agreed to the published version of the manuscript.

Funding: This research received no external funding.

Institutional Review Board Statement: The study was conducted in accordance with the Declaration of Helsinki, and approved by the local Ethics Committee of the state of Upper Austria (Study number 1167/2020).

Informed Consent Statement: Informed consent was obtained from all subjects involved in the study.

Data Availability Statement: All data relevant to the study are included in the article. Details regarding where data supporting reported results can be asked at the following e-mail address: emil.noschaj@yahoo.de.

Conflicts of Interest: The authors declare no conflict of interest.

References

1. Kim, S.H.; Wise, B.L.; Zhang, Y.; Szabo, R.M. Increasing incidence of shoulder arthroplasty in the United States. *J. Bone Jt. Surg.* **2011**, *93*, 2249–2254. [CrossRef] [PubMed]
2. Best, M.J.; Aziz, K.T.; Wilckens, J.H.; McFarland, E.G.; Srikumaran, U. Increasing incidence of primary reverse and anatomic total shoulder arthroplasty in the United States. *J. Shoulder Elb. Surg.* **2021**, *30*, 1159–1166. [CrossRef] [PubMed]
3. Wiater, J.M.; Fabing, M.H. Shoulder arthroplasty: Prosthetic options and indications. *J. Am. Acad. Orthop. Surg.* **2009**, *17*, 415–425. [CrossRef] [PubMed]
4. Bonnevialle, N.; Melis, B.; Neyton, L.; Favard, L.; Mole, D.; Walch, G.; Boileau, P. Aseptic glenoid loosening or failure in total shoulder arthroplasty: Revision with glenoid reimplantation. *J. Shoulder Elb. Surg.* **2013**, *22*, 745–751. [CrossRef] [PubMed]
5. Somerson, J.S.; Hsu, J.E.; Neradilek, M.B.; Matsen, F.A., 3rd. Analysis of 4063 complications of shoulder arthroplasty reported to the US Food and Drug Administration from 2012 to 2016. *J. Shoulder Elb. Surg.* **2018**, *27*, 1978–1986. [CrossRef] [PubMed]
6. Kim, D.M.; Aldeghaither, M.; Alabdullatif, F.; Shin, M.J.; Kholinne, E.; Kim, H.; Jeon, I.H.; Koh, K.H. Loosening and revision rates after total shoulder arthroplasty: A systematic review of cemented all-polyethylene glenoid and three modern designs of metal-backed glenoid. *BMC Musculoskelet. Disord.* **2020**, *21*, 114. [CrossRef] [PubMed]
7. Gustas-French, C.; Petscavage-Thomas, J.; Bernard, S.A. Imaging of Shoulder Arthroplasties. *AJR Am. J. Roentgenol.* **2018**, *211*, 485–495. [CrossRef] [PubMed]
8. Castagna, A.; Garofalo, R. Journey of the glenoid in anatomic total shoulder replacement. *Shoulder Elb.* **2019**, *11*, 140–148. [CrossRef] [PubMed]
9. Fuchs, B.; Weishaupt, D.; Zanetti, M.; Hodler, J.; Gerber, C. Fatty degeneration of the muscles of the rotator cuff: Assessment by computed tomography versus magnetic resonance imaging. *J. Shoulder Elb. Surg.* **1999**, *8*, 599–605. [CrossRef]
10. Walch, G.; Badet, R.; Boulahia, A.; Khoury, A. Morphologic study of the glenoid in primary glenohumeral osteoarthritis. *J. Arthroplast.* **1999**, *14*, 756–760. [CrossRef]
11. Alolabi, B.; Youderian, A.R.; Napolitano, L.; Szerlip, B.W.; Evans, P.J.; Nowinski, R.J.; Ricchetti, E.T.; Iannotti, J.P. Radiographic assessment of prosthetic humeral head size after anatomic shoulder arthroplasty. *J. Shoulder Elb. Surg.* **2014**, *23*, 1740–1746. [CrossRef] [PubMed]
12. Lazarus, M.D.; Jensen, K.L.; Southworth, C.; Matsen, F.A., 3rd. The radiographic evaluation of keeled and pegged glenoid component insertion. *J. Bone Jt. Surg.* **2002**, *84*, 1174–1182. [CrossRef] [PubMed]
13. Molé, D.; Roche, O.; Riand, N.; Lévigne, C.; Walch, G. Cemented glenoid component: Results in osteoarthritis and rheumatoid arthritis. In *Shoulder Arthroplasty*; Springer: Berlin/Heidelberg, Germany, 1999; pp. 163–171.
14. Gallacher, S.; Williams, H.L.M.; King, A.; Kitson, J.; Smith, C.D.; Thomas, W.J. Clinical and radiologic outcomes following total shoulder arthroplasty using Arthrex Eclipse stemless humeral component with minimum 2 years' follow-up. *J. Shoulder Elb. Surg.* **2018**, *27*, 2191–2197. [CrossRef]
15. Gregory, T.M.; Boukebous, B.; Gregory, J.; Pierrart, J.; Masemjean, E. Short, Medium and Long Term Complications After Total Anatomical Shoulder Arthroplasty. *Open Orthop. J.* **2017**, *11*, 1133–1141. [CrossRef] [PubMed]
16. Gauci, M.O.; Bonnevialle, N.; Moineau, G.; Baba, M.; Walch, G.; Boileau, P. Anatomical total shoulder arthroplasty in young patients with osteoarthritis: All-polyethylene versus metal-backed glenoid. *Bone Jt. J.* **2018**, *100-B*, 485–492. [CrossRef] [PubMed]
17. Boileau, P.; Moineau, G.; Morin-Salvo, N.; Avidor, C.; Godenèche, A.; Lévigne, C.; Baba, M.; Walch, G. Metal-backed glenoid implant with polyethylene insert is not a viable long-term therapeutic option. *J. Shoulder Elb. Surg.* **2015**, *24*, 1534–1543. [CrossRef] [PubMed]
18. Fox, T.J.; Cil, A.; Sperling, J.W.; Sanchez-Sotelo, J.; Schleck, C.D.; Cofield, R.H. Survival of the glenoid component in shoulder arthroplasty. *J. Shoulder Elb. Surg.* **2009**, *18*, 859–863. [CrossRef]
19. Papadonikolakis, A.; Matsen, F.A.I. Metal-Backed Glenoid Components Have a Higher Rate of Failure and Fail by Different Modes in Comparison with All-Polyethylene Components: A Systematic Review. *J. Bone Jt. Surg.* **2014**, *96*, 1041–1047. [CrossRef] [PubMed]
20. Boileau, P.; Baba, M.; Moineau, G.; Morin-Salvo, N.; Avidor, C.; Godenèche, A.; Lévigne, C.; Walch, G. Response to Katz et al: The weak link in metal-backed glenoid implants is the polyethylene. *J. Shoulder Elb. Surg.* **2016**, *25*, e396–e398. [CrossRef] [PubMed]
21. Taunton, M.J.; McIntosh, A.L.; Sperling, J.W.; Cofield, R.H. Total shoulder arthroplasty with a metal-backed, bone-ingrowth glenoid component. Medium to long-term results. *J. Bone Jt. Surg.* **2008**, *90*, 2180–2188. [CrossRef]
22. Khazzam, M.; Sager, B.; Box, H.N.; Wallace, S.B. The effect of age on risk of retear after rotator cuff repair: A systematic review and meta-analysis. *JSES Int.* **2020**, *4*, 625–631. [CrossRef] [PubMed]
23. Rasmussen, J.V.; Olsen, B.S. Previous surgery for instability is a risk factor for a worse patient-reported outcome after anatomical shoulder arthroplasty for osteoarthritis: A Danish nationwide cohort study of 3,743 arthroplasties. *Acta Orthop.* **2022**, *93*, 588–592. [CrossRef] [PubMed]

24. Schrumpf, M.; Maak, T.; Hammoud, S.; Craig, E.V. The glenoid in total shoulder arthroplasty. *Curr. Rev. Musculoskelet. Med.* **2011**, *4*, 191–199. [CrossRef] [PubMed]
25. Clement, N.D.; Mathur, K.; Colling, R.; Stirrat, A.N. The metal-backed glenoid component in rheumatoid disease: Eight- to fourteen-year follow-up. *J. Shoulder Elb. Surg.* **2010**, *19*, 749–756. [CrossRef] [PubMed]
26. Fucentese, S.F.; Costouros, J.G.; Kühnel, S.P.; Gerber, C. Total shoulder arthroplasty with an uncemented soft-metal-backed glenoid component. *J. Shoulder Elb. Surg.* **2010**, *19*, 624–631. [CrossRef] [PubMed]
27. Kany, J.; Jose, J.; Katz, D.; Werthel, J.D.; Sekaran, P.; Amaravathi, R.S.; Valenti, P. The main cause of instability after unconstrained shoulder prosthesis is soft tissue deficiency. *J. Shoulder Elb. Surg.* **2017**, *26*, e243–e251. [CrossRef] [PubMed]
28. Kany, J.; Amouyel, T.; Flamand, O.; Katz, D.; Valenti, P. A convertible shoulder system: Is it useful in total shoulder arthroplasty revisions? *Int. Orthop.* **2015**, *39*, 299–304. [CrossRef] [PubMed]
29. Boileau, P.; Avidor, C.; Krishnan, S.G.; Walch, G.; Kempf, J.F.; Molé, D. Cemented polyethylene versus uncemented metal-backed glenoid components in total shoulder arthroplasty: A prospective, double-blind, randomized study. *J. Shoulder Elb. Surg.* **2002**, *11*, 351–359. [CrossRef] [PubMed]
30. Magosch, P.; Lichtenberg, S.; Tauber, M.; Martetschläger, F.; Habermeyer, P. Prospective midterm results of a new convertible glenoid component in anatomic shoulder arthroplasty: A cohort study. *Arch. Orthop. Trauma Surg.* **2021**, *141*, 717–724. [CrossRef] [PubMed]
31. Magosch, P.; Habermeyer, P.; Vetter, P. Radiologic midterm results of cemented and uncemented glenoid components in primary osteoarthritis of the shoulder: A matched pair analysis. *Arch. Orthop. Trauma Surg.* **2021**, 1–11. [CrossRef] [PubMed]
32. Castagna, A.; Randelli, M.; Garofalo, R.; Maradei, L.; Giardella, A.; Borroni, M. Mid-term results of a metal-backed glenoid component in total shoulder replacement. *J. Bone Jt. Surg.* **2010**, *92*, 1410–1415. [CrossRef] [PubMed]
33. Keener, J.D.; Wei, A.S.; Kim, H.M.; Steger-May, K.; Yamaguchi, K. Proximal humeral migration in shoulders with symptomatic and asymptomatic rotator cuff tears. *J. Bone Jt. Surg.* **2009**, *91*, 1405–1413. [CrossRef] [PubMed]
34. Montoya, F.; Magosch, P.; Scheiderer, B.; Lichtenberg, S.; Melean, P.; Habermeyer, P. Midterm results of a total shoulder prosthesis fixed with a cementless glenoid component. *J. Shoulder Elb. Surg.* **2013**, *22*, 628–635. [CrossRef] [PubMed]
35. Ammarullah, M.I.; Afif, I.Y.; Maula, M.I.; Winarni, T.I.; Tauviqirrahman, M.; Jamari, J. Tresca stress evaluation of Metal-on-UHMWPE total hip arthroplasty during peak loading from normal walking activity. *Mater. Today Proc.* **2022**, *63*, S143–S146. [CrossRef]
36. Jamari, J.; Ammarullah, M.I.; Saad, A.P.M.; Syahrom, A.; Uddin, M.; van der Heide, E.; Basri, H. The Effect of Bottom Profile Dimples on the Femoral Head on Wear in Metal-on-Metal Total Hip Arthroplasty. *J. Funct. Biomater.* **2021**, *12*, 38. [CrossRef] [PubMed]

Article

Clinical and Radiological Results of Hemiarthroplasty and Total Shoulder Arthroplasty for Primary Avascular Necrosis of the Humeral Head in Patients Less than 60 Years Old

Anthony Hervé [1,*], Mickael Chelli [2], Pascal Boileau [2], Gilles Walch [3], Luc Favard [4], Christophe Levigne [5], François Sirveaux [6], Philippe Clavert [7], Nicolas Bonnevialle [8] and Philippe Collin [9]

1. Rennes Ortho Sport, Polyclinique St Laurent Rennes, 35000 Rennes, France
2. Institut de Chirurgie Réparatrice Locomoteur et Sports, 06004 Nice, France; mickael.chelli@gmail.com (M.C.); boileau.pascal@wanadoo.fr (P.B.)
3. Clinique Santy, 69008 Lyon, France; gilleswalch15@gmail.com
4. CHU Tours, 37000 Tours, France; luc.favard@wanadoo.fr
5. Clinique du Parc, 69006 Lyon, France; dr.levigne@cliniqueduparclyon.fr
6. CHU Nancy, 54000 Nancy, France; francois.sirveaux@wanadoo.fr
7. CHU Strasbourg, 67200 Strasbourg, France; philippe.clavert@chru-strasbourg.fr
8. CHU Toulouse Pierre Paul Ricquet, 31300 Tolouse, France; nicolasbonnevialle@wanadoo.fr
9. Institut Locomoteur de l'Ouest, CHP St Grégoire, 35760 Saint Grégoire, France; docphcollin@gmail.com
* Correspondence: drhervebuard@gmail.com; Tel.: +33-0299256740

Abstract: Background: Total shoulder arthroplasty (TSA) and hemiarthroplasty (HA) have shown good clinical outcomes in primary avascular necrosis of the humeral head (PANHH) both in short and long terms. The purpose of this study was to assess the complications, the clinical and radiological outcomes of shoulder arthroplasty in young patients with PANHH. Methods: One hundred and twenty-seven patients aged under 60 years old and suffering from PANHH were operated with arthroplasty. Patients were assessed clinically and radiographically before surgery with a minimum of 2 years of follow up (FU). Results: HA was performed on 108 patients (85%). Two patients were revised for painful glenoid wear after 2 and 4 years. TSA was performed on 19 patients (15%). Five TSA had to be revised for glenoid loosening ($n = 4$) or instability ($n = 1$). Revision rate was 26% with TSA and 2% with HA. There were no significant differences between HA and TSA in terms of clinical outcomes. Conclusions: With a mean FU of 8 years, HA and TSA improved clinical outcomes of patients with PANHH. HA revisions for painful glenoid wear were rare (2%). The revision rate was excessively high with TSA (26%).

Keywords: shoulder arthroplasty; glenohumeral osteoarthritis; avascular necrosis of the humeral head; hemi arthroplasty; total shoulder arthroplasty; young patients

1. Introduction

Primary avascular necrosis of the humeral head (PANHH) is the result of the necrosis of the bone tissue and bone marrow of the humeral head. It often affects patients in their 4th or 5th decade. While many etiologies are linked to corticosteroid therapy or alcohol abuse, most of the time no causes are identified. Several studies have investigated the results of shoulder arthroplasty for PANHH. Total shoulder arthroplasty (TSA) [1–5] and hemiarthroplasty (HA) [1,6–11] have shown satisfactory clinical outcomes in short-, mid- and long-term follow-up (FU). It has been well demonstrated that post-traumatic necrosis resulted in inferior outcomes than PANHH [1,12,13]. Only two studies [1,4] have compared the results of HA and TSA but gathered primary and post-traumatic AVHH [1] or the two groups were not comparative in terms of age and age related factor [4]. Therefore, our aim was to assess the complications, the clinical and radiological outcomes of shoulder arthroplasty for PANHH in patients aged 60 years old or younger at the time of the surgery. The hypotheses were that HA and TSA would (1) both improve clinical outcomes during the FU midterm (2) but would differ with TSA having a higher rate of complication than HA.

2. Materials and Methods

2.1. Patients

A multicenter retrospective study among 9 centers was conducted. Inclusion criteria were patients suffering from PANHH operated with total shoulder arthroplasty (TSA) or hemiarthroplasty (HA), aged 60 years old or under at the time of the surgery. Exclusion criteria were post-traumatic avascular necrosis, and less than 2 years between surgery and last follow-up (FU) for clinical and radiological analysis.

One hundred and twenty-seven patients were operated between 1991 and 2015 with a mean age of 46 years old (SD 10, range 19–60): 108 HA and 19 TSA. The etiologies of PANHH were Churg and Strauss disease (n = 2), corticotherapy for Hodgkin lymphoma (n = 2), drepanocytosis (n = 1) and post-radiotherapy (n = 1). For the other 121 patients (95%), no specific etiologies were found, and osteonecrosis was therefore classified as idiopathic. Five patients had undergone conservative treatment prior to arthroplasty: micro-fractures (n = 3), arthroscopic suprasupinatus repair (n = 1) and acromioplasty (n = 1).

We evaluated clinical outcomes with passive and active range of motion using the Constant score [14] and Subjective shoulder value [15] (SSV). Radiographic evaluation consisted of true anteroposterior radiographs of the gleno-humeral joint using a standardized protocol during the preoperative evaluation and the last follow-up. The osteonecrosis severity was assessed with Ficat's [16] classification modified by Cruess [17] (Table 1).

Table 1. Pre-operative radiographs assessed by Ficat's classification modified by Cruess.

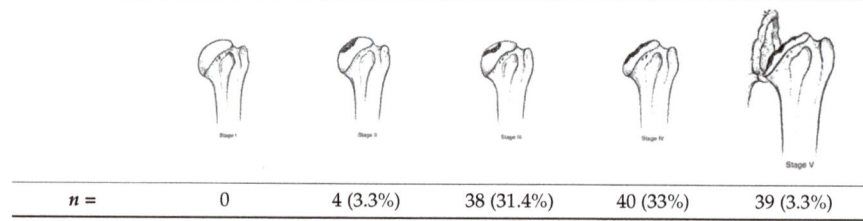

n =	0	4 (3.3%)	38 (31.4%)	40 (33%)	39 (3.3%)

Radiographs were evaluated by a senior and a resident orthopedic surgeon. Pre-operative radiographs were missing for 6 patients. Radiolucent lines (RLL) around the humeral stem and the glenoid component (of TSA) were assessed with Mole score [18]. All patients provided informed consent for their participation in this study, which had been approved by the institutional review board.

2.2. Operative Technique

The operative technique was performed in a beach-chair position under general anesthesia with an inter-scalene block. The surgical approach was almost exclusively deltopectoral and anterosuperior in 2 cases (2%). Tenodesis and subscapularis repair were systematic. For 2 patients (2 HA), the cuff tear was also repaired while undergoing the arthroplasty. The type of arthroplasty was left to the operator's choice and to the severity of the osteoarthritis.

2.3. Hemiarthroplasty Group

Hemiarthroplasty was performed on 108 patients (85%). On pre-operative radiographs, Ficat and Cruess classification stages were in 12 times stage 2, in 36 times stage 3, in 37 times stage 4 and in 21 times stage 5. Two pre-operative radiographs were missing (1, 8%). Hemi-metal implants were implanted 67 times (62%), 6 (5%) hemi pyrocarbone, 19

(18%) pyrocarbone interposition (PI) sphere and 16 (15%) resurfacing. Overall a stem was used in 67% of times. Hemi-metal implants included 63 Aequalis Anatomic (Tornier SAS-Wright Medical, Bloomington, MN, USA). Among them 6 were uncemented. Otherwise 4 uncemented Ascend flex anatomic were used (Tornier SAS-Wright Medical). Hemi-pyrocarbone implants were uncemented Ascend Flex anatomic stems (Tornier SAS-Wright Medical). PI spheres corresponded to Inspyre implant (Tornier SAS-Wright Medical). Resurfacing and stemless implants consisted of 6 Aequalis Resurfacing Head (Tornier SAS-Wright Medical), 4 Copeland (Biomet, Inc., Warsaw, IN, USA), 2 Global Cap Resurfacing (DePuy Orthopaedics, Warsaw, IN, USA), 2 TESS (Total Evolutive Shoulder System) (Biomet, Inc., Warsaw, IN, USA), 1 HemiCAP-Arthrosurface® system (Arthrosurface, Inc., Franklin, MA, USA) and 1 Affinis stemless (Mathys, Bettlach, Switzerland).

2.4. Total Anatomic Arthroplasty

Total anatomic arthroplasty was performed on 19 patients (15%). On pre-operative radiographs, Ficat and Cruess classification was in 1 time stage 3 and in 14 times stage 5. Four pre-operative radiographs were missing. On the glenoid side, 3 (16%) metal-backed and 16 (84%) keeled full polyethylene (PE) components were used. Humeral stems consisted of Aequalis anatomic for 17 (Tornier SAS-Wright Medical) and Ascend flex stems (Tornier SAS-Wright Medical) for 2. The stem was cemented for 78% of the procedures.

2.5. Statistical Analysis

Data collection and statistical analysis were investigated with the free online software EasyMedStat (www.easymedstat.com; Neuilly-Sur-Seine; France). Continuous data were expressed as mean (standard deviation, minimum–maximum) and categorical data were given as absolute and relative frequencies (%). To compare differences between preoperative and last FU data, the Student t-test for paired data or the Wilcoxon signed-rank test were used accordingly. Survival rate without a revision surgery and its 5% pointwise confidence intervals were estimated with the method of Kaplan Meier. The significance level was set at $p < 0.05$.

3. Results

3.1. Postoperative Complications

Thirteen patients (9%) suffered from postoperative complications: 6 (6%) in the HA group and 7 (37%) in the TSA group (OR = 9.9; 95% CI = (2.9; 34.4); $p < 0.001$). In the HA group, 2 painful glenoid wear complications were observed as well as 1 humeral shaft fracture, 1 coagulase-negative Staphylococcus infection, 1 cuff tear involving supraspinatus and subscapularis, and 1 ulnar nerve palsy which recovered in 3 months. In the TSA group, one patient had an immediate posterior dislocation with a metal-back glenoid.

3.2. Reoperations

Three HA were reoperated without a humeral stem revision: One patient suffered from a humerus shaft fracture after a trauma and was treated by plating. Another patient had a massive cuff tear type A [19] after a severe trauma in a motor bike accident and was repaired with an open approach. The last patient had an arthroscopic biopsy due to acute pain which appeared one year after the surgery. Bacterial cultures were negatives. During the last FU (116 months after), this last patient's range of motion was excellent. Nevertheless, Constant score was 61, especially because the patient was still in pain. None of the TSA that needed to be reoperated had to undergo a revision of prosthetic components.

3.3. Revisions

Revision surgery was required for 7 patients (6%) including 2 HA (2%) and 5 TSA (26%) (OR = 20; 95% CI = 4–116); $p < 0.001$). Survival rate without revision at 5 years was 97% (89–99%) for HA and 97% (89–99%) for TSA. At 10 years, survival rate without revision was 95% (68–99%) for HA and 57% (19–82%) for TSA ($p < 0.001$) (Figure 1).

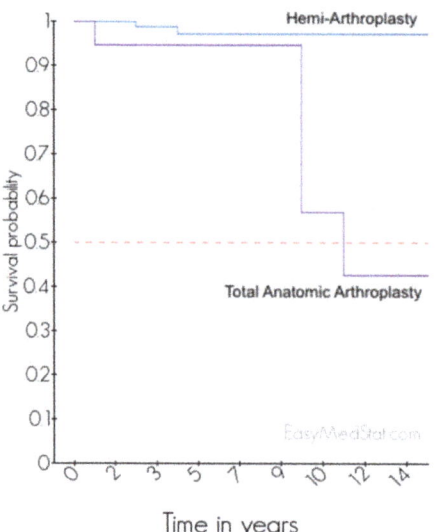

Figure 1. Survival curve of HA and TSA after PANHH.

In the HA group, 2 were revised for glenoid wear. The stage of Ficat's classification in pre-operative radiographs was stage 3. The first one was a resurfacing HA (Figure 2) complicated with painful glenoid wear at 49 months and reoperated with a pyrocarbone HA. During the final FU, 2 years after the revision surgery, the Constant score was 55 and SSV 80%.

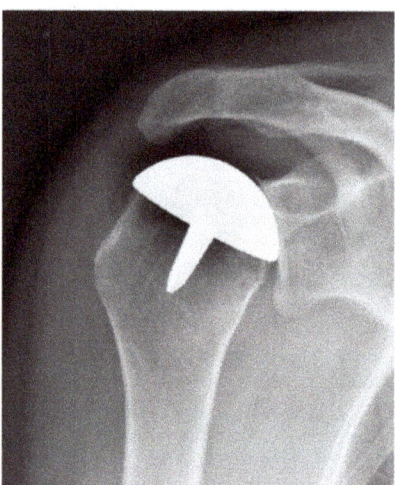

Figure 2. Resurfacing complicated by glenoid wear at 49 months of FU.

The second case was a metal HA where glenoid wear occurred at 25 months of FU (Figure 3). The humeral stem was unchanged and a cemented full PE glenoid was implanted. During the final FU, 3 years after the revision surgery, the Constant score was 57 and SSV 70%.

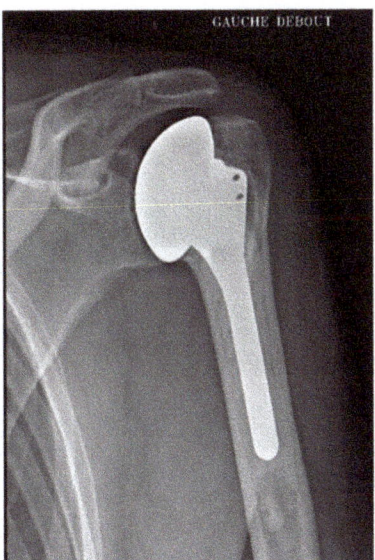

Figure 3. HA metal complicated by glenoid wear at 25 months of FU.

In the TSA group, one patient who had a posterior instability underwent a full-PE implant but due to a glenoid loosening 5 years later, it lead to a definitive explanation of both humeral and glenoid components with a poor functional result (CS = 15). Three patients with glenoid loosening were reoperated using HA (Figure 4).

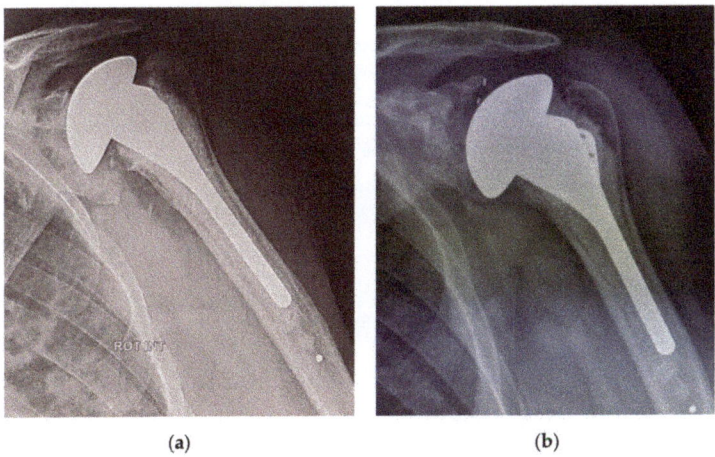

(a) (b)

Figure 4. (a) TSA complication due to glenoid loosening at 9 years FU and (b) reoperated using an HA.

3.4. Clinical Outcomes

For clinical and radiological analysis, patients who had their FU within 2 years, and those who sustained a revision of their primary arthroplasty were excluded, leaving 92 patients: 83 HA with a mean FU of 8.2 years (SD: 5.2, range: 2–26) and 9 TSA with a mean FU of 8.8 years (SD: 5.6, range: 2–18) ($p = 0.84$). At the last FU, both HA and TSA were significantly improved regarding CS, and SSV ($p < 0.01$) with a mean CS of 76 for HA and 71 for TSA ($p = 0.35$). Details and range of motion are provided in Table 2.

Table 2. Clinical outcomes in hemi-arthroplasty and total anatomic arthroplasty surgeries.

	Forward Elevation (°)	External Rotation (°)	Internal Rotation (/10)	CS (/100)	SSV (%)
	Hemi-arthroplasty (n = 83)				
Preoperative	105 ± 37 (30–180)	22 ± 18 (−10–70)	4.7 ± 2.5 (0–10)	37 ± 14 (10–71)	39 ± 17 (5–70)
Last FU	154 ± 23 (90–180)	39 ± 19 (−10–85)	7.1 ± 1.9 (2–10)	76 ± 11 (50–96)	87 ± 13 (60–100)
p-Value [a]	<0.001 *	<0.001 *	<0.001 *	<0.001 *	<0.001 *
	Total Anatomic Arthroplasty (n = 9)				
Preoperative	112 ± 29 (80–160)	14 ± 19 (−10–45)	4.2 ± 2.9 (0–10)	43 ± 11 (28–55)	33 ± 14 (20–50)
Last FU	142 ± 33 (90–170)	39 ± 18 (10–60)	6.2 ± 2.9 (2–10)	71 ± 20 (43–94)	73 ± 6 (70–80)
p-Value [a]	0.055	<0.01 *	0.022 *	<0.01 *	<0.001 *

[a] p-Value for the difference between preoperative and last FU (Wilcoxon signed-rank test * $p < 0.05$).

3.5. Radiological Analysis

At last FU, the mean humeral RLL score was 0.02 (range 0–1) for HA and 2.0 (range 0–6) for TSA ($p = 0.002$). In the HA group, there was no significant trend between glenoid bone wear and the pre-operative stage of Ficat and Cruess classification ($p > 0.05$). In the TSA group, the mean glenoid RLL score was 5.2 (range 0–18) with 2 migrated glenoid implants, considered as loosened but no revision surgery had been done (CS = 49 and 67). After 7 to 10 years postoperatively, glenoid loosening was observed in 6 patients who had not received revision surgery. There was no significant trend between glenoid loosening and the pre-operative stage of Ficat and Cruess classification ($p > 0.05$).

3.6. Comparison between Different Hemi-Arthroplasties

There were no significant differences between HA regarding postoperative complications, revision surgery and clinical outcomes (Table 3).

Table 3. Comparison of complications, revision surgery and clinical outcomes among different hemi-arthroplasties.

	Metal-Head (n = 67)	Pyrocarbon (n = 6)	Resurfacing (n = 16)	Interposition Sphere (n = 19)	p-Value
Postoperative Complication (%)	6%	0%	6%	5%	1
Revision surgery (%)	1%	0%	6%	0%	0.40
	Metal-Head (n = 47)	Pyrocarbon (n = 5)	Resurfacing (n = 13)	Interposition Sphere (n = 18)	p-Value
Forward Elevation (°)	155 ± 22 (90–180)	148 ± 27 (110–170)	149 ± 27 (100–180)	154 ± 23 (110–180)	0.98
External Rotation (°)	35 ± 18 (−10–70)	53 ± 15 (45–80)	44 ± 16 (20–70)	42 ± 21 (−10–85)	0.09
Internal Rotation (/10)	6.6 ± 2.0 (2–10)	8.4 ± 1.7 (6–10)	6.8 ± 2.4 (4–10)	7.7 ± 1.5 (4–10)	0.14
Constant Score (/100)	73 ± 14 (30–91)	75 ± 10 (61–89)	75 ± 13 (54–96)	78 ± 10 (61–95)	0.79
SSV (%)	82 ± 21 (40–100)	86 ± 9 (80–100)	82 ± 11 (60–100)	89 ± 12 (65–100)	0.46

4. Discussion

The purpose of our study was to evaluate clinically and radiographically the outcomes of shoulder arthroplasty in young patients with PANHH. Both HA and TSA improved the clinical function of affected patients significantly after 8.2 years (mean FU). Revision surgeries for glenoid wear were low (2%). Complications after TSA were excessively high with 32% exhibiting glenoid loosening and 26% receiving revision surgery.

Mansat et al. [2] reported outcomes on 19 HA with a mean FU of 7 years. Mean Constant score (58 points) was significantly improved at last FU. Post-irradiation PANHH yielded the worst results. At long term, with a mean FU set at 12 years, Smith et al. [6] confirmed in 31 HA that mean motion range had still improved significantly ($p < 0.001$).

In our study, two hemi-metal implants (2%) had revision surgery for glenoid wear at 2.4 and 4.1 years postoperatively, with pre-operative Ficat classification at stage 3. Mansat et al. [2] related painful glenoid wear developed in 2 of the 14 HA (14%) at 6.2 and 9.6 years of FU. Only one patient with low Constant score (33 points) had revision surgery. At long term, Smith et al. [6] noted 14 glenoid erosions out of 23 shoulders (61%), but only 2 patients had revision surgery for TSA (7%). The estimated survival rate for HA in their study was 100% after 5 years and 92% after 10 and 15 years.

In our study, survival rate without revision surgery was 97% (89–99%) and 95% (68–99%) at 5 and 10 years. No significant differences between different types of HA, regarding postoperative complication, revision surgery or clinical outcomes were observed. Nevertheless, anatomic cemented stems with metal head (Aequalis, Tornier SAS-Wright Medical) were the device which had the longest follow up and excellent treatment outcomes.

In Herschel et al. [20] study, valgus position of the prosthetic humeral and glenoid cysts were identified as risk factors for glenoid erosion after HA. The size of the humeral head component was not correlated with glenoid erosion in the study of Al-Hadithy et al. [21].

TSA gave excellent results at short and middle term but it exposed patients to glenoid implant loosening.

In our study, glenoid loosening occurred in 6 of 19 TSA (31.6%) between 7 and 10 years FU but this cohort was small. Four TSA had been reoperated. Two glenoids components considered as loosened did not undergo a new surgery (CS = 49 and 67).

Schoch et al. [4] followed 71 TSA after PANHH with a mean follow up of 7.7 years. Pain and range of motion were significantly improved. Among them, 11 (15%) underwent reoperation at a mean time of 4.4 years (range, 0.6–11 years) after index arthroplasty. Four patients (5%) needed to be reoperated for aseptic glenoid loosening.

In a prospective study, Parch et al. [3] prospectively evaluated 13 TSA at a mean follow-up of 30.2 months (range, 14–49 months). Shoulder function assessed by the Constant score improved from 18 (adjusted score, 24%) to 51 (adjusted score, 69%; $p < 0.001$). They observed that patients younger than 65 years obtained lower adjusted Constant scores (mean, 58%; $n = 7$) than patients older (mean, 82%; $n = 6$; $r_s = -0.73$, $p = 0.02$). During follow up, the patient with the lowest adjusted Constant scores was the one with progressive glenoid erosion preoperatively.

Relatively few studies compared the outcomes between HA and TSA for PANHH in the literature. Recently, a study by Ristow et al. [5] assessed 10 TSA and 19 HA and showed no significant differences in clinical outcomes with a mean follow-up of 3.9 years (range, 1–8.5 years). Mean age at surgery was 49.2 years (range, 16–77 years). It demonstrated a trend of better outcome scores with TSA but without statistical significance. Traumatic cases concerned 20% of their patients which impacted the results.

Feeley et al. [1] compared 26 HA vs. 17 TSA with 4.8 years of FU. TSA was associated with lower ASES score and decreased forward flexion compared to hemiarthroplasty ($p < 0.05$). There were significantly more reoperations in the TSA group (22%) among which 4 exhibited glenoid loosening. Schoch et al. [4] compared 67 HA vs. 71 TSA with a mean FU of 9.3 years. At the time of final follow-up, active elevation was significantly higher in the HA group ($p = 0.04$).

In our study, despite a shorter follow up with HA, 2 HA had revision surgery for glenoid wear with a mean follow up of 11.9 years. Twenty years later, the percentage of reoperation-free patients was calculated to be 87%. Fifteen percent of TSA had revision surgery with a mean time of 4.4 years at index surgery. Four of eleven patients were reoperated for aseptic glenoid loosening. Reoperation-free survival rate was calculated to be 79% (CI, 67–92).

Our study has inherent limitations due to its retrospective and multicentric design. It mixed different kinds of hemiarthroplasties with a heterogeneous follow-up. Moreover, the cohort of TSA was smaller with a smaller FU than HA. Nevertheless, it analyses one of the longest FU in the literature about shoulder arthroplasty for PANHH. There were no statistical differences between clinical outcomes and post-operative complications with the stage of the osteonecrosis. Glenoid wear occurred rarely after HA. TSA seemed to be complicated by glenoid loosening more. Humeral metal-head implants gave excellent results and are still a good option for HA.

5. Conclusions

With a mean follow-up of 8 years, HA and TSA improved significantly clinical outcomes in patients with PANHH. Revision surgeries of HA for painful glenoid wear were rare (2%), but the revision rate for glenoid loosening was high with TSA (26%).

Author Contributions: Conceptualization and methodology, P.B., M.C.; software, M.C., L.F., C.L., F.S., N.B., A.H., M.C., G.W., P.C. (Philippe Clavert); investigation, A.H.; writing—original draft preparation, P.C. (Philippe Collin), M.C.; writing—review and editing, P.C. (Philippe Collin); supervision. All authors have read and agreed to the published version of the manuscript.

Funding: This research received no external funding.

Institutional Review Board Statement: The study was conducted according to the guidelines of the Declaration of Helsinki, and approved by the Institutional Review Board (or Ethics Committee) of University Institute of Locomotion and Sports at the date of 3 March 2017.

Informed Consent Statement: Informed consent was obtained from all subjects involved in the study.

Data Availability Statement: The data can be found at www.easymedstat.com.

Conflicts of Interest: The authors declare no conflict of interest.

References

1. Feeley, B.T.; Fealy, S.; Dines, D.M.; Warren, R.F.; Craig, E.V. Hemiarthroplasty and Total Shoulder Arthroplasty for Avascular Necrosis of the Humeral Head. *J. Shoulder Elb. Surg.* **2008**, *17*, 689–694. [CrossRef] [PubMed]
2. Mansat, P.; Huser, L.; Mansat, M.; Bellumore, Y.; Rongières, M.; Bonnevialle, P. Shoulder Arthroplasty for Atraumatic Avascular Necrosis of the Humeral Head: Nineteen Shoulders Followed up for a Mean of Seven Years. *J. Shoulder Elb. Surg.* **2005**, *14*, 114–120. [CrossRef] [PubMed]
3. Parsch, D.; Lehner, B.; Loew, M. Shoulder Arthroplasty in Nontraumatic Osteonecrosis of the Humeral Head. *J. Shoulder Elb. Surg.* **2003**, *12*, 226–230. [CrossRef]
4. Schoch, B.S.; Barlow, J.D.; Schleck, C.; Cofield, R.H.; Sperling, J.W. Shoulder Arthroplasty for Atraumatic Osteonecrosis of the Humeral Head. *J. Shoulder Elb. Surg.* **2016**, *25*, 238–245. [CrossRef]
5. Ristow, J.J.; Ellison, C.M.; Mickschl, D.J.; Berg, K.C.; Haidet, K.C.; Gray, J.R.; Grindel, S.I. Outcomes of Shoulder Replacement in Humeral Head Avascular Necrosis. *J. Shoulder Elb. Surg.* **2019**, *28*, 9–14. [CrossRef] [PubMed]
6. Smith, R.G.; Sperling, J.W.; Cofield, R.H.; Hattrup, S.J.; Schleck, C.D. Shoulder Hemiarthroplasty for Steroid-Associated Osteonecrosis. *J. Shoulder Elb. Surg.* **2008**, *17*, 685–688. [CrossRef] [PubMed]
7. Raiss, P.; Kasten, P.; Baumann, F.; Moser, M.; Rickert, M.; Loew, M. Treatment of Osteonecrosis of the Humeral Head with Cementless Surface Replacement Arthroplasty. *J. Bone Jt. Surg. Am.* **2009**, *91*, 340–349. [CrossRef]
8. Ohl, X.; Nérot, C.; Saddiki, R.; Dehoux, E. Shoulder Hemi Arthroplasty Radiological and Clinical Outcomes at More than Two Years Follow-Up. *Orthop. Traumatol. Surg. Res.* **2010**, *96*, 208–215. [CrossRef] [PubMed]
9. Uribe, J.W.; Botto-van Bemden, A. Partial Humeral Head Resurfacing for Osteonecrosis. *J. Shoulder Elb. Surg.* **2009**, *18*, 711–716. [CrossRef] [PubMed]
10. Sweet, S.J.; Takara, T.; Ho, L.; Tibone, J.E. Primary Partial Humeral Head Resurfacing: Outcomes with the HemiCAP Implant. *Am. J. Sports Med.* **2015**, *43*, 579–587. [CrossRef] [PubMed]
11. Soudy, K.; Szymanski, C.; Lalanne, C.; Bourgault, C.; Thiounn, A.; Cotten, A.; Maynou, C. Results and Limitations of Humeral Head Resurfacing: 105 Cases at a Mean Follow-up of 5 Years. *Orthop. Traumatol. Surg. Res.* **2017**, *103*, 415–420. [CrossRef] [PubMed]

12. Sowa, B.; Thierjung, H.; Bülhoff, M.; Loew, M.; Zeifang, F.; Bruckner, T.; Raiss, P. Functional Results of Hemi- and Total Shoulder Arthroplasty According to Diagnosis and Patient Age at Surgery. *Acta Orthop.* **2017**, *88*, 310–314. [CrossRef] [PubMed]
13. Orfaly, R.M.; Rockwood, C.A.; Esenyel, C.Z.; Wirth, M.A. Shoulder Arthroplasty in Cases with Avascular Necrosis of the Humeral Head. *J. Shoulder Elb. Surg.* **2007**, *16*, S27–S32. [CrossRef] [PubMed]
14. Constant, C.R.; Murley, A.H. A Clinical Method of Functional Assessment of the Shoulder. *Clin. Orthop. Relat. Res.* **1994**, 160–164. [CrossRef]
15. Gerber, C.; Vinh, T.S.; Hertel, R.; Hess, C.W. Latissimus Dorsi Transfer for the Treatment of Massive Tears of the Rotator Cuff. A Preliminary Report. *Clin. Orthop. Relat. Res.* **1992**, *232*, 51–61. [CrossRef]
16. Ficat, P.; Arlet, J. Pre-radiologic stage of femur head osteonecrosis: Diagnostic and therapeutic possibilities. *Rev. Chir. Orthop. Reparatrice Appar. Mot.* **1973**, *59* (Suppl. S1), 26–38.
17. Cruess, R.L. Steroid-Induced Avascular Necrosis of the Head of the Humerus. Natural History and Management. *J. Bone Jt. Surg. Br.* **1976**, *58*, 313–317. [CrossRef] [PubMed]
18. Molé, D.; Roche, O.; Riand, N.; Lévigne, C.; Walch, G. Cemented Glenoid Component: Results in Osteoarthritis and Rheumatoid Arthritis. In *Shoulder Arthroplasty*; Springer: Berlin/Heidelberg, Germany, 1999; pp. 163–171. ISBN 978-3-642-63554-0.
19. Collin, P.; Matsumura, N.; Lädermann, A.; Denard, P.J.; Walch, G. Relationship between Massive Chronic Rotator Cuff Tear Pattern and Loss of Active Shoulder Range of Motion. *J. Shoulder Elb. Surg.* **2014**, *23*, 1195–1202. [CrossRef] [PubMed]
20. Herschel, R.; Wieser, K.; Morrey, M.E.; Ramos, C.H.; Gerber, C.; Meyer, D.C. Risk Factors for Glenoid Erosion in Patients with Shoulder Hemiarthroplasty: An Analysis of 118 Cases. *J. Shoulder Elb. Surg.* **2017**, *26*, 246–252. [CrossRef]
21. Al-Hadithy, N.; Domos, P.; Sewell, M.D.; Naleem, A.; Papanna, M.C.; Pandit, R. Cementless Surface Replacement Arthroplasty of the Shoulder for Osteoarthritis: Results of Fifty Mark III Copeland Prosthesis from an Independent Center with Four-Year Mean Follow-Up. *J. Shoulder Elb. Surg.* **2012**, *21*, 1776–1781. [CrossRef] [PubMed]

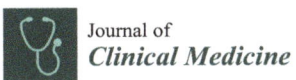

Article

Shoulder Replacement in the Elderly with Anatomic versus Reverse Total Prosthesis? A Prospective 2-Year Follow-Up Study

Maciej J. K. Simon [1,2], Jennifer A. Coghlan [1,3] and Simon N. Bell [1,3,*]

[1] Melbourne Shoulder and Elbow Centre, 1/80 Beach Road, Sandringham, Melbourne, VIC 3191, Australia; maciej.simon@gmail.com (M.J.K.S.); coghlan@bigpond.net.au (J.A.C.)
[2] Department of Orthopaedics and Trauma Surgery, Campus Kiel, University Medical Center Schleswig-Holstein, Arnold-Heller-Str. 3, 24105 Kiel, Germany
[3] Department of Surgery, School of Clinical Sciences, Monash Health, Monash University, Clayton, Melbourne, VIC 3168, Australia
* Correspondence: snbell@bigpond.net.au

Abstract: Background: In older patients requiring a total shoulder replacement (TSR) and with an intact rotator cuff, there is currently uncertainty on whether an anatomic TSR (aTSR) or a reverse TSR (rTSR) is best for the patient. This comparison study of same-aged patients aims to assess clinical and radiological outcomes of older patients ($\geq$75 years) who received either an aTSR or an rTSR. Methods: Consecutive patients with a minimum age of 75 years who received an aTSR (n = 44) or rTSR (n = 51) were prospectively studied. Pre- and post-operative clinical evaluations included the ASES score, Constant score, SPADI score, DASH score, range of motion (ROM) and pain and patient satisfaction for a follow-up of 2 years. Radiological assessment identified glenoid and humeral component osteolysis, including notching with an rTSR. Results: We found postoperative improvement for ROM and all clinical assessment scores for both groups. There were significantly better patient reported outcome scores (PROMs) in the aTSR group compared with the rTSR patients ($p < 0.001$). Both groups had only minor osteolysis on radiographs. No revisions were required in either group. The main complications were scapular stress fractures for the rTSR (n = 11) patients and acromioclavicular joint pain for both groups (aTSR = 2; rTSR = 6). Conclusions: This study of older patients ($\geq$75 years) demonstrated that an aTSR for a patient with good rotator cuff muscles can lead to a better clinical outcome and less early complications than an rTSR. Level of evidence: Level II—prospective cohort study.

Keywords: anatomic total shoulder replacement; reverse total shoulder replacement; Lazarus score; Sirveaux score; older patients; clinical scores

1. Introduction

In shoulder replacement, the type of shoulder prosthesis chosen for a particular patient is based on the underlying pathology, in particular the status of the rotator cuff, the degree of bony erosion, and the biological age of the patient.

Rotator cuff tendons degenerate progressively with increasing age and with secondary wasting of the muscle belly [1,2], and rotator cuff tears are present in almost 50% of the population in their 8th or 9th decade of life [3]. In the other 50% of older patients with an arthritic glenohumeral joint but an intact rotator cuff requiring a total shoulder replacement (TSR), there is at present uncertainty as to which patients would do better with an aTSR. There is a currently an increasing tendency to recommend a reverse total shoulder replacement (rTSR) in patients older than 70 years with an intact rotator cuff [4], which seems to assume that the result of an aTSR vs. an rTSR in this age group is similar.

This study aims to compare the results both clinically and radiologically, and the rate of complications, between a group of patients 75 years or over who had either an aTSR or an rTSR. The hypothesis is that patients with an aTSR have better clinical outcomes than same age patients receiving an rTSR.

2. Materials and Methods

2.1. Study Protocol and Patients' Eligibility

The nested study interrogated two existing databases from the same department. These included consecutive patients 75 years or older with either advanced primary glenohumeral osteoarthritis (OA) with or without an intact rotator cuff (RC), or an irreparable rotator cuff tear with minor osteoarthritis, who had a TSR.

Decision on prosthesis type (aTSR or rTSR) depended on the rotator cuff's status. Initial assessment was made clinically and radiologically with an X-ray and CT scan. If the integrity of the rotator cuff was uncertain, these cases were further assessed with an MRI scan to assess the rotator cuff status, including, if present, tear type (full or partial thickness), extent of muscle atrophy, and degeneration [5,6]. If the patient had osteoarthritis but the RC was intact and not degenerated, with no major muscle atrophy, the decision was made for an aTSR. If the patient had osteoarthritis and the RC was torn or degenerated, including severe fatty atrophy, the decision was made for an rTSR. If imaging demonstrated a massive irreparable RC tear with minor arthritis, an rTSR was indicated.

Inclusion criteria for the group receiving an aTSR were glenohumeral OA and an intact rotator cuff. The criteria for inclusion for the group receiving an rTSR were glenohumeral arthritis with an inadequate rotator cuff for an aTSR (n = 25), or a massive irreparable rotator cuff tear (n = 26).

Exclusion criteria were age under 75 years before the operation, post fracture/traumatic osteoarthritis, abnormal neurology or inability to comply with the study requirements. Exclusion criterion for performing an aTSR was a full-thickness rotator cuff tear, or inadequate rotator cuff function based on clinical examination and MRI findings. Therefore, all patients with glenohumeral arthritis who had a good rotator cuff had an aTSR, despite their age.

Eligible consecutive patients gave written consent and were prospectively enrolled in the study over the same time period. An identical prospective study protocol was set up for both groups. All patients had a minimum age of 75 years at the time of operation and a minimum follow-up time of 2 years. Written consent for study participation and publication was obtained from all patients. All studies were carried out in accordance with the World Medical Association most recent Declaration of Helsinki.

2.2. Clinical Assessments

Preoperatively, patient-reported outcome measures (PROMs), including the American shoulder and elbow surgeons (ASES) score [7,8], shoulder pain and disability index (SPADI) [9,10], disability of the arm, shoulder and hand (DASH) scores [9,11], pain (VAS 0 = no pain-10 = severe pain), were recorded, together with the Constant score (CS) [12,13], and clinical range of motion (ROM) for all patients in the study.

Postoperatively, patients were clinically reviewed at 2-week, 6-week, 3-month, 6-month, 1-year, and 2-year time points. Pain levels and ROM were documented at 3 months, 1 year and 2 years. Active and passive ROM, CS, and PROMs were recorded at 1-year and 2-year follow-up. Satisfaction (scored from 0%—dissatisfied to 100%—totally satisfied) was also recorded.

2.3. Radiological Assessments

Radiological assessments were carried out preoperatively (Walch and Favard classification), and postoperatively at day 1, 12 weeks and yearly [14–16]. In order to assess both the humeral and glenoid components, radiographs were taken according to a standardized protocol in multiple planes (axillary, true lateral, standard anteroposterior (AP) and true AP view of glenoid with the arm in 20° external and internal rotation). Radiographs were assessed independently and separately by two orthopaedic surgeons (MJKS and MC) not involved in the patient surgeries. Disagreements were referred to a third independent experienced surgeon (HC) for final decision.

The aTSR was radiologically evaluated and assessed in a standard technique for perihumeral component osteolysis with assessment of five zones, as previously described [17]. The glenoid component was assessed using the Lazarus classification quantifying radiolucent lines (RLL) between the cement surrounding the glenoid pegs and bone interface [18].

The rTSR was radiologically assessed in a standard technique for scapular notching according to the classification by Sirveaux et al. for the glenoid component [19,20]. The humeral component was assessed for RLL around the implant in seven different zones as previously described by Levigne et al. and Bell et al. [16,21,22].

2.4. Implants and Postoperative Rehabilitation

All shoulders were replaced via a standard deltopectoral approach. For the aTSR, a stemless Affinis® short humeral ceramic head component was utilized in all cases. This was articulated with a double-pegged, cemented, all-polyethylene glenoid component made of standard, not cross-linked, polyethylene (Mathys AG, Bettlach, Switzerland) in 34 cases and more recently in 11 cases with a highly cross-linked polyethylene (HXLPE)—Affinis® Glenoid Vitamys prosthesis (Mathys AG, Bettlach, Switzerland).

For rTSR, a Grammont-style humeral prosthesis was used—Aequalis Reversed II Shoulder System (Tornier SAS (Montbonnot Saint Martin, France) part of Stryker). For the glenoid, a 25 mm baseplate was utilized in all cases, together with either a 36 mm or 42 mm glenosphere made of cobalt–chromium alloy. An appropriately sized humeral liner of standard polyethylene was utilized.

Post operation, all patients wore a sling for 5 to 6 weeks. A structured physiotherapy programme was commenced on the first postoperative day.

2.5. Statistical Methods

The data were analysed using a mixture of parametric procedures (*t*-tests and general linear models, including analysis of covariance) and nonparametric procedures (Mann–Whitney test, sign test, Fisher's exact test and logistic regression), as appropriate. Analyses were conducted using either Minitab statistical software version 18 (Minitab, Inc., State College, PA, USA) or R (R Core Team) [23].

3. Results

The more than 2-year results of 44 patients with aTSR and 51 patients with rTSR were analysed (Figure 1). The two groups were fairly similar demographically, in particular they had similar preoperative VAS, ASES, SPADI, DASH, and CS scores. The average age of aTSR patients was 77.33 ± 1.97 and of rTSR 82.10 ± 3.93 years (Table 1). In the aTSR group, 72% were female compared with 90% in the rTSR group. In the aTSR group, glenoid morphology from the Walch classification was 16 A1, 11 A2, 12 B1 and 5 B2. There were no B3 or C or D glenoids. Glenoid assessment from the Favard classification for the rTSR showed 17 E0, 11 E1, 6 E2, 15 E3 and 2 E4.

All 44 included patients for aTSR completed the 2-year follow-up (Figure 1). In the rTSR group, eight patients were not available at 2 years, resulting in 43 patients at this time point.

Prospectively collected preoperative and 2-year postoperative clinical assessments, ROM, and postsurgery satisfaction, are presented in Table 2. The preoperative and 2-year postoperative VAS pain scores, CS, and PROMs are presented in Table 3.

Table 1. Patient demographics and preoperative radiographic glenoid scores (Walch [14,15] and Favard [16] classification).

Anatomic TSR		Reverse TSR	
	n = 44		n = 51
Age (years ± SD)	77.37 ± 1.97	Age (years ± SD)	82.10 ± 3.93
(min; max)	(75; 81)	(min; max)	(76; 91)
BMI (% ± SD)	29.03 ± 4.82	BMI (% ± SD)	26.95 ± 4.01
(min; max)	(20.7; 40.8)	(min; max)	(18; 37)
Gender		Gender	
male	12 (27.27%)	male	5 (9.80%)
female	32 (72.73%)	female	46 (90.20%)
Operated arm		Operated arm	
right	29	right	31
left	15	left	20
Dominant arm		Dominant arm	
right	40	right	47
left	4	left	4
Walch classification		Favard classification	
A1	16	E0	17
A2	11	E1	11
B1	12	E2	6
B2	5	E3	15
B3, C, D	0	E4	2
Missing	0	Missing	0

Table 2. Clinical range of motion assessment—external rotation (ER), active elevation (AE), stabilized scapular glenohumeral abduction (GH)—preoperative and at the 2-year follow-up mark and postsurgery satisfaction. The difference for each category from preoperative to 2-year postoperative is demonstrated with a delta (Δ). (Mann–Whitney and two-sample t-test: * $p < 0.05$; ** $p < 0.01$; *** $p < 0.001$).

	Anatomic TSR			Reverse TSR		
	Mean ± SD (min; max)	n	Missing	Mean ± SD (min; max)	n	Missing
preOP ER [°]	17.79 ± 13.49 (−5; 50)	34	10	25.95 ± 22.09 (0; 80)	42	9
preOP GH [°]	52.32 ± 19.91 (10; 90)	41	3	55.54 ± 18.26 (10; 90)	46	5
preOP AE [°]	84.42 ± 31.80 (15; 150)	43	1	71.67 ± 32.90 (0; 130)	48	3
Y2 ER [°]	61.14 ± 14.10 (30; 90) ***	44	0	39.08 ± 15.50 (10; 70)	49	2
Y2 GH [°]	75.68 ± 12.32 (50; 90)	44	0	75.20 ± 10.05 (45; 90)	51	0
Y2 AE [°]	146.93 ± 18.84 (100;175) ***	44	0	125.29 ± 21.85 (90; 160)	51	0
Satisfaction (%)	97.5 ± 7.35 (60; 100) ***	44	0	90.09 ± 13.23 (50; 100)	45	6
ΔER (Y2—preOP)	42.50 ± 19.55 (0; 90) ***	34	10	12.50 ± 24.23 (−40; 50)	40	11
ΔGH (Y2—preOP)	23.05 ± 23.37 (−30; 80)	42	3	19.89 ± 17.56 (−10; 50)	46	5
ΔAE (Y2—preOP)	61.98 ± 33.19 (0; 135)	43	1	55.42 ± 30.94 (0; 140)	48	3

At 2 years, while the final scores had improved for both groups, the aTSR group had better results. The final VAS pain scores for both groups were less than one on the pain scale, with the aTSR group having slightly less pain. The ROM had improved ($p = < 0.001$) with active elevation up to 147 degrees for aTSR and 125 degrees for rTSR. Patient satisfaction was significantly higher for aTSR than for the rTSR group, at 97.5% versus 90.09% ($p < 0.001$), respectively. The improvement from the preoperative scores was overall better in the aTSR than the rTSR group (Table 3). The final CS in the aTSR group had improved 46 points to 75 compared with the rTSR group's improvement of 33 points to 56. The ASES showed comparative results (Tables 3 and 4).

Table 3. Patient assessment with VAS pain levels, ASES, DASH, SPADI and Constant scores preoperative and 2 years postoperative. The difference for each category from preoperative to 2 years postoperative is demonstrated with a delta (Δ). (Mann–Whitney and two-sample t-test: * $p < 0.05$; ** $p < 0.01$; *** $p < 0.001$).

	Anatomic TSR			Reverse TSR		
	Mean ± SD (min; max)	n	Missing	Mean ± SD (min; max)	n	Missing
preOP VAS pain (0–10)	5.62 ± 2.57 (1; 10)	42	2	5.73 ± 2.29 (2; 10)	51	0
preOP ASES Total	39.58 ± 20.03 (3; 73.33)	42	2	35.50 ± 17.38 (0; 63.33)	50	1
preOP SPADI Total	65.05 ± 20.96 (23.85; 97.69)	40	4	69.59 ± 15.94 (34.60; 100)	34	17
preOP DASH Total	49.80 ± 19.08 (15; 95) ***	40	4	64.16 ± 15.47 (30.83; 89.17)	38	13
preOP Constant Total	28.20 ± 12.93 (4; 60)	41	3	22.59 ± 13.40 (2; 58)	39	12
Y2 VAS pain (0–10)	0.29 ± 0.85 (0; 5)	44	0	0.56 ± 1.08 (0; 4)	45	6
Y2 ASES Total	90.58 ± 9.88 (63.33; 100) ***	44	0	73.50 ± 16.71 (30; 100)	39	12
Y2 SPADI Total	5.33 ± 8.25 (0; 36.92) ***	44	0	26.03 ± 19.83 (0; 84.62)	40	11
Y2 DASH Total	10.42 ± 10.65 (0; 48.33) ***	44	0	35.01 ± 22.35 (1.79; 80)	39	12
Y2 Constant Total	75.20 ± 11.41 (42; 96) ***	44	0	56.14 ± 11.48 (25; 76)	37	14
ΔVAS pain (Y2—preOP)	−5.33 ± 2.68 (−10; −1)	42	2	−5.13 ± 2.38 (−10; −1)	45	6
ΔASES (Y2—preOP)	50.99 ± 20.67 (7; 90.33) **	42	2	39.17 ± 17.78 (0; 71.67)	38	13
ΔSPADI (Y2—preOP)	−59.56 ± 21.28 (−95.85; −18.23) **	40	4	−44.34 ± 22.27 (−93.85; 4.62)	30	21
ΔDASH (Y2—preOP)	−38.80 ± 18.86 (−89.33; −0.81)	40	4	−30.11 ± 22.16 (−79.17; 13.40)	33	18
ΔConstant (Y2—preOP)	46.20 ± 17.44 (7; 77) **	41	3	33.39 ± 15.31 (4; 70)	33	18

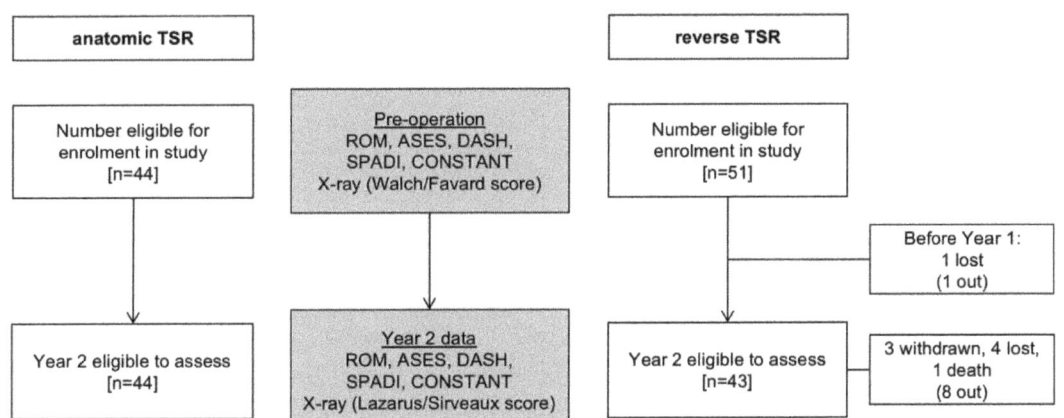

Figure 1. The CONSORT flowchart of the study. Pre- and post-operative assessment of range of motion (ROM), ASES, DASH, SPADI and Constant scores, and radiologic assessments.

3.1. Radiologic Assessment

Radiolucency on the humeral side was only minor and did not differ between the groups. It was detected in three cases for the rTSR group and in four cases for the aTSR group at the 2-year mark (Table 5). The glenoid component demonstrated more surrounding radiolucency/notching signs for the rTSR ($n = 10$) than the aTSR group ($n = 6$) after 2 years. There was no significant component loosening in either group, and no dislocations, hence no revision surgery was required in either group.

Table 4. Overview and comparison of 2-year follow-up outcomes (radiological and clinical outcomes, patient satisfaction and complication rates). The "+" (plus sign) represents higher values in comparison with the other category, whereas "=" (equal sign) represents no significant differences. (External rotation (ER), active elevation (AE), stabilized scapular glenohumeral abduction (GH)).

Categories	Anatomic TSR	Reverse TSR
Glenoid radiolucency/notching		=
Humeral radiolucency		=
ASES	+	
SPADI	+	
DASH	+	
Constant	+	
VAS pain		=
ER	+	
GH		=
AE	+	
Satisfaction	+	
Complication rate		+

Table 5. Postoperative radiologic assessment for the glenoid and humeral components for the anatomic and reverse TSR. Radiolucency for the glenoid component of aTSR is scored according to Lazarus [18], whereas for the rTSR, glenoid notching is scored according to Sirveaux [20].

Anatomic TSR			Reverse TSR		
X-ray—Lazarus glenoid radiolucency score	Y1	Y2	X-ray—Sirveaux glenoid notching score	Y1	Y2
Total eligible	44	44	Total eligible	50	43
0	39	38	0—No defect	43	33
1	5	6	1—Defect only concerns the pillar	6	8
2			2—Contact with the lower screw	1	2
3			3—Extension over the lower screw		
4			4—Extension under baseplate		
5					
Missing	0	0	Missing	0	0
X-ray—humeral radiolucency score (zones)	Y1	Y2	X-ray—humeral radiolucency score (zones)	Y1	Y2
Total eligible	44	44	Total eligible	51	43
No radiolucency	41	40	No radiolucency	49	40
Radiolucency cases (all zones)	3	4	Radiolucency cases (all zones)	2	3
Zone 1	1	2	Zone 1	0	1
Zone 2	0	0	Zone 2	0	0
Zone 3	0	0	Zone 3	0	0
Zone 4	0	0	Zone 4	0	0
Zone 5	2	2	Zone 5	0	0
			Zone 6	0	0
			Zone 7	2	3
Missing	0	0	Missing	0	0
Drop-outs	**0**	**0**	**Drop-outs**	**1**	**8**

3.2. Complications

There were no readmissions in either group. Complication rates were higher for the rTSR (n = 18 in 14 patients) than for the aTSR group (n = 3 in 3 patients) (Table 6).

Table 6. Postoperative complications for both types of shoulder replacements. Acromioclavicular joint (ACJ) pain is common among aTSR and rTSR, and can be resolved by injections or arthroscopic excision of the distal clavicle (EDC). The main complications for rTSR are stress fractures (#) of the acromion or the scapular spine. The category "Other" reports one case with an avulsion fracture of the triceps. Percentages (%) are based on total number of patients available at 2-year follow-up (aTSR $n = 44$; rTSR $n = 43$).

	Anatomic TSR				Reverse TSR		
n	%	Time ± SD after Surgery (Months)	Complications	n	%	Time ± SD after Surgery (Months)	
2	4.54	18 ± 8.5	ACJ pain	6	13.95	13.5 ± 9.7	
1	2.27	12	resolved by injection	5	11.62	11.4 ± 9.2	
1	2.27	24	resolved by EDC	1	2.32	24	
0	-	-	acromial and scapular stress #	11	25.58	9.9 ± 7.0	
0	-	-	Instability	0	-	-	
1	2.27	10	Cuff failure	0	-	-	
0	-	-	Infection	0	-	-	
0	-	-	Other	1	2.32	10	
3	6.81	10.0 ± 9.3	**Total patients**	14	32.55	11.7 ± 8.1	

One common complication seen in both groups was acromioclavicular joint (ACJ) pain. This occurred in two shoulders with an aTSR and in six shoulders with an rTSR. Most patients recovered well after a steroid injection, however in two cases (one case in each group), an arthroscopic excision of distal clavicle (EDC) was necessary with a good result.

One patient with an aTSR (Table 6) developed cuff failure. The MRI scan demonstrated a massively retracted and atrophied supraspinatus tendon by the time of presentation. As the shoulder joint was stable, AE was good (>90°) and there was no pain throughout the 2-year follow-up period, no revision surgery was undertaken.

Apart from the ACJ pain, the main other complication for the rTSR group was a stress fracture of the acromion or the scapular spine ($n = 11$), which mostly occurred within the first year, after patients began unrestricted use of the arm (Table 6). All cases resolved nonoperatively with rest for up to 3 months in an abduction pillow. One rTSR case had an avulsion fracture of the posterior inferior glenoid by the long head of the triceps 10 months after surgery. There was no functional deficit and only mild pain, which resolved after 2 months with nonoperative treatment.

4. Discussion

The current study compares patients following an aTSR versus an rTSR aged 75 years and older. The baseline demographics of the two groups were similar, including PROMs. The overall outcomes in the 2-year follow-up period confirm our original hypothesis, as better ROM, clinical outcome scores including patient satisfaction, and less complications were demonstrated for the aTSR group than the rTSR group, as shown in Table 4.

These results differ to Kiet et al. who looked at outcomes of aTSR and rTSR results after 2 years [24]. They demonstrated no differences in the complication or revision rates, nor ASES and pain scores. The ROM in both groups was similar except for a slightly better external rotation in the aTSR group, which was also found in our study. In addition, in our study, the AE was also significantly better in the aTSR group ($p < 0.001$). It is difficult to compare our results with Kiet's study, as the average age of the patients is not documented, and further, they used a stemmed anatomic humeral prosthesis which was cemented and a metal humeral head [24].

Another study by Wright et al. compared aTSR with rTSR in patients aged 70 years and older with an intact rotator cuff [25]. They were able to identify similar postoperative ROM and outcome scores for both prostheses. Although they reported no significant differences in complication rates for the two prostheses types, they did identify that rotator cuff tears were the principal complication in the aTSR group leading to conversion to an rTSR, which occurred within an average of 28 months postsurgery. In the current study, there was one early cuff failure following an aTSR within 24 months follow-up, but revision of the prosthesis was not required.

An additional problem with an rTSR is that the medical complication rate has been reported to be significantly higher than with an aTSR [26]. The factor of age and complications was analysed by Koh et al. [27]. They assessed patients at 30 days postoperation and demonstrated that the older age group (>80 years) had significantly more complications and readmissions than younger patients for any type of shoulder arthroplasty [27].

Although all patients were 75 years of age and older, the rTSR patients were slightly older and a slightly lower ROM preoperatively, however, the PROMs and CS were very similar. Therefore, both groups started from a similar basepoint for all indices. However, the overall improvement in most indices and scores was greater in the aTSR group than the rTSR group. This resulted in the rTSR group having lower final postoperative clinical scores and a worse ROM than the aTSR group. It was not possible to analyse males' versus females' results due to the relatively few male patients.

Friedman and colleagues demonstrated that older patients with an rTSR had better outcome scores (ASES and SPADI) despite smaller improvement in abduction and forward flexion than younger patients [28]. Triplet et al. were able to demonstrate good improvements in motion (ER and AE), pain and function (ASES) in a smaller cohort of older patients (>80 years) for both types of shoulder replacements (aTSR n = 18 and rTSR n = 33). However, they did detect more postoperative complications and higher transfusion rates for rTSR patients [29]. This was different to Anakwenze and colleagues, who looked at the effect of age and outcomes in aTSR and rTSR [30]. They identified a higher odds ratio (OR) for patients older than 75 years for readmissions and an increased 1-year mortality in patients with an aTSR (OR 1.75 and 3.34) versus rTSR (OR 0.68 and 0.92). Furthermore, their hazard ratios (HR) for risk of revision were significantly lower for rTSR vs. aTSR patients in patients older than 75 years versus patients 75 years or younger, at HR 0.45 versus 1.24, respectively [30]. In our study there were no revisions. Another study from Wagner et al. demonstrated that no matter what sort of shoulder prosthesis is implanted, the risk of revision for mechanical failure, aseptic loosening or infection decreased with age 65 years and above [31]. According to their data, only instability remained an age-independent complication.

Stress fractures were the main complications seen in our rTSR group (21.6%), while none of the above-mentioned studies reported acromial or scapular stress fractures [25,26,32,33]. However, Zmistowski et al. reported an incidence of 10.5% for acromial stress fractures and reactions following rTSR, with an average follow-up of 407 days [34]. There was also no mention in the previous studies of acromioclavicular joint pain, as was seen in some cases in our study [25,26,32–34].

In our study, component loosening was not an issue in this short-term follow-up period. On radiographic evaluation of the humeral component side, there was no difference between prosthesis types, with only minor osteolysis seen for both the stemless aTSR and the long-stem rTSR. On the glenoid side, osteolysis for both types of component was again only minor, but there was a slight tendency towards more osteolysis with the rTSR than the aTSR, although it is difficult to compare in such different prostheses as notching is only seen with rTSR and radiolucent lines with aTSR.

Shields and Wiater [33] compared aTSRs which were revised to rTSRs because of rotator cuff failure or component loosening to matched patients with primarily an rTSR. They demonstrated that patients with a revision surgery for a failed aTSR not only had a lower satisfaction but also significantly poorer subjective outcome scores and more complications than the primary rTSR group. However, revision of a primary aTSR to an rTSR solely due to cuff failure has also been shown by Flury et al. to be a good salvaging procedure, as it improves ROM, clinical scores and patients' satisfaction when comparing pre- and post-operative scores [32]. The latter study results support a surgeon's decision to continue using an aTSR in older patients, especially as with a stemless prosthesis, revision of the components to an rTSR is relatively easy.

Despite prospective data collection, our study has limitations. The follow-up time is limited to 2 years, which is less than the average time of secondary rotator cuff failure in aTSR [25,35]. Despite this, during this short follow-up time, the rTSR demonstrated more complications, in particular stress fractures of the scapula, than aTSR. Patients receiving an rTSR were slightly older than the aTSR patients, skewing the data slightly, as there is a naturally increased chance with age of a later rotator cuff tear, which requires an rTSR rather than an aTSR [36]. Another limiting factor is the relatively small cohort size and the predominance of female patients, both of which are probably related to the increased age of the patients. Further research and longer follow-up studies need to be performed in order to address these issues.

5. Conclusions

Our results suggest that judicious patient selection in the older-aged patient (75+ years) for the type of shoulder replacement needs to be performed individually and not merely on the basis of patient age. This process can then lead to higher selection towards aTSR, which demonstrated in the current setting significantly better ROM and clinical outcomes than same-aged patients with an rTSR. Additionally, the complication rate is less for an aTSR in the first 2 years following shoulder replacement, making this an acceptable surgical option despite increased age. However, this study only has a short follow-up of 2 years, therefore the outcomes are to be judged carefully and preliminarily, as further prolonged research is necessary.

Author Contributions: Conceptualization: M.J.K.S., J.A.C. and S.N.B.; Methodology: M.J.K.S., J.A.C. and S.N.B.; Validation: M.J.K.S., J.A.C. and S.N.B.; Formal analysis: J.A.C.; Investigation: M.J.K.S. and J.A.C.; Resources: J.A.C. and S.N.B.; Data curation: M.J.K.S., J.A.C. and S.N.B.; Writing—original draft preparation: M.J.K.S., J.A.C. and S.N.B.; Writing—review and editing: M.J.K.S., J.A.C. and S.N.B.; Visualization: M.J.K.S., J.A.C. and S.N.B.; Supervision: S.N.B.; Project administration: M.J.K.S., J.A.C. and S.N.B.; Funding acquisition: J.A.C. and S.N.B. All authors have read and agreed to the published version of the manuscript.

Funding: Mathys and Stryker received financial assistance for data collection and statistical support from the University of Melbourne.

Institutional Review Board Statement: The study was conducted in accordance with the Declaration of Helsinki, and approved by the Ethics Committee of Monash University (CF10/0378—2010000170; 26 February 2010) and was registered in Australian New Zealand Clinical Trials Registry (AC-TRN12613001183774; 29 October 2013).

Informed Consent Statement: Informed consent was obtained from all subjects involved in the study.

Data Availability Statement: Data available on reasonable request due to privacy and ethics board restrictions. The data presented in this study are available on reasonable request from the corresponding author. The data are not publicly available due to privacy and ethics board restrictions.

Acknowledgments: The authors wish to acknowledge Richard J Dallalana, Jeff Hughes, Richard Page and Warwick Wright for submitting patients for the study. We thank Maxim Christmas (MC) for reading the radiographs, Harry Clitherow (HC) for adjudicating the radiographs and Kelli Gray and Caroline Thomas for their database management. We would like to thank Ken Sharpe from the Statistical Consulting Centre, School of Mathematics and Statistics, University of Melbourne for statistical analysis and advice and assistance.

Conflicts of Interest: Maciej Simon: This author, their immediate family, and any research foundation with which they are affiliated did not receive any financial payments or other benefits from any commercial entity related to the subject of this article. Jennifer Coghlan: Receives funds for data collection, entry and storage through her Department of Monash University from Mathys Bettlach, Switzerland, Mathys Australia and Wright Medical, Australia. Simon Bell: Has a consultancy agreement with Mathys Ltd. Bettlach, Switzerland, and Wright Medical, Australia.

References

1. Milgrom, C.; Schaffler, M.; Gilbert, S.; van Holsbeeck, M. Rotator-cuff changes in asymptomatic adults. The effect of age, hand dominance and gender. *J. Bone Jt. Surg. Br.* **1995**, *77*, 296–298. [CrossRef]
2. Teunis, T.; Lubberts, B.; Reilly, B.T.; Ring, D. A systematic review and pooled analysis of the prevalence of rotator cuff disease with increasing age. *J. Shoulder Elb. Surg.* **2014**, *23*, 1913–1921. [CrossRef]
3. Yamamoto, A.; Takagishi, K.; Osawa, T.; Yanagawa, T.; Nakajima, D.; Shitara, H.; Kobayashi, T. Prevalence and risk factors of a rotator cuff tear in the general population. *J. Shoulder Elb. Surg.* **2010**, *19*, 116–120. [CrossRef]
4. Mellano, C.R.; Chalmers, P.N.; Mascarenhas, R.; Kupfer, N.; Forsythe, B.; Romeo, A.A.; Nicholson, G.P. Reverse total shoulder arthroplast for the treatment of osteoarthritis without rotator cuff tear. *Orthop. Proc.* **2016**, *98-B*, 9. [CrossRef]
5. Goutallier, D.; Postel, J.M.; Bernageau, J.; Lavau, L.; Voisin, M.C. Fatty muscle degeneration in cuff ruptures. Pre- and postoperative evaluation by CT scan. *Clin. Orthop. Relat. Res.* **1994**, *304*, 78–83. [CrossRef]
6. Thomazeau, H.; Rolland, Y.; Lucas, C.; Duval, J.M.; Langlais, F. Atrophy of the supraspinatus belly. Assessment by MRI in 55 patients with rotator cuff pathology. *Acta Orthop. Scand.* **1996**, *67*, 264–268. [CrossRef]
7. Richards, R.R.; An, K.N.; Bigliani, L.U.; Friedman, R.J.; Gartsman, G.M.; Gristina, A.G.; Iannotti, J.P.; Mow, V.C.; Sidles, J.A.; Zuckerman, J.D. A standardized method for the assessment of shoulder function. *J. Shoulder Elb. Surg.* **1994**, *3*, 347–352. [CrossRef]
8. Schmidt, S.; Ferrer, M.; Gonzalez, M.; Gonzalez, N.; Valderas, J.M.; Alonso, J.; Escobar, A.; Vrotsou, K.; EMPRO Group. Evaluation of shoulder-specific patient-reported outcome measures: A systematic and standardized comparison of available evidence. *J. Shoulder Elb. Surg.* **2014**, *23*, 434–444. [CrossRef]
9. Angst, F.; Schwyzer, H.K.; Aeschlimann, A.; Simmen, B.R.; Goldhahn, J. Measures of adult shoulder function: Disabilities of the Arm, Shoulder, and Hand Questionnaire (DASH) and its short version (QuickDASH), Shoulder Pain and Disability Index (SPADI), American Shoulder and Elbow Surgeons (ASES) Society standardized shoulder assessment form, Constant (Murley) Score (CS), Simple Shoulder Test (SST), Oxford Shoulder Score (OSS), Shoulder Disability Questionnaire (SDQ), and Western Ontario Shoulder Instability Index (WOSI). *Arthritis Care Res.* **2011**, *63* (Suppl. 11), S174–S188. [CrossRef]
10. Roach, K.E.; Budiman-Mak, E.; Songsiridej, N.; Lertratanakul, Y. Development of a shoulder pain and disability index. *Arthritis Care Res.* **1991**, *4*, 143–149. [CrossRef] [PubMed]
11. Hudak, P.L.; Amadio, P.C.; Bombardier, C. Development of an upper extremity outcome measure: The DASH (disabilities of the arm, shoulder and hand) [corrected]. The Upper Extremity Collaborative Group (UECG). *Am. J. Ind. Med.* **1996**, *29*, 602–608. [CrossRef]
12. Constant, C.R.; Gerber, C.; Emery, R.J.; Sojbjerg, J.O.; Gohlke, F.; Boileau, P. A review of the Constant score: Modifications and guidelines for its use. *J. Shoulder Elb. Surg.* **2008**, *17*, 355–361. [CrossRef]
13. Constant, C.R.; Murley, A.H. A clinical method of functional assessment of the shoulder. *Clin. Orthop. Relat. Res.* **1987**, *214*, 160–164. [CrossRef]
14. Bercik, M.J.; Kruse, K., 2nd; Yalizis, M.; Gauci, M.O.; Chaoui, J.; Walch, G. A modification to the Walch classification of the glenoid in primary glenohumeral osteoarthritis using three-dimensional imaging. *J. Shoulder Elb. Surg.* **2016**, *25*, 1601–1606. [CrossRef]
15. Walch, G.; Badet, R.; Boulahia, A.; Khoury, A. Morphologic study of the glenoid in primary glenohumeral osteoarthritis. *J. Arthroplast.* **1999**, *14*, 756–760. [CrossRef]
16. Levigne, C.; Boileau, P.; Favard, L.; Garaud, P.; Mole, D.; Sirveaux, F.; Walch, G. Scapular notching in reverse shoulder arthroplasty. *J. Shoulder Elb. Surg.* **2008**, *17*, 925–935. [CrossRef]
17. Bell, S.N.; Coghlan, J.A. Short stem shoulder replacement. *Int. J. Shoulder Surg.* **2014**, *8*, 72–75. [CrossRef]
18. Lazarus, M.D.; Jensen, K.L.; Southworth, C.; Matsen, F.A., 3rd. The radiographic evaluation of keeled and pegged glenoid component insertion. *J. Bone Jt. Surg.* **2002**, *84-A*, 1174–1182. [CrossRef] [PubMed]
19. Sirveaux, F. Grammont Prosthesis in the Treatment of Shoulder Arthropathies with Massive Cuff Tear. Multicenter Series of 42 Cases. Ph.D. Thesis, Nancy I University, Nancy, France, 1997. (In French)
20. Sirveaux, F.; Favard, L.; Oudet, D.; Huquet, D.; Walch, G.; Mole, D. Grammont inverted total shoulder arthroplasty in the treatment of glenohumeral osteoarthritis with massive rupture of the cuff. Results of a multicentre study of 80 shoulders. *J. Bone Jt. Surgery. Br. Vol.* **2004**, *86*, 388–395. [CrossRef]
21. Bell, S.N.; Christmas, M.; Coghlan, J.A. Proximal humeral osteolysis and glenoid radiolucent lines in an anatomic shoulder arthroplasty: A comparison of a ceramic and a metal humeral head component. *J. Shoulder Elb. Surg.* **2020**, *29*, 913–923. [CrossRef] [PubMed]
22. Levigne, C.; Garret, J.; Boileau, P.; Alami, G.; Favard, L.; Walch, G. Scapular notching in reverse shoulder arthroplasty: Is it important to avoid it and how? *Clin. Orthop. Relat. Res.* **2011**, *469*, 2512–2520. [CrossRef]
23. R Core Team. *R: A Language and Environment for Statistical Computing*; R Foundation for Statistical Computing: Vienna, Austria, 2018; Available online: https://www.R-project.org (accessed on 29 July 2021).
24. Kiet, T.K.; Feeley, B.T.; Naimark, M.; Gajiu, T.; Hall, S.L.; Chung, T.T.; Ma, C.B. Outcomes after shoulder replacement: Comparison between reverse and anatomic total shoulder arthroplasty. *J. Shoulder Elb. Surg.* **2015**, *24*, 179–185. [CrossRef] [PubMed]
25. Wright, M.A.; Keener, J.D.; Chamberlain, A.M. Comparison of Clinical Outcomes After Anatomic Total Shoulder Arthroplasty and Reverse Shoulder Arthroplasty in Patients 70 Years and Older with Glenohumeral Osteoarthritis and an Intact Rotator Cuff. *J. Am. Acad. Orthop. Surg.* **2020**, *28*, e222–e229. [CrossRef] [PubMed]

26. Ponce, B.A.; Oladeji, L.O.; Rogers, M.E.; Menendez, M.E. Comparative analysis of anatomic and reverse total shoulder arthroplasty: In-hospital outcomes and costs. *J. Shoulder Elb. Surg.* **2015**, *24*, 460–467. [CrossRef] [PubMed]
27. Koh, J.; Galvin, J.W.; Sing, D.C.; Curry, E.J.; Li, X. Thirty-day Complications and Readmission Rates in Elderly Patients After Shoulder Arthroplasty. *J. Am. Acad. Orthop. Surg. Glob. Res. Rev.* **2018**, *2*, e068. [CrossRef]
28. Friedman, R.J.; Cheung, E.V.; Flurin, P.H.; Wright, T.; Simovitch, R.W.; Bolch, C.; Roche, C.P.; Zuckerman, J.D. Are Age and Patient Gender Associated with Different Rates and Magnitudes of Clinical Improvement After Reverse Shoulder Arthroplasty? *Clin. Orthop. Relat. Res.* **2018**, *476*, 1264–1273. [CrossRef] [PubMed]
29. Triplet, J.J.; Everding, N.G.; Levy, J.C.; Formaini, N.T.; O'Donnell, K.P.; Moor, M.A.; Virraroel, L.D. Anatomic and Reverse Total Shoulder Arthroplasty in Patients Older Than 80 Years. *Orthopedics* **2015**, *38*, e904–e910. [CrossRef] [PubMed]
30. Anakwenze, O.A.; Yehyawi, T.; Dillon, M.T.; Paxton, E.; Navarro, R.; Singh, A. Effect of Age on Outcomes of Shoulder Arthroplasty. *Perm. J.* **2017**, *21*, 16-056. [CrossRef]
31. Wagner, E.R.; Houdek, M.T.; Schleck, C.D.; Harmsen, W.S.; Sanchez-Sotelo, J.; Cofield, R.; Elhassan, B.T.; Sperling, J.W. The role age plays in the outcomes and complications of shoulder arthroplasty. *J. Shoulder Elb. Surg.* **2017**, *26*, 1573–1580. [CrossRef]
32. Flury, M.P.; Frey, P.; Goldhahn, J.; Schwyzer, H.K.; Simmen, B.R. Reverse shoulder arthroplasty as a salvage procedure for failed conventional shoulder replacement due to cuff failure–midterm results. *Int. Orthop.* **2011**, *35*, 53–60. [CrossRef]
33. Shields, E.; Wiater, J.M. Patient Outcomes after Revision of Anatomic Total Shoulder Arthroplasty to Reverse Shoulder Arthroplasty for Rotator Cuff Failure or Component Loosening: A Matched Cohort Study. *J. Am. Acad. Orthop. Surg.* **2019**, *27*, e193–e198. [CrossRef] [PubMed]
34. Zmistowski, B.; Gutman, M.; Horvath, Y.; Abboud, J.A.; Williams, G.R., Jr.; Namdari, S. Acromial stress fracture following reverse total shoulder arthroplasty: Incidence and predictors. *J. Shoulder Elb. Surg.* **2020**, *29*, 799–806. [CrossRef] [PubMed]
35. Young, A.A.; Walch, G.; Pape, G.; Gohlke, F.; Favard, L. Secondary rotator cuff dysfunction following total shoulder arthroplasty for primary glenohumeral osteoarthritis: Results of a multicenter study with more than five years of follow-up. *J. Bone Jt. Surg.* **2012**, *94*, 685–693. [CrossRef]
36. Codding, J.L.; Keener, J.D. Natural History of Degenerative Rotator Cuff Tears. *Curr. Rev. Musculoskelet. Med.* **2018**, *11*, 77–85. [CrossRef] [PubMed]

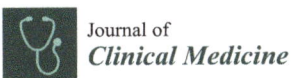 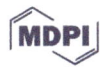

Article

Reverse Shoulder Arthroplasty for Proximal Humerus Head-Split Fractures—A Retrospective Cohort Study

Jan-Philipp Imiolczyk [1,*], Ulrich Brunner [2], Tankred Imiolczyk [3], Florian Freislederer [4], David Endell [4] and Markus Scheibel [1,4,*]

1. Center for Musculoskeletal Surgery, Charité-Universitaetsmedizin, 13353 Berlin, Germany
2. Department of Trauma and Orthopedic Surgery, Krankenhaus Agatharied, 83734 Hausham, Germany; ulrich.brunner@khagatharied.de
3. Department of Mathematics, University of Mannheim, 68131 Mannheim, Germany; imiolczyktankred@gmail.com
4. Department of Shoulder and Elbow Surgery, Schulthess Clinic, 8008 Zurich, Switzerland; florian.freislederer@kws.ch (F.F.); david.endell@kws.ch (D.E.)
* Correspondence: jan-philipp.imiolczyk@charite.de (J.-P.I.); markus.scheibel@kws.ch (M.S.)

Abstract: Head-split fractures are proximal humerus fractures (PHF) that result from fracture lines traversing the articular surface. While head-split fractures are rare, surgical treatment of these complex injuries can be extremely challenging and is associated with high rates of complications. Treatment using primary reverse shoulder arthroplasty (RSA) has been associated with moderate complication rates and reproducible clinical results. The aim of this study was to evaluate clinical and radiographic outcomes, and complication rates of RSA for head-split PHF. Twenty-six patients were evaluated based on Constant Score (CS) and range of motion of both shoulders and Subjective Shoulder Value (SSV). Radiographic analysis evaluated tuberosity healing, prosthetic loosening and scapular notching. Patients achieved good clinical results with a CS of 73.7 points and SSV of 82% after a mean follow-up of 50 months. The relative CS comparing operated versus the unaffected shoulder was 92%. Greater tuberosity healing was achieved in 61%. Patients who suffered a high-energy trauma reached a significantly greater functional outcome. Patients who suffered multifragmentation to the humeral head performed the worst. There were no cases of loosening; scapular notching was visible in two cases. The complication rate was 8%. RSA is an adequate treatment option with for head-split PHF in elderly patients.

Keywords: head split; splitting; tuberosity; healing; union; trauma; humerus; trauma; low; high; energy; double shadow; pelican sign

Citation: Imiolczyk, J.-P.; Brunner, U.; Imiolczyk, T.; Freislederer, F.; Endell, D.; Scheibel, M. Reverse Shoulder Arthroplasty for Proximal Humerus Head-Split Fractures— A Retrospective Cohort Study. J. Clin. Med. 2022, 11, 2835. https://doi.org/10.3390/jcm11102835

Academic Editor: Patrick Joel Denard

Received: 15 April 2022
Accepted: 12 May 2022
Published: 17 May 2022

Publisher's Note: MDPI stays neutral with regard to jurisdictional claims in published maps and institutional affiliations.

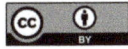

Copyright: © 2022 by the authors. Licensee MDPI, Basel, Switzerland. This article is an open access article distributed under the terms and conditions of the Creative Commons Attribution (CC BY) license (https:// creativecommons.org/licenses/by/ 4.0/).

1. Introduction

Proximal humerus fractures (PHF) account for approximately 6% of all fractures [1]. The so-called head-split fracture describes a rare phenomenon (accounting for less than 5% of all PHF) that results from fracture lines traversing the articular surface of the humeral head [2]. This occurs when the impaction force of trauma acts in a vertical direction against the glenoid or acromion, such that shearing forces lead to humeral head cleavage.

This type of fracture was originally diagnosed by a double shadow visible on plain anteroposterior (AP) radiographs, although it was usually regarded as a subtype of posterior dislocation fractures because of its rare occurrence [3–5]. Furthermore, the double shadow sign was easily missed on plain AP views of three patients in the first consecutive series including eight PHF patients [4]. Chesser et al. recommended the need for additional axillary radiographs and computed tomography (CT) scans to thoroughly diagnose these rare yet devastating fractures, which require early treatment to restore shoulder function [6]. If the pelican sign is detected on axillary views, a type II head-split fracture is diagnosed.

The first arc represents the lesser tuberosity and the second arc a part of the articular surface which remained attached to the lesser tuberosity [2,7].

Therefore, a most recent attempt has been made to classify these specific fractures on CT scans by Scheibel et al. [7]. With the extension of CT for diagnosis or surgery planning, the event of fracture lines through the articular face can be diagnosed far better than on two-dimensional radiographs.

Head-split PHF were first described in young male patients with high-energy trauma (i.e., a bicycle, motor or car accident) or epileptic seizures, where open reduction and internal fixation (ORIF) was considered the adequate treatment solution whenever closed reduction was not possible [6]. While these patients usually have good bone quality and the best potential for revascularization, it is important that these fractures are surgically fixed early after trauma in order to lower the risk of avascular necrosis and potential cartilage and joint degeneration [5,6,8]. Head-split fractures have also been reported in older, mainly female, patients involved in low-energy trauma (i.e., a simple fall from height) who typically have poorer bone quality and limited regenerative potential [2,7]. Conservative treatment for these particular fractures that are often misdiagnosed on plain radiographs has shown unsatisfactory results; in this instance, hemiarthroplasty (HA) was considered as a salvage procedure [6].

Reverse shoulder arthroplasty (RSA) has proven a reliable treatment option for severely displaced three- or four-part PHF in the older population, which offers encouraging mid-term results regarding pain loss, good return in range of motion and good functional outcome [9–14]. While ORIF and HA are both associated with high rates of complications (50% and 100%, respectively), and often followed by consecutive revision surgery, RSA may present as a potential treatment option even for relatively young patients aged below 70 years [15].

Given the sparse knowledge on the ideal treatment for this particular PHF and the accompanying high complication rates after HA and ORIF, the aim of this study was to evaluate clinical and radiological results as well as occurrence of complications in a unique consecutive series of head-split PHF patients treated with RSA.

2. Materials and Methods

2.1. Study Population

Between December 2009 and September 2020, 45 consecutive patients (m = 10, f = 35, mean age 75.8; range: 56–92 years at time of surgery) were identified with a head-split PHF. Of 45, 5 had sustained an additional glenoid rim fracture. All patients underwent RSA at one of two hospitals by one of three specialized shoulder surgeons. The indication for RSA was an unreconstructable PHF in an elderly patient population. All patients were retrospectively recruited via telephone invitation to attend a clinical follow-up examination. When patients could not be reached because the original contact details were no longer valid, we used the emergency contact details from medical records to gain further information on the patient's current location and ensure follow-up assessment of these cases. For those patients unable to attend the clinical assessment because of age, poor health and/or the inability to travel to one of our clinics, we evaluated shoulder function and status only via telephone and postal contact.

2.2. Implant Description, Surgical Procedure and Postoperative Rehabilitation Protocol

Patients were treated in a beach chair position using a deltopectoral approach. For all RSA patients, a Grammont type of prosthesis (155° humeral inclination) was used with either a conventional ($n = 5$) or fracture-specific stem design ($n = 40$) and open metaphysis to allow bone ingrowth (AEQUALIS™ REVERSED II or AEQUALIS™ REVERSED FX, Tornier/Stryker Inc., Kalamazoo, MI, USA) (Figure 1). In addition, we applied a hybrid cementing technique to enable bone ingrowth at the metaphysis. In each case, both the greater and lesser tuberosities were anatomically reattached using FiberWire® #5 sutures (Arthrex Inc., Naples, FL, USA) against the fin of the metaphyseal neck of the prosthesis as previously described [14]. After surgery, the shoulder was immobilized in a sling for 14 days. Passive mobilization began on postoperative day 15 and active mobilization was undertaken six weeks post-RSA. All patients completed the same standardized rehabilitation protocol.

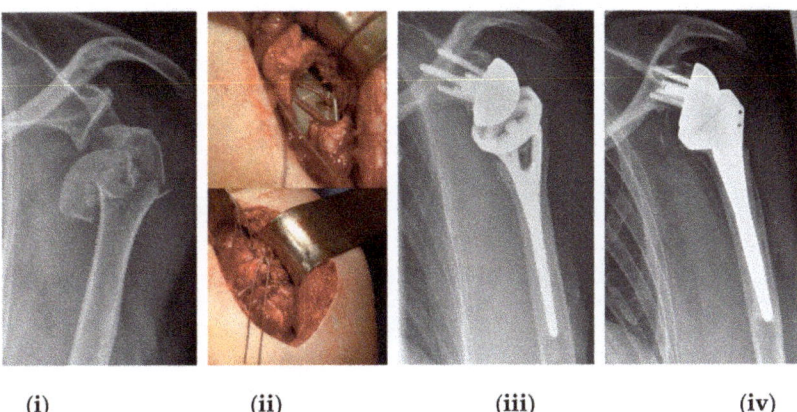

Figure 1. This figure shows a severe head-split PHF that has been treated with a RSA (**i**). All patients have received the same surgical treatment with a tuberosity refixation (**ii**). One year postoperatively, the greater tuberosity shows complete consolidation (**iii**). The *Fracture* stem (**iii**) shows a metaphyseal window to encourage bone ingrowth, whereas the *Reverse II* (**iv**) displays two holes for suturing the tuberosities. After 7 years of follow-up in another patient, however, the greater tuberosity has resorbed completely (**iv**).

2.3. Clinical Assessment

Patients were questioned about their history of trauma (low or high energy). In addition, the absolute as well as age- and gender-modified Constant-Murley score (CS), American Shoulder and Elbow Surgeons Assessment Form (ASES) score, Subjective Shoulder Value (SSV), Simple Shoulder Test (SST) and Activities of Daily Living requiring active External Rotation (ADLER) score were evaluated [16–21]. Abduction strength was measured using an Isobex 3.0 dynamometer (Veribor, Germany); pain was assessed using a scale of 0 to 15 points (15 = no pain; 0 = excruciating pain) and patient satisfaction (1 = unsatisfied; 2 = somewhat satisfied; 3 = satisfied; 4 = very satisfied) was also evaluated at the final follow-up examination.

Active range of motion (ROM), including anterior forward elevation, abduction, internal and external rotation, the Hornblower and external rotation lag signs (ERLS) were documented. Furthermore, ROM and CS were determined for the contralateral shoulder to assess the outcome of relative CS (i.e., the ratio of absolute CS of the affected versus contralateral shoulders).

2.4. Radiographic Evaluation

Preoperative radiographic assessments were made on standardized true AP, axillary and Y-view images. A CT scan was also performed to classify the head-split fracture type [7] and determine the presence of any additional glenoid rim fractures. The arrangement of patterns depends on the involvement of the head-split component adjacent tuberosity (Figure 2).

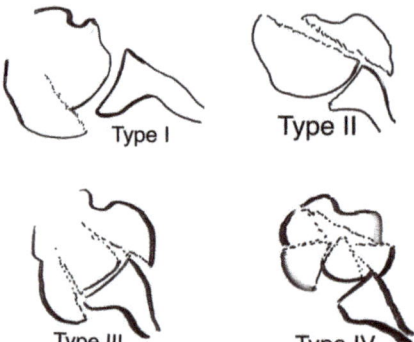

Figure 2. Four different types of head-split fracture patterns depending on involvement of the head-split component adjacent tuberosity (**Type I**: greater tuberosity; **Type II**: lesser tuberosity), whether fracture fragments split into disconnecting pieces that may lead to a stamp-like fracture pattern resulting in both greater and lesser tuberosity fragments connected to the articular face (**Type III**) or the multifragmentation of the disconnection of split pieces (**Type IV**) [7]. (Reproduced, with modification, under Creative Commons Attribution 4.0 International. License [https://creativecommons.org/licenses/by/4.0/] (accessed on 1 January 2022)], from: [7].

Postoperative evaluations were also made on true AP, axillary and Y-view radiographs to identify osteolysis, prosthetic loosening, heterotopic ossification and calcification, and scapular notching as well as tuberosity healing or migration. All radiographic examinations were evaluated by two independent surgeons, one of which was not involved in the surgical procedure.

2.5. Complication

All patients' medical records were scanned for any shoulder-related complication or reoperation until the final follow-up examination.

2.6. Statistical Analysis

Due to the nature of this retrospective cohort study without a control group, all data are presented using standard descriptive statistics. Due to the small sample size, we applied the Wilcoxon rank-sum test to compare the clinical function of tuberosity healing, the presence of the ER lag sign and the difference in outcome after fracture pattern types I and IV. Analysis of variance (ANOVA) testing was applied to investigate any clinical differences among the various fracture types. Due to the small and nonrepresentational sample sizes for fracture types II and III (n = 3 each), we have used ANOVA testing just for investigation of tendencies. In addition, we also compared the outcomes of the "classic" type I fracture to those with comminution (type IV) to achieve a more reliable statistical analysis.

All statistical analyses were completed using SPSS 27 (IBM, Armonk, NY, USA) and the significance level was set to 0.05.

3. Results

Twenty-six patients (20 females, 6 males) with a mean age of 73.4 years were available for clinical and radiographic follow-up. The average postoperative follow-up occurred at 50 months (range: 12–142 months). A total of 19 patients dropped out of the study either because of death (n = 11), multimorbidity (n = 2) or severe dementia (n = 3) that hindered adequate examination of shoulder function; one patient suffered from paralysis following a severe stroke (n = 1), while two more dropped out either because of a SARS-COVID-19 infection (n = 1) or they were lost to follow-up (n = 1). There was no radiographic follow-up available for 3 of the 26 patients. Fracture morphologies and patient demographics are displayed in Table 1.

Table 1. Baseline patient demographics.

N (women in %)	26 (77%)	
Age at surgery (years) (mean ± SD) (range)	73.4 ± 7.8 56–91	
Follow-up period (months) (mean ± SD) (range)	50 ± 22 12–142	
Trauma mechanism	Low energy	High energy
N	13 (50%)	13 (50%)
(Women in %)	85%	69%
Age at surgery (years) (mean ± SD) (range)	77.8 ± 7.8 (64–91)	68.5 ± 7.3 (56–78)
Follow-up period (months) (mean ± SD) (range)	52.6 ± 36.7 (14–142)	46.8 ± 22.0 (12–93)
Head-split classification * (n)		
I	3	7
II	3	0
III	2	1
IV	5	5
Additional glenoid rim fracture (n)	2	0

SD—standard deviation. * according to Scheibel et al. [7].

3.1. Clinical Results

Our patient cohort achieved excellent clinical results based on all measured shoulder function scores and ROM (Table 2, Figure 3). The average SSV was 82% (range: 50–100%) and the absolute CS was 80% (range: 58–97 points). Most patients were pain free and reached full points in ADLER score and satisfaction. Patients in our cohort reached on average a flexion of 148° (range 100–175), external rotation of 15° (range: −10–60) and internal rotation up to L3 vertebra (range: thigh–scapula). Compared to the healthy, unaffected shoulder, the RSA shoulder reached 92% (range: 67–141%) of the contralateral function on average.

Table 2. Final postoperative clinical scores and range of motion.

	Mean (SD)	Range
Absolute CS (points)	73.7 (11.2)	43–92
Absolute CS of opposite shoulder (points)	80.3 (10.4)	58–97
Relative CS compared to opposite shoulder (%)	92.4 (14.1)	67–141
Age- and gender-modified CS (%)	79.1 (10.0)	53–95
ASES score (points)	89.1 (13.8)	53–100
SSV (%)	82.0 (13.0)	50–100
SST (%)	77.3 (19.4)	33–100
ADLER score (0–30 points)	27.7 (4.0)	12–30
Pain scale (0–15 points)	14.3 (2.0)	8–15
Abduction strength (kg)	4.0 (1.9)	0–8.7
Range of motion		
Anterior forward elevation (°)	148 (25)	100–175
Abduction (°)	144 (27)	80–180
External rotation in 0° abduction (°)	15 (16)	−10–60
Internal rotation (CS points)	6.1 (2.7)	0–10
Satisfaction (1–4)	3.8 (0.4)	3–4

SD—standard deviation; CS—constant score; ASES—American shoulder and elbow surgeons assessment form; SSV—subjective shoulder score; SST—Simple Shoulder Test; ADLER—activities of daily living requiring active external rotation.

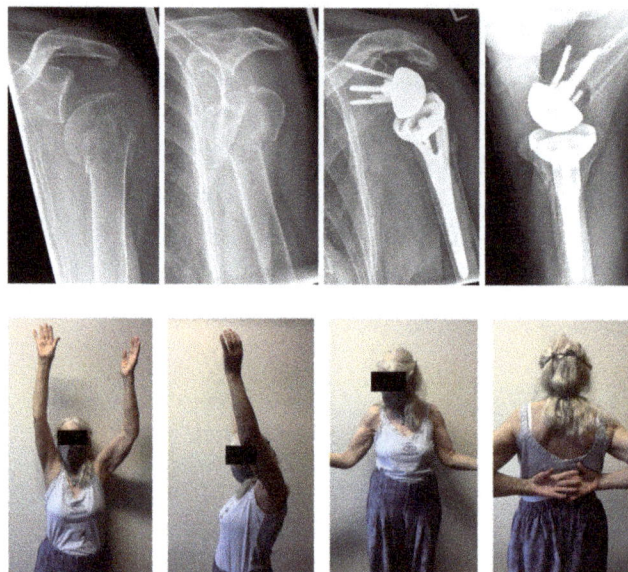

Figure 3. This 77-year-old woman sustained a type III fracture in preoperative radiographs (**upper two left**) after a fall onto her left shoulder while hiking. At 50 months post-RSA, the patient was very satisfied with excellent function (**lower bottom**) and a CS of 81 points, a relative CS of 99%, and a SSV of 95%. Both the greater and lesser tuberosities show healing and no scapular notching is visible on post-op (**upper two right**) images.

Patients who suffered a high-energy trauma performed significantly better and showed a greater absolute CS (79 vs. 69 points; $p = 0.010$), ASES (94 vs. 84 points; $p = 0.044$), ADLER score (30 vs. 26 points; $p < 0.001$) and SST score (87 vs. 68 points; $p = 0.005$) as well as abduction strength (5.0 vs. 2.9 kg; $p = 0.005$). With regard to ROM, patients after high-energy trauma reached greater anterior forward elevation (157° vs. 141°; $p = 0.011$), abduction (151° vs. 139°; $p = 0.042$) and external rotation (19° vs. 12°; $p = 0.047$) at final follow-up.

A total of seven patients presented with a positive ERLS, two of which also presented with a positive Hornblower sign. The presence of a positive ERLS coincided with significantly worse outcomes for SSV (72% vs. 84%; $p = 0.023$), the ADLER score (29 vs. 24 points; $p = 0.002$) and external rotation (1° vs. 21°; $p = 0.002$). Healing of both the greater ($p = 0.02$) and lesser tuberosities ($p = 0.004$) was observed when the ERLS was absent.

3.2. Radiographic Results

There were no cases of osteolysis or prosthetic loosening at final follow-up in all patients with radiographic follow-up ($n = 23$). There were two patients with calcification of the posterosuperior cuff and another with heterotopic ossification around both the scapular neck and humerus. Scapular notching (Grade 1) was documented in two patients (8.7%).

Greater tuberosity (GT) healing was present in 14 patients (61%) and the GT migrated superiorly and presented as a nonunion in five patients (22%). Four patients exhibited GT resorption at final follow-up (17%). Greater tuberosity healing was associated with greater ER ($p = 0.03$). Healing of the lesser tuberosity (LT) occurred in 18 patients (78%). There was no impact of LT healing on any clinical outcome measurement. However, higher rates of tuberosity healing were documented after a high-energy trauma.

3.3. Comparison of Head-Split Types

There were some differences in the absolute and modified CS, ASES score and internal rotation among the four fracture patterns (Table 3). Type 1 fractures seem to present the most favorable outcome, whereas fractures patterns with impairment of the LT (Type II–IV) seem to perform worse. In particular, LT head-split fragmentation seems to impact internal rotation the most.

Table 3. Clinical scores with regard to head-split fracture pattern types.

c	Type 1	Type 2	Type 3	Type 4	p-Value *	p-Value ** Type 1 vs. 4
	Mean (SD) Range					
n	10	3	3	10		
Age at surgery	77 (6.1) 68–87	76 (7.8) 70–85	71 (7.9) 62–77	69 (10.7) 56–91		
Follow-up period	43 (25.4) 14–95	80 (55.0) 37–142	47 (12.8) 33–58	49 (27.3) 12–93		
High-energy (n)/low-energy trauma setting (n)	7/3	0/3	1/2	5/5		
Age and gender modified CS (%)	87 (4.8) 80–95	73 (11.8) 60–81	78 (10.1) 67–86	74 (9.3) 53–86	0.010	>0.001
Absolute CS (points)	81 (6.3) 72–92	68 (10.0) 57–75	75 (7.8) 66–81	68 (12.7) 43–84	0.033	0.006
Relative CS to opposite shoulder (%)	100 (15.0) 91–141	82 (8.1) 73–88	90 (12.8) 75–99	89 (13.0) 67–112	0.2	0.06
ASES score (points)	98 (1.7) 88–100	86 (16.4) 68–100	77 (20.4) 62–100	85 (14.2) 53–98	0.047	0.002
SSV (%)	88 (9.5) 70–100	78 (25.7) 50–100	73 (19) 60–95	80 (9.1) 70–90	0.3	0.03
SST (%)	90 (12.3) 67–100	72 (21.0) 50–92	72 (17.5) 58–92	68 (20.6) 33–92	0.2	0.1
ADLER score (0–30 points)	29 (1.7) 26–30	24 (10.4) 12–30	25 (3.8) 21–28	28 (2.2) 24–30	0.053	0.050
Anterior forward elevation (°)	154 (23) 110–170	142 (28) 110–160	162 (3) 160–165	140 (28) 100–175	0.5	0.1
Abduction (°)	155 (22) 120–180	150 (17) 130–160	157 (23) 130–170	128 (29) 80–165	0.1	0.04
External rotation in 0° abduction (°)	16 (21) 0–60	13 (12) 0–20	10 (15) −5–25	16 (14) 100–175	0.9	0.4
Internal rotation (CS points)	8.2 (1.4) 6–10	3.3 (2.3) 2–6	6.7 (2.3) 4–8	4.6 (2.7) 0–8	0.002	<0.001
Abduction strength (kg)	4.9 (1.9) 2.5–8.7	2.7 (1.0) 1.5–3.4	3.9 (0.8) 3.3–4.8	3.5 (2.2) 0–7.2	0.3	0.08
GT healing	4 out of 8 (50%)	1 out of 3 (33%)	2 out of 3 (67%)	7 out of 9 (78%)	0.5	0.3
LT healing	7 out of 8 (88%)	2 out of 3 (67%)	2 out of 3 (67%)	7 out of 9 (78%)	0.9	0.3
Scapular notching	0%	1 × Grade 1 (33%)	0%	1 × Grade 1 (11%)	0.02	0.5

SD—standard deviation; CS—constant score; ASES—American shoulder and elbow surgeons assessment form; SST – Simple Shoulder Test; SSV—subjective shoulder score; ADLER—activities of daily living requiring active external rotation; GT—greater tuberosity; LT—lesser tuberosity. * ANOVA for comparison of all four fracture types. ** Wilcoxon rank-sum test.

When comparing the "classic" fracture type I with the GT adjacent head-split fragment to that with a comminuted articular face, type IV exhibited worse function in all clinical outcome measurements, particularly for internal rotation ($p < 0.001$). Although the GT healing rate was higher for type IV fractures, this did not reach statistical significance.

3.4. Complications

Of 26 patients, we reported a total of two (8%) complications throughout the post-RSA follow-up, one (4%) of which required revision surgery.

The first reported complication involved one patient who encountered instability 7 weeks post-RSA while undergoing physiotherapy. During a reoperation, the inlay liner was exchanged and a larger one was implanted. At 43 months after the secondary intervention, no further dislocations were encountered and a CS of 76 points and SSV of 70% was documented. The second complication was an acromion stress fracture reported at 39 months post-RSA. The affected patient declined the possibility of undergoing a reoperation after being informed of the potential risks associated with further surgery and opted for conservative treatment. This patient achieved the worst clinical outcome in our cohort with a CS of 52 points and forward flexion of 80°, but remained satisfied with their outcome despite a SSV of 70%.

After further investigations into our medical records, an additional patient was documented with a posterior dislocation 6 weeks post-RSA and underwent early revision surgery to increase the inlay liner. This patient was excluded from this analysis based on the diagnosis of severe dementia and inability to comply with the required follow-up examination.

4. Discussion

Patients with RSA after head-split PHF showed very good clinical and radiographic results, and the revision rate was 4% for those patients with clinical follow-up. Our cohort shows that patients who sustained a head-split fractures resulting from high-impact trauma had better results regardless of tuberosity healing. In addition, patients with a classic type 1 GT adjacent head-split showed better outcomes over those with multifragmentation of the articular face.

A current meta-analysis including 1303 PHF patients found the average anterior forward elevation flexion of about 122° with an average CS of 59 points and a total complication rate of 11% [22]. In our population, we achieved a similar complication rate, but our patients scored 74 points, on average, for the CS and achieved 148° elevation.

Healing of the GT led to favorable external rotation. Although GT healing was achieved in 61% of our cohort, this factor did not influence anterior forward elevation or any other functional outcome parameter besides external rotation, in contrast to a current meta-analysis [23]. This result could be biased by the small sample size in our cohort. However, the presence of the ER lag sign seems to be a prognostic factor not only for poorer external rotation but for subjective performance (SSV) since external rotation is involved in many activities of daily life.

Since our study population is older than 50 years, this study presents the advantages of RSA treatment for older patients. While complication rates for joint-preserving therapy options are high, young patients should be treated as soon as possible to minimize the risk of avascular necrosis [8,15]. High-impact trauma resulted in humeral head splitting that was first documented in dislocation fractures [4,6,8,24], yet we observed a collateral glenoid rim fracture in 5 out of 45 patients. We hypothesize that this is due to the trauma mechanism of the humeral head being forced against the glenoid, which causes the head-split fracture but may also result in glenoid rim fractures due to either extremely high shearing forces or poor bone quality.

The first published consecutive cohort included eight patients (3x ORIF, 3x missed, 1x CRIF, 1x HA): the oldest patient was a 56-year-old female who sustained a low-energy trauma fracture that was initially missed on radiographic examination and left untreated [6].

The outcome was a stiff and painful shoulder with extremely poor function. Conversely, younger patients (19- and a 21-year-old males) within the cohort who both suffered high-energy traumas achieved excellent functional results after early open or closed reduction and internal fixation (CS was 89 and 100 points, respectively) [6,8].

Although our study population is older by far, this finding concurs with our data including patients who had experienced a high-energy trauma and achieved a better outcome post-RSA. We hypothesize that head-split fractures resulting from high-impact and low-impact injuries are two different entities. Active patients who are confident to cycle or ski regularly can anticipate an increased risk of experiencing a high-impact accident. These patients could be considered biologically young as their active lifestyle results in good bone quality according to Wolff's law [25]. In such cases, high shearing forces result in head-splitting fractures, but due to the great regenerative potential of vital tissue, patients can achieve better outcomes after RSA. Patients that sustain head-split fractures due to a fall from standing height were, on average, ten years older in our cohort and were not participating in an active lifestyle. For these cases, the fracture patterns are the result of poor bone quality and poor bone density due to immobility or osteoporosis.

Based on our cohort, articular-faced comminution of the humerus presents a serious treatment challenge for surgeons because very poor postoperative outcome can be expected. Our type IV patients had significantly poorer outcomes in all clinical scores measured. In addition, abduction and internal rotation were significantly lower for type IV fractures; external rotation was not affected by fracture type.

Although HA offers comparable results for head-split fractures (diagnosed on radiographs) compared to conventional three- or four-part PHF at short- to long-term follow-up [2,26], the complication rate of 36% and a revision rate of 12.5% should not be underestimated [2]. Compared to the cohort that has been treated with HA ($n = 8$), short-term results are comparable even though patients with RSA perform better in flexion but worse in external rotation [2]. Nowadays, RSA has limited the use of HA for PHF due to the current development and progress in shoulder arthroplasty [27,28].

Our study has several limitations, such as the retrospective design of this study as well as its small cohort. Differences between the different fracture types should not be considered as significant results; rather as trends. Our cohort analysis showed that head-split fracture patients were quite old with many in their mid-70s at the time of surgery, which resulted in a high rate of loss to follow-up due to death alone (24%). A strength of this study was that all patients were treated by only one of two senior surgeons in the same operative technique and that the head-split fracture was diagnosed on CT scans.

Finally, while joint-preserving therapy is the precedent for young patients with unreconstructable PHF, the high complication rates of 44% in cases aged under 55 years and up to 50% in general dictate the greater likelihood for secondary surgery due to osteonecrosis or nonunion [15,29]. As RSA techniques develop and push the boundaries of age due to good results in complicated fracture situations, long-term studies must continue to monitor whether young patients benefit more from early primary or later secondary RSA treatment.

5. Conclusions

RSA is a very good and reliable treatment option with low complication rates for proximal humerus head-split fractures in the older patient population. Patients who sustain a head-split fracture due to high-impact trauma have greater biological and regenerative potential that can lead to more promising outcomes. Comminution or multifragmentation of the articular face presents as a prognostic indicator for significantly poorer outcome.

Author Contributions: Conceptualization, J.-P.I., U.B. and M.S.; methodology, J.-P.I., U.B. and M.S.; formal analysis, T.I.; investigation, J.-P.I.; data curation, M.S., U.B.; writing—original draft preparation, J.-P.I.; writing—review and editing, U.B., F.F., D.E., M.S.; visualization, J.-P.I., T.I.; supervision, M.S. All authors have read and agreed to the published version of the manuscript.

Funding: This research received no external funding.

Institutional Review Board Statement: The study was conducted according to the guidelines of the Declaration of Helsinki and approved by the Institutional Review Board (or Ethics Committee) of Charité—Universitaetsmedicine Berlin (EA1/167/18; date of approval: 11 November 2018) and Ludwig-Maximilians-Universitaet Muenchen (22-0178; date of approval: 6 April 2022).

Informed Consent Statement: Informed consent was obtained from all subjects involved in the study.

Data Availability Statement: Data available on request due to ethical restrictions. The data presented in this study are available on request from the corresponding author. The data are not publicly available.

Acknowledgments: The authors thank M. Wilhelmi, (medical writer at Schulthess Clinic) for manuscript proofreading.

Conflicts of Interest: J.-P.I., T.I., F.F. and D.E. declare no conflict of interest. M.S. and U.B. are consultants for Stryker Corporation.

References

1. Aaron, D.; Shatsky, J.; Paredes, J.C.; Jiang, C.; Parsons, B.O.; Flatow, E.L. Proximal Humeral Fractures: Internal Fixation. *Instr. Course Lect.* **2013**, *62*, 143–154.
2. Greiwe, R.M.; Vargas-Ariza, R.; Bigliani, L.U.; Levine, W.N.; Ahmad, C.S. Hemiarthroplasty for head-split fractures of the proximal humerus. *Orthopedics* **2013**, *36*, e905–e911. [CrossRef] [PubMed]
3. Rowe, C.R.; Zarins, B. Chronic unreduced dislocations of the shoulder. *J. Bone Jt. Surg. Am.* **1982**, *64*, 494–505. (In English) [CrossRef]
4. Randelli, M. La Fracture-Luxation Postérieure de L'épaule: Noveux Éléments de Classification et Thérapeutiques. In Proceedings of the 2nd Congrés de la Société Européenne de Chirurgie de l'éPaule et du Coude, Berné, France, 1–2 October 1988.
5. Walch, G.; Boileau, P.; Martin, B.; Dejour, H. Unreduced Posterior Luxations and Fractures-Luxations of the Shoulder. Apropos of 30 cases. *Revue Chir. Orthop. Reparatrice L'appareil Mot.* **1990**, *76*, 546–558.
6. Chesser, T.J.; Langdon, I.J.; Ogilvie, C.; Sarangi, P.P.; Clarke, A.M. Fractures Involving Splitting of the Humeral Head. *J. Bone Jt. Surg. Br.* **2001**, *83*, 423–426. [CrossRef]
7. Scheibel, M.; Peters, P.; Moro, F.; Moroder, P. Head-split fractures of the proximal humerus. *Obere Extremität* **2019**, *14*, 93–102. [CrossRef]
8. Gokkus, K.; Agar, E.; Sagtas, E.; Aydin, A.T. Proximal humerus head-splitting fracture associated with single-part anterior dislocation. *BMJ Case Rep.* **2014**, *2014*, bcr2013202188. [CrossRef]
9. Bufquin, T.; Hersan, A.; Hubert, L.; Massin, P. Reverse shoulder arthroplasty for the treatment of three- and four-part fractures of the proximal humerus in the elderly: A prospective review of 43 cases with a short-term follow-up. *J. Bone Jt. Surg. Br.* **2007**, *89*, 516–520. [CrossRef] [PubMed]
10. Cazeneuve, J.F.; Cristofari, D.J. Grammont reversed prosthesis for acute complex fracture of the proximal humerus in an elderly population with 5 to 12 years follow-up. *Orthop. Traumatol. Surg. Res.* **2014**, *100*, 93–97. [CrossRef]
11. Chalmers, P.N.; Slikker, W., III; Mall, N.A.; Gupta, A.K.; Rahman, Z.; Enriquez, D.; Nicholson, G.P. Reverse total shoulder arthroplasty for acute proximal humeral fracture: Comparison to open reduction-internal fixation and hemiarthroplasty. *J. Shoulder Elb. Surg.* **2014**, *23*, 197–204. [CrossRef]
12. Cuff, D.J.; Pupello, D.R. Comparison of hemiarthroplasty and reverse shoulder arthroplasty for the treatment of proximal humeral fractures in elderly patients. *J. Bone Jt. Surg. Am.* **2013**, *95*, 2050–2055. [CrossRef] [PubMed]
13. Mata-Fink, A.; Meinke, M.; Jones, C.; Kim, B.; Bell, J.E. Reverse shoulder arthroplasty for treatment of proximal humeral fractures in older adults: A systematic review. *J. Shoulder Elb. Surg.* **2013**, *22*, 1737–1748. [CrossRef] [PubMed]
14. Imiolczyk, J.P.; Moroder, P.; Scheibel, M. Fracture-Specific and Conventional Stem Designs in Reverse Shoulder Arthroplasty for Acute Proximal Humerus Fractures-A Retrospective, Observational Study. *J. Clin. Med.* **2021**, *10*, 175. [CrossRef]
15. Peters, P.-M.; Plachel, F.; Danzinger, V.; Nove, M.; Märdian, S.; Scheibel, M.; Moroder, P. Clinical and Radiographic Outcomes After Surgical Treatment of Proximal Humeral Fractures with Head-Split Component. *J. Bone Jt. Surg. Am.* **2020**, *102*, 68–75. [CrossRef] [PubMed]
16. Constant, C.R.; Murley, A.H. A Clinical Method of Functional Assessment of the Shoulder. *Clin. Orthop. Relat. Res.* **1987**, *214*, 160–164. [CrossRef]
17. Michener, L.A.; McClure, P.W.; Sennett, B.J. American Shoulder and Elbow Surgeons Standardized Shoulder Assessment Form, patient self-report section: Reliability, validity, and responsiveness. *J. Shoulder Elb. Surg.* **2002**, *11*, 587–594. [CrossRef]
18. Gilbart, M.K.; Gerber, C. Comparison of the subjective shoulder value and the Constant score. *J. Shoulder Elb. Surg.* **2007**, *16*, 717–721. [CrossRef]
19. Godfrey, J.; Hamman, R.; Lowenstein, S.; Briggs, K.; Kocher, M. Reliability, validity, and responsiveness of the simple shoulder test: Psychometric properties by age and injury type. *J. Shoulder Elb. Surg.* **2007**, *16*, 260–267. [CrossRef]

20. Boileau, P.; Chuinard, C.; Roussanne, Y.; Bicknell, R.T.; Rochet, N.; Trojani, C. Reverse shoulder arthroplasty combined with a modified latissimus dorsi and teres major tendon transfer for shoulder pseudoparalysis associated with dropping arm. *Clin. Orthop. Relat. Res.* **2008**, *466*, 584–593. [CrossRef]
21. Tavakkolizadeh, A.; Ghassemi, A.; Colegate-Stone, T.; Latif, A.; Sinha, J. Gender-specific Constant score correction for age. *Knee Surg. Sports Traumatol. Arthrosc.* **2009**, *17*, 529–533. [CrossRef]
22. Kennedy, J.; Klifto, C.S.; Ledbetter, L.; Bullock, G.S. Reverse total shoulder arthroplasty clinical and patient-reported outcomes and complications stratified by preoperative diagnosis: A systematic review. *J. Shoulder Elb. Surg.* **2021**, *30*, 929–941. [CrossRef] [PubMed]
23. Jain, N.P.; Mannan, S.S.; Dharmarajan, R.; Rangan, A. Tuberosity healing after reverse shoulder arthroplasty for complex proximal humeral fractures in elderly patients-does it improve outcomes? A systematic review and meta-analysis. *J. Shoulder Elb. Surg.* **2019**, *28*, e78–e91. (In English) [CrossRef]
24. Gokkus, K.; Sagtas, E.; Kara, H.; Aydin, A.T. Posterior Shoulder Dislocation Associated with the Head (Splitting) and Humeral Neck Fracture: Impact of Understanding Radiologic Signs and Experience With an Extended Deltopectoral Approach. *Tech. Hand Up. Extrem. Surg.* **2018**, *22*, 57–64. [CrossRef] [PubMed]
25. Wolff, J. Das Gesetz der Transformation des Knochen. *DMW Dtsch. Med. Wochenschr.* **1893**, *19*, 1222–1224. [CrossRef]
26. Antuña, S.A.; Sperling, J.W.; Cofield, R.H. Shoulder hemiarthroplasty for acute fractures of the proximal humerus: A minimum five-year follow-up. *J. Shoulder Elb. Surg.* **2008**, *17*, 202–209. (In English) [CrossRef]
27. Shukla, D.R.; McAnany, S.; Kim, J.; Overley, S.; Parsons, B.O. Hemiarthroplasty versus reverse shoulder arthroplasty for treatment of proximal humeral fractures: A meta-analysis. *J. Shoulder Elb. Surg.* **2016**, *25*, 330–340. [CrossRef]
28. Bonnevialle, N.; Tournier, C.; Clavert, P.; Ohl, X.; Sirveaux, F.; Saragaglia, D. Hemiarthroplasty versus reverse shoulder arthroplasty in 4-part displaced fractures of the proximal humerus: Multicenter retrospective study. *Orthop. Traumatol. Surg. Res.* **2016**, *102*, 569–573. [CrossRef]
29. Gavaskar, A.S.; Tummala, N.C. Locked plate osteosynthesis of humeral head-splitting fractures in young adults. *J. Shoulder Elb. Surg.* **2015**, *24*, 908–914. [CrossRef]

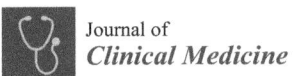

Article

Reverse Shoulder Arthroplasty with Bony and Metallic versus Standard Bony Reconstruction for Severe Glenoid Bone Loss. A Retrospective Comparative Cohort Study

Marko Nabergoj [1,2], Lionel Neyton [3], Hugo Bothorel [4], Sean W. L. Ho [5], Sidi Wang [6], Xue Ling Chong [6] and Alexandre Lädermann [6,7,8,*]

1. Valdoltra Orthopaedic Hospital, 6280 Ankaran, Slovenia; mmarkoj@gmail.com
2. Faculty of Medicine, University of Ljubljana, 1000 Ljubljana, Slovenia
3. Ramsay Générale de Santé, Hôpital Privé Jean Mermoz, Centre Orthopédique Santy, 69008 Lyon, France; neyton.lionel@gmail.com
4. Research Department, La Tour Hospital, 1217 Meyrin, Switzerland; hugo.bothorel@latour.ch
5. Department of Orthopaedic Surgery, Tan Tock Seng Hospital, Singapore 308433, Singapore; Sean_WL_HO@ttsh.com.sg
6. Division of Orthopaedics and Trauma Surgery, La Tour Hospital, 1217 Meyrin, Switzerland; sidi99.wang@gmail.com (S.W.); chongxueling@gmail.com (X.L.C.)
7. Faculty of Medicine, University of Geneva, 1211 Geneva 4, Switzerland
8. Division of Orthopaedics and Trauma Surgery, Department of Surgery, Geneva University Hospitals, 1205 Geneva, Switzerland
* Correspondence: alexandre.laedermann@gmail.com; Tel.: +41-22-719-75-55; Fax: +41-22-719-60-77

Citation: Nabergoj, M.; Neyton, L.; Bothorel, H.; Ho, S.W.L.; Wang, S.; Chong, X.L.; Lädermann, A. Reverse Shoulder Arthroplasty with Bony and Metallic versus Standard Bony Reconstruction for Severe Glenoid Bone Loss. A Retrospective Comparative Cohort Study. *J. Clin. Med.* **2021**, *10*, 5274. https://doi.org/10.3390/jcm10225274

Academic Editors: Emmanuel Andrès and Nicola Fabbri

Received: 21 September 2021
Accepted: 9 November 2021
Published: 13 November 2021

Publisher's Note: MDPI stays neutral with regard to jurisdictional claims in published maps and institutional affiliations.

Copyright: © 2021 by the authors. Licensee MDPI, Basel, Switzerland. This article is an open access article distributed under the terms and conditions of the Creative Commons Attribution (CC BY) license (https://creativecommons.org/licenses/by/4.0/).

Abstract: There are different techniques to address severe glenoid erosion during reverse shoulder arthroplasty (RSA). This study assessed the clinical and radiological outcomes of RSA with combined bony and metallic augment (BMA) glenoid reconstruction compared to bony augmentation (BA) alone. A review of patients who underwent RSA with severe glenoid bone loss requiring reconstruction from January 2017 to January 2019 was performed. Patients were divided into two groups: BMA versus BA alone. Clinical outcome measurements included two years postoperative ROM, Constant score, subjective shoulder value (SSV), and the American Shoulder and Elbow Surgeons Shoulder (ASES) score. Radiological outcomes included radiographic evidence of scapular complications and graft incorporation. The BMA group had significantly different glenoid morphology ($p < 0.001$) and greater bone loss thickness than the BA group (16.3 ± 3.8 mm vs. 12.0 ± 0.0 mm, $p = 0.020$). Both groups had significantly improved ROM (anterior forward flexion and external rotation) and clinical scores (Constant, SSV and ASES scores) at 2 years. Greater improvement was observed in the BMA group in terms of anterior forward flexion (86.3° ± 27.9° vs. 43.8° ± 25.6°, $p = 0.013$) and Constant score (56.6 ± 10.1 vs. 38.3 ± 16.7, $p = 0.021$). The BA group demonstrated greater functional and clinical improvements with higher postoperative active external rotation and ASES results (active external rotation, 49.4° ± 17.0° vs. 29.4° ± 14.7°, $p = 0.017$; ASES, 89.1 ± 11.3 vs. 76.8 ± 11.0, $p = 0.045$). The combination use of bone graft and metallic augments in severe glenoid bone loss during RSA is safe and effective and can be considered in cases of severe glenoid bone loss where bone graft alone may be insufficient.

Keywords: shoulder; prosthesis; defect; reconstruction; autologous graft; survivorship; loosening; integration

1. Introduction

Addressing severe glenoid deficiency during shoulder arthroplasty is technically challenging. Glenoid deficiencies have been reported in up to 39% of patients undergoing reverse shoulder arthroplasty (RSA). Such glenoid bone loss may occur in any part of the glenoid, including the posterior aspect (18%), superior aspect (9%), anterior aspect (4%), or as a global erosion (6%) in patients undergoing RSA [1,2].

Implantation of RSA in patients with advanced deformity of the glenoid may lead to several problems due to malpositioning of the glenoid baseplate. Excessive medialization of the glenoid baseplate causes muscle shortening with decreased tension resulting in poorer function [3,4]. Diminished deltoid wrapping around the greater tuberosity can also increase the risk of prosthetic instability and cosmetic deformity [5]. Additionally, the excessive medialization results in increased scapular notching with inferomedial glenoid bone erosion and polyethylene wear [6]. In superior glenoid bone loss, there is a risk of placing the glenoid baseplate in superior inclination. This has been shown to be an important risk factor for aseptic loosening as it increases shear forces and decreases compressive forces that otherwise stabilize RSA [7,8].

To avoid these negative outcomes, surgeons often attempt to reconstruct the glenoid bone loss, allowing for an optimal positioning of the baseplate. The common approach is to use the humeral head autograft to fill glenoid defects. However, there are some technical considerations. Firstly, the amount of humeral head autograft available is not always sufficient to fully compensate for the bone defect. Secondly, it should be noted that in such complicated glenoid reconstruction, graft incorporation requires stabilization through a peg inserted in a native glenoid [9]. These factors add to the technical difficulties. One alternative is to use a metallic augment to compensate for the glenoid bone loss [10]. However, in severe glenoid deficiencies, the available metallic augments may not be adequately thick enough to fully reconstruct the glenoid bone loss. In these cases, a combination of both metallic augment and bone graft can be utilized to sufficiently build up the bone loss. To our knowledge, no study has evaluated the combination of an augmented baseplate with bone grafting for RSA with severe glenoid defects.

The aim of this study was to assess the clinical and radiological outcomes of a combined bony and metallic augmented baseplate for RSA with severe glenoid defects. The hypothesis was that the combined use of bone graft and metallic augments in severe glenoid bone loss during RSA is safe and effective.

2. Materials and Methods

2.1. Study Design, Data Collection, and Ethical Committee Approval

Between January 2017 and January 2019, all patients who had an RSA by either a combination of bony and metallic augments or bony augments alone were considered potentially eligible for inclusion in this retrospective analysis of data prospectively collected during the SHOUT (Shoulder OUTcome) multi-center study. The inclusion criteria were a severe glenoid defect, defined by a need to use a graft thicker than 1 cm to restore inclination and version at acceptable values (0 degree and <20 degrees, respectively) using a 3D planning software (Blueprint™ I Wright Medical Group, Memphis, TN, USA). The exclusion criteria included avascular necrosis of the humeral head, neurological conditions affecting the upper limb, and patients with less than two years follow-up. Two groups of patients were defined: Group 1 were patients who had only bone graft for glenoid reconstruction during RSA, and Group 2 were patients who had a combination of bone graft and metallic augments for glenoid reconstruction during RSA. The study received ethics committee approval from both centers (CCER 14-227 and COS-RGDS-2021-06-009-NEYTON-L). All the patients gave informed consent for participation in this study.

2.2. Surgical Technique and Implant Design

All operations were performed by two experienced [10] shoulder surgeons (A.L. and L.N.) who had performed more than 250 RSAs before the study period. A standard deltopectoral approach was used. A humeral head autograft was harvested and prepared to match the size and location of the glenoid defect. The graft was either temporarily fixed to the native glenoid or held by the post during impaction or screw insertion (Figure 1). The only difference between the two techniques was the baseplate: in the bony-metallic augmentation (BMA) group, a 15 degrees full wedge augmented baseplate (Aequalis™ Perform™ Reversed Glenoid I Wright Medical Group, Memphis, TN, USA) was screwed at the edge of the glenoid with the greatest bone loss (Figure 2). In the bony augmentation (BA) group, a 25-mm-long central peg baseplate (Aequalis Reversed II Glenoid™ | Wright Medical Group, Memphis, TN, USA) was impacted into the native glenoid (Figure 2). The type of glenosphere (size and eccentricity) depended on the bone defect, the morphology of the patient, and the tension of the soft tissues. In both groups, the same curved, monoblock short-stem system was used (Aequalis™ Ascend Flex™ | Wright Medical Group, Memphis, TN, USA). With this onlay device, the placement of the offset tray affects both humerus lateralization and distalization [11,12]. A 145° neck-shaft angle was used in this study, acquired by using a stem inclination of 132.5° combined with an asymmetric 12.5° polyethylene insert. Stems were cemented if rotational stability was not obtained intra-operatively after insertion of a cement restrictor plug.

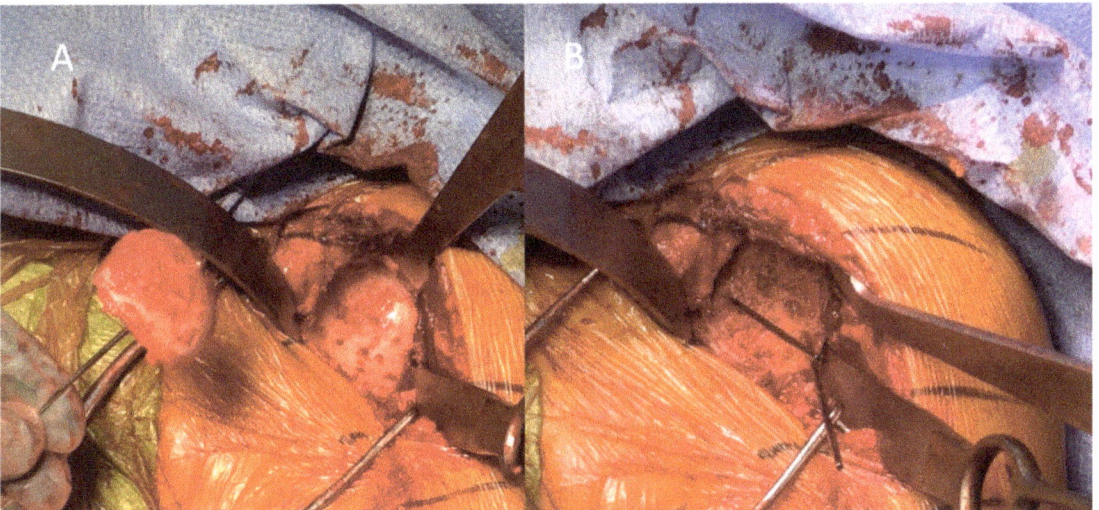

Figure 1. Sagittal view of a left glenoid with severe bone loss. (**A**) The glenoid is prepared with multiple small holes to promote bone healing and graft incorporation. (**B**) The graft is temporarily fixed to the native glenoid before screw insertion. In this case, bone graft alone is able to sufficiently restore the glenoid bone loss.

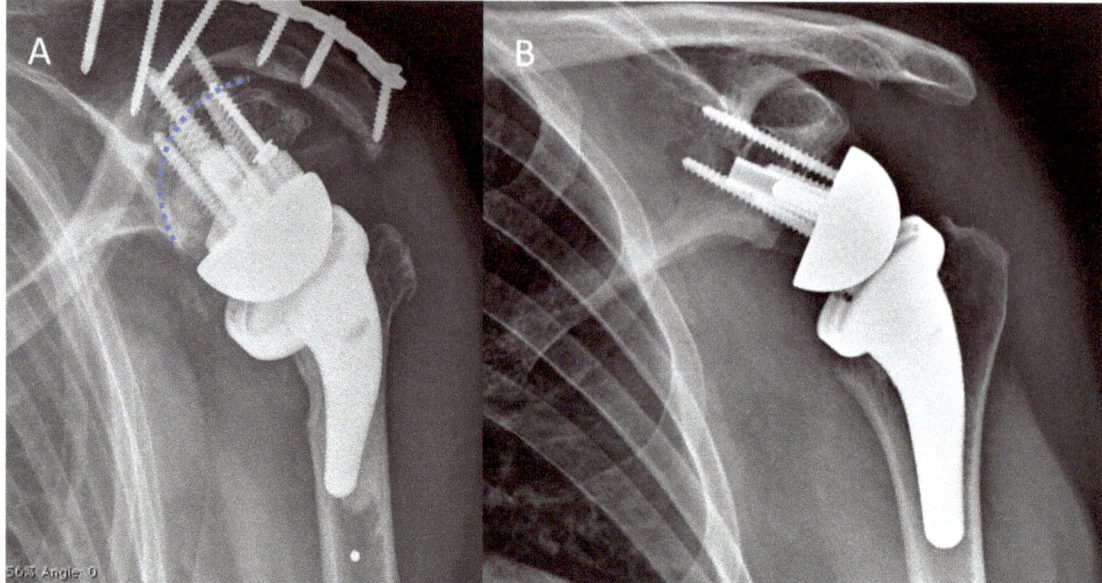

Figure 2. Postoperative anteroposterior X-ray of left shoulders. (**A**) Reconstruction of the glenoid with BMA and a 15 degrees full wedge augmented central screw baseplate. The dotted blue line represents the native glenoid. There is concurrent plate fixation of a preoperative fatigue fracture of the spine of the scapula. (**B**) Reconstruction of the glenoid with BA and a 25-mm-long central peg baseplate.

2.3. Postoperative Rehabilitation

All patients followed the same postoperative rehabilitation protocol. Postoperatively, the arm was placed in an abduction pillow sling for six weeks to promote compression instead of shear forces. After six weeks, the immobilization was discontinued, and active ROM was initiated. Activities of daily living were progressed, but strengthening was not specifically recommended [13].

2.4. Study Variables

Patient demographics such as age, gender, diagnosis, side of pathology, hand dominance, body mass index, and tobacco use were collected. Clinical outcomes and radiological outcomes were collected as described below.

2.5. Clinical Evaluation

The Constant score, SSV, and ASES were used for clinical assessment. These scores were used for their ease of administration and well-validated data [11,12]. All the patients completed all three scores at the preoperative time point and at the final follow-up of two years. For clinical assessment of ROM, a goniometer was used for the active evaluation of anterior forward flexion and rotations. The external rotation was measured with the arm by the side of the body, whereas internal rotation by the highest vertebral spinous process reached by the patient's extended thumb.

2.6. Radiological Assessment

The initial glenoid bone loss was measured on preoperative CT scans, recorded and classified according to Walch et al. classification [14,15]. The standard anteroposterior view in neutral, external and internal rotation, and axillary lateral view were obtained under fluoroscopic control preoperatively and postoperatively. Using Osirix (Pixmeo, Geneva, Switzerland), postoperative radiographs were assessed for bone graft incorporation defined by the absence of lucent lines observed between the humeral bone graft and the native glenoid, inferior notching at the native glenoid, radiolucent lines (around the peg, screws, and humeral stem), and a shift in the position of the components. The severity of the inferior notching was graded according to Sirveaux classification [16]. Glenoid loosening was confirmed following the criteria of Mélis et al. [17], the criteria being the presence of a radiolucent line >2 mm thick.

2.7. Statistical Analysis

The Shapiro–Wilk test was used to check the normality of distributions. Descriptive statistics were presented in terms of means, standard deviations (SD) and ranges for continuous variables and percentages for categorical variables. The significance of pre- vs. postoperative differences within each group was determined using the Wilcoxon signed-rank test for non-normally distributed data and the paired Student's t-test for normally distributed data. The significance of differences between groups was determined using the Mann–Whitney U test (Wilcoxon rank sum test) for non-normally distributed quantitative data and using the Student's unpaired t-test for normally distributed data. For categorical data, the significance of differences between groups was determined using the Fisher exact test. Statistical analyses were performed using R version 3.6.2 (R Foundation for Statistical Computing, Vienna, Austria). p values < 0.05 were considered statistically significant.

3. Results

There was no significant difference in the demographic data of patients in both groups. Patient characteristics showed no significant differences in terms of patient age, gender, BMI, tobacco usage, or affected side. There was also no significant difference in the preoperative surgical variables such as history of prior surgery, primary diagnosis, glenoid inclination, or glenoid version (Table 1). Patients in the BMA group presented a different glenoid morphology ($p < 0.001$) and a greater bone loss thickness than patients in the bony augmentation (BA) group (16.3 ± 3.8 mm vs. 12.0 ± 0.0 mm, $p = 0.020$). All patients in the BA group had a B2 glenoid defect. In the BMA group, one patient had a glenoid type B1, one patient had a glenoid type B3 and two patients each had a glenoid type D, E3, and C. Preoperative radiological data of each patient are summarized in Table 2. Compared to the BA group, BMA patients had a lower preoperative anterior forward flexion (55.0° ± 38.5° vs. 101.3° ± 31.8°, $p = 0.010$) and worse preoperative Constant scores (18.8 ± 7.4 vs. 34.5 ± 11.7, $p = 0.013$).

Table 1. Patient characteristics between the Bony-metallic augmentation (BMA) and Bony augmentation (BA) groups.

	Bony-Metallic Augmentation (n = 8 Patients)			Bony Augmentation (n = 8 Patients)			p-Value
	N	(%)		N	(%)		
	Mean	±SD	(Range)	Mean	±SD	(Range)	
Male sex	3	(37.5%)		5	(62.5%)		0.619
Operation on dominant side	7	(87.5%)		3	(37.5%)		0.119
Prior surgery	1	(12.5%)		0	(0.0%)		1.000
Tobacco use	1	(12.5%)		0	(0.0%)		1.000
Primary diagnosis							0.200
Primary OA	5	(62.5%)		8	(100.0%)		
Post-traumatic arthritis	1	(12.5%)		0	(0.0%)		
Dislocation arthropathy	1	(12.5%)		0	(0.0%)		
Revision	1	(12.5%)		0	(0.0%)		
Glenoid morphology							<0.001
B1	1	(12.5%)		0	(0.0%)		
B2	0	(0.0%)		8	(100.0%)		
B3	1	(12.5%)		0	(0.0%)		

Table 1. Cont.

	Bony-Metallic Augmentation (n = 8 Patients)				Bony Augmentation (n = 8 Patients)				p-Value
	N	(%)			N	(%)			
	Mean	±SD	(Range)		Mean	±SD	(Range)		
C	2	(25.0%)			0	(0.0%)			
D	2	(25.0%)			0	(0.0%)			
E3	2	(25.0%)			0	(0.0%)			
Age at index operation (yrs)	72.1	±11.7	(51.9	−83.9)	73.2	±6.8	(61.5	−84.1)	0.721
Body mass index	25.4	±4.1	(20.4	−31.6)	26.6	±3.0	(23.7	−31.0)	0.400
Weight (kg)	70.0	±11.1	(60.0	−85.0)	74.8	±11.2	(60.0	−95.0)	0.461
Height (cm)	166.6	±13.1	(140.0	−180.0)	167.5	±7.9	(155.0	−175.0)	0.635
Follow-up (months)	28.1	±15.0	(11.0	−51.0)	30.7	±10.8	(24.0	−55.4)	0.752
Inclination (°)	15.1	±12.0	(0.0	−34.0)	9.3	±7.5	(−7.0	−17.0)	0.528
Ante retroversion (°)	−22.5	±21.1	(−41.0	−12.0)	−26.1	±4.7	(−36.0	−−21.0)	0.494
Bone loss thickness (mm)	16.3	±3.8	(11.0	−21.0)	12.0	±0.0	(12.0	−12.0)	**0.020**

BMA—bony-metallic augmentation, BA—bony augmentation, OA—Osteoarthrosis. Underlined p-values indicate those below 0.05.

Table 2. Radiological data of each patient.

Patient	Glenoid Morphology	Inclination (°)	Ante/Retroversion (°)	Bone Loss Thickness (mm)
Patient 1	B2	10	−27	12
Patient 2	B2	9	−27	12
Patient 3	B2	−7	−21	12
Patient 4	B2	17	−36	12
Patient 5	B2	9	−23	12
Patient 6	B2	7	−23	12
Patient 7	B2	13	−28	12
Patient 8	B2	16	−24	12
Patient 9	D	5	12	11
Patient 10	E3	0	−36	14
Patient 11	B1	10	−10	12
Patient 12	C	16	−40	16
Patient 13	B3	27	−37	21
Patient 14	D	34	−41	20
Patient 15	E3	23	3	20
Patient 16	C	6	−31	16

Both the BMA and BA groups completed at least two years of follow-up, with a mean follow-up of 28.1 ± 15.0 and 30.7 ± 10.8 months, respectively. At the final follow-up, both the BMA and BA groups significantly improved their ROM (anterior forward flexion and external rotation) and clinical scores (Constant, SSV, and ASES scores) (Table 3). A greater improvement could be observed in the BMA group in terms of anterior forward flexion (86.3° ± 27.9° vs. 43.8° ± 25.6°, $p = 0.013$) and Constant score (56.6 ± 10.1 vs. 38.3 ± 16.7, $p = 0.021$), probably due to their lower preoperative scores compared to BA patients. However, in the absence of significant preoperative differences, the BA group demonstrated greater functional and clinical improvements than BMA patients with higher postoperative active external rotation and ASES results (active external rotation, 49.4° ± 17.0° vs. 29.4° ± 14.7°, $p = 0.017$; ASES, 89.1 ± 11.3 vs. 76.8 ± 11.0, $p = 0.045$).

At two years follow-up, a bony scapular spur and three inferior graft resorptions were noted in the BA group. In the BMA group, a bony scapular spur, two ossifications in the glenohumeral space, and a grade 1 scapular notching were observed.

Table 3. Pre- and postoperative data between the Bony-metallic augmentation (BMA) and Bony augmentation (BA) groups.

	Bony-Metallic Augmentation (n = 8 Patients)				Bony Augmentation (n = 8 Patients)				p-Value
	N	(%)			N	(%)			
	Mean	±SD	(Range)		Mean	±SD	(Range)		
Internal rotation									
preoperative									0.022
Thigh	5	(62.5%)			0	(0.0%)			
Buttock	3	(37.5%)			4	(50.0%)			
Sacrum	0	(0.0%)			3	(37.5%)			
Th12	0	(0.0%)			1	(12.5%)			
postoperative									0.220
Buttock	0	(0.0%)			1	(12.5%)			
Sacrum	0	(0.0%)			3	(37.5%)			
L5/L3	4	(50.0%)			3	(37.5%)			
Th12	2	(25.0%)			1	(12.5%)			
Th7	2	(25.0%)			0	(0.0%)			
p-value *		0.014				0.090			
Anterior forward flexion (°)									
preoperative	55.0	±38.5	(0.0	−95.0)	101.3	±31.8	(40.0	−150.0)	0.010
postoperative	141.3	±22.2	(90.0	−160.0)	145.0	±12.0	(130.0	−160.0)	0.915
improvement	86.3	±27.9	(55.0	−130.0)	43.8	±25.6	(10.0	−90.0)	0.013
p-value *		0.014				0.014			
Active external rotation (°)									
preoperative	14.4	±15.5	(0.0	−40.0)	10.6	±22.4	(−20.0	−45.0)	0.545
postoperative	29.4	±14.7	(15.0	−60.0)	49.4	±17.0	(30.0	−80.0)	0.017
improvement	15.0	±12.0	(−10.0	−30.0)	38.8	±16.2	(5.0	−60.0)	0.009
p-value *		0.027				0.014			
Constant score									
preoperative	18.8	±7.4	(6.0	−30.0)	34.5	±11.7	(12.0	−49.0)	0.013
postoperative	75.4	±10.4	(55.0	−87.0)	72.8	±14.8	(54.0	−91.0)	0.792
improvement	56.6	±10.1	(38.0	−72.0)	38.3	±16.7	(17.0	−69.0)	0.021
p-value *		0.014				0.008			
SSV									
preoperative	34.4	±21.9	(15.0	−70.0)	36.3	±14.1	(10.0	−50.0)	0.630
postoperative	83.8	±11.6	(65.0	−100.0)	85.5	±9.2	(70.0	−99.0)	0.915
improvement	49.4	±24.4	(10.0	−80.0)	49.3	±16.8	(35.0	−85.0)	0.958
p-value*		0.008				0.014			
ASES score									
preoperative	28.6	±14.1	(3.0	−47.0)	22.9	±11.8	(10.0	−35.0)	0.426
postoperative	76.8	±11.0	(57.0	−95.0)	89.1	±11.3	(67.0	−100.0)	0.045
improvement	48.1	±12.2	(31.0	−66.0)	66.3	±11.9	(45.0	−83.0)	0.027
p-value *		0.014				0.008			

* Between pre- and postoperative measurements; SSV, Subjective Shoulder Value; ASES, American Shoulder and Elbow surgeons. Underlined p-values indicate those below 0.05.

4. Discussion

This study demonstrates that the combination of bone graft and metallic augmentation of the glenoid baseplate is a safe and effective option to treat severe glenoid deformities during RSA, confirming our hypothesis. Both the BMA and BA groups attained significantly better postoperative functional outcomes (SSV, Constant and ASES scores). Both groups also attained significantly better clinical ROM postoperatively (anterior forward flexion and external rotation). There was a greater improvement in the BMA group with regard to anterior forward flexion (86.3° ± 27.9° vs. 43.8° ± 25.6°, $p = 0.013$) and Constant score (56.6 ± 10.1 vs. 38.3 ± 16.7, $p = 0.021$), but that might be attributed to the significant preoperative differences. Simovitch et al. reported on the minimal clinically important difference (MCID) for different shoulder outcome metrics and ROM after shoulder arthroplasty. They noted that the MCID in terms of active external rotation is 3° ± 2° [18]. Werner et al. showed that patients undergoing reverse shoulder arthroplasty due to rotator cuff arthropathy or glenohumeral arthritis experience a clinically important change if they have at least a nine-point improvement in ASES score [19]. These studies further confirm that in both the BA and BMA groups, the MCID was achieved in both active external rotation and ASES scores.

Current surgical options that address severe bone loss include preferentially using bone grafting (autograft or allograft) or the use of metallic augmented baseplates (wedge compensation or patient matched implant) [20]. Bone graft can be obtained as an autograft from the autologous humeral head [21–24] and iliac crest [23], or as a femoral head allograft [21,22,25,26]. However, the quantity or the quality of the graft might not be adequate. Furthermore, the price of allografts or patient matched implants may be unaffordable. Jones et al. directly compared bone grafting versus augmented baseplate and reported similar outcomes in both groups. However, they observed a higher complication percentage in the group with bone graft [27]. To the best of our knowledge, combining an augmented baseplate with a bone graft has not been published yet. The present study shows that integrating a metallic compensation into a bony compensation (compared to native glenoid) is a viable option for extreme bone loss cases. This technique has several advantages. It allows the surgeon to compensate for massive bone defects while avoiding excessive donor-site morbidity by not harvesting an additional bone graft from the iliac crest. It can also relativize the auto- or allograft quality and risk of partial integration. Additionally, we also achieve glenoid lateralization with this technique which decreases scapular notching, and increases ROM and soft tissue tension [9,28,29]. Lastly, adding a full wedge baseplate on a graft creates more inferior tilt, which is key to transforming shear forces into compression ones and promoting graft healing (Figure 3) [5,7,30,31].

In patients with severe glenoid bone loss, integration of the graft is a crucial factor. Recent studies analyzing the use of bone graft in RSA described a satisfactory rate of bone graft incorporation [21,32–36]. However, a systematic review by Malahias et al. still reported a rate of radiographic non-union at 5.2% [37]. In addition, it is important to note that despite evidence of radiological union, true integration of the graft is rarely complete [38], as confirmed in the present study. Given this finding, the authors recommend that as much of the bony defect as possible should be covered by the graft in order to maximize the surface of contact and, consequently, the potential of healing.

The use of a central screw baseplate to fix massive grafts is debatable. It is thought that screws do not provide bone ingrowth possibilities like it is the case around a central peg [38]. The minimal central peg length proposed in the literature that should be inserted in the native bone stock to avoid loosening varies between 8 to 10 mm [21,39]. However, we did not observe signs of glenoid loosening or migration when using a central screw after two years, confirming sufficient stability and the biomechanical findings of Bonnevialle et al. [40]. This observation can be explained by the tremendous compression obtained at the insertion of screw devices and the additional inferior tilt provided by the full wedge baseplate.

The restoration of global lateralization is also essential to improve postoperative function. Humeral offset is heavily influenced by prosthetic design. The use of a curved stem, an eccentric reverse tray with a high offset (3.3 mm), and a 145° neck-shaft angle provides around 10 mm of humeral lateralization that also help to balance the glenoid side [4].

In this study, both the BMA and BA groups achieved significantly better clinical and functional outcomes postoperatively. Regarding active external rotation and ASES scores, there was no significant difference between the groups preoperatively, but the BA group achieved significantly better external rotation and ASES scores postoperatively. As such, the authors recommend that isolated bone grafting be performed for glenoid loss during RSA where possible. In cases where the glenoid bone loss appears too severe for bone grafting alone, a combination of bone graft and metallic augments is a safe and effective option for glenoid reconstruction.

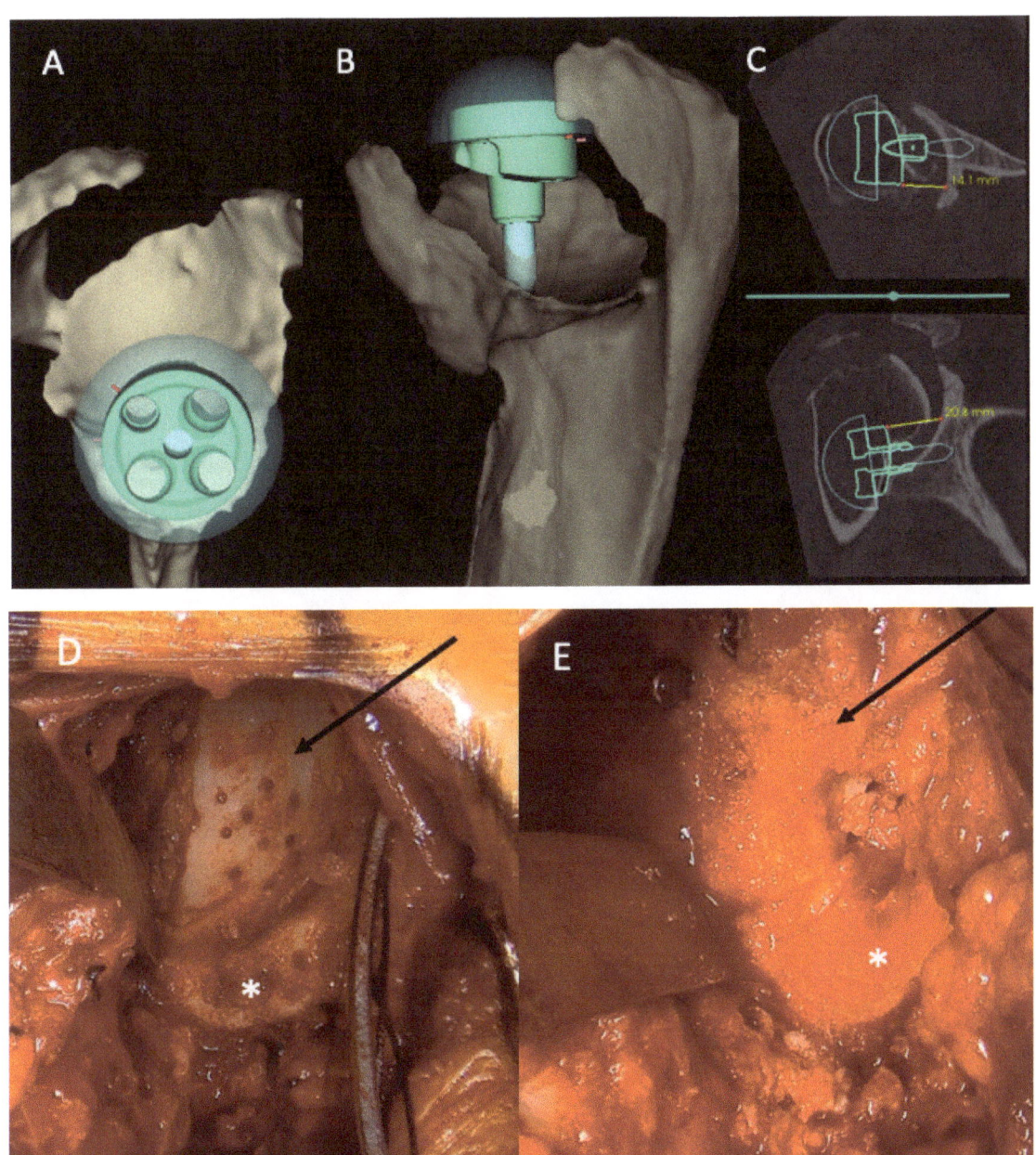

Figure 3. Cont.

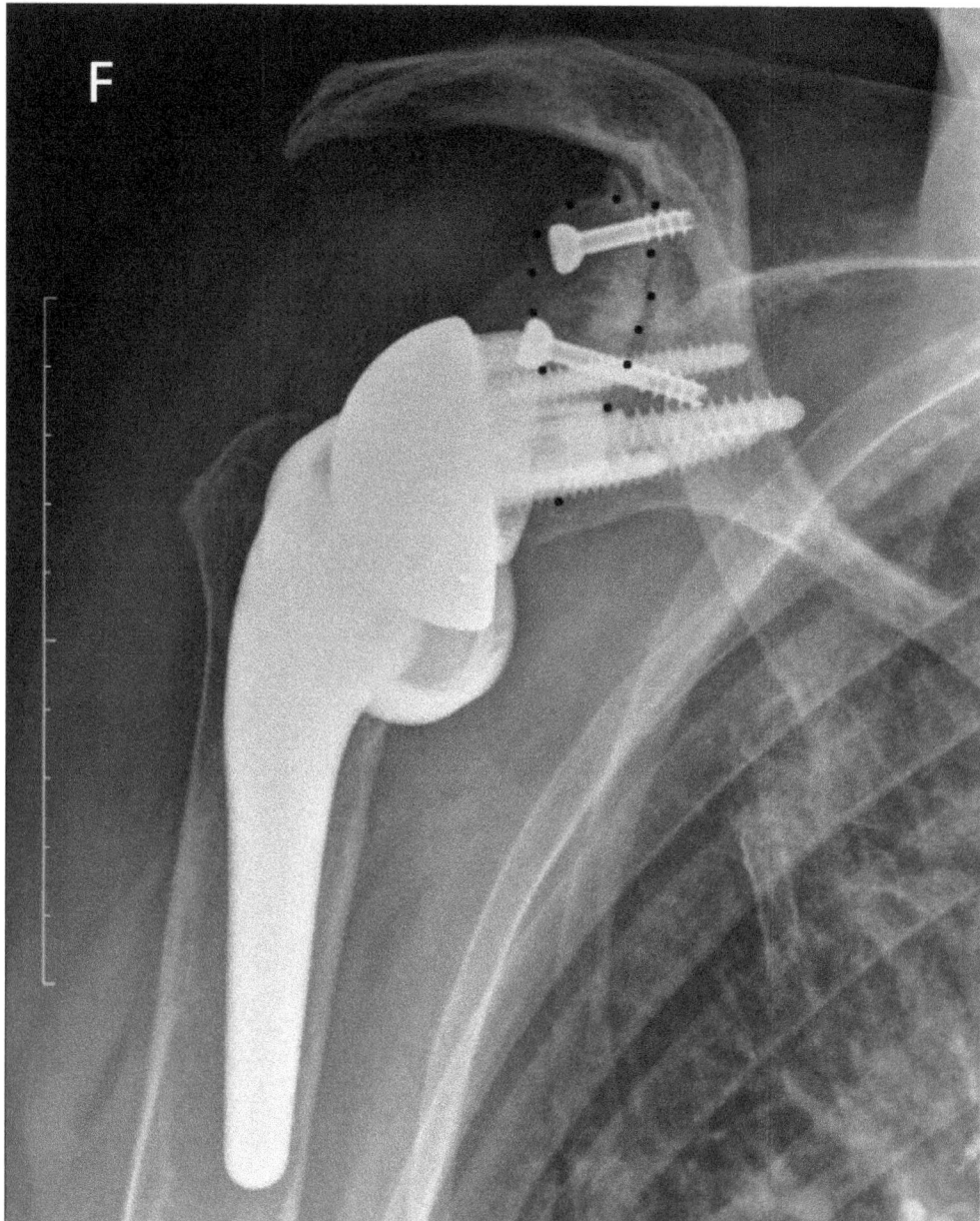

Figure 3. This technique compensates for massive bone defects and creates a more inferior tilt, transforming shear forces into compression ones. (**A**) Sagittal and (**B**) superior views of a 3-dimensional (3D) reconstruction of a right shoulder. Note the massive posterosuperior bone loss. (**C**) Planification reveals that metallic augmentation alone would not achieve optimal joint line restoration. (**D**) Intraoperative anterior view of the paleoglenoid (white asterix) and superior bone erosion (black line). (**E**) Glenoid reconstruction after humeral bone autograft (black arrow). The entire humeral head is hardly sufficient to compensate for the bony erosion. *: paleoglenoid. (**F**) Postoperative anteroposterior X-ray confirms that BMA allows for a large area of bony contact between the autograft (complete humeral head, dotted black line) and the native glenoid, correcting massive bone loss.

Strengths and Limitations

To our knowledge, this is the first study that explicitly analyzes the success of a combination of bone grafting and metallic baseplate augmentation with RSA in severe glenoid deformities. The surgeries were performed by experienced, shoulder-fellowship-trained surgeons. This study had several limitations. Firstly, the sample size is small and as such, the analysis may be underpowered. Secondly, the sustained long-term improvement of clinical outcomes and ROM of both surgical techniques remains unclear. Thirdly, the assessment of bone graft incorporation could have been more accurate using a CT compared to the radiograph. Lastly, our study is heterogeneous as different types of glenoid bone erosion were present in each group. Future work should assess a larger population with longer follow-up.

5. Conclusions

Combining bone graft and metallic augments in severe glenoid bone loss during RSA is safe and effective, resulting in significantly improved clinical outcomes and ROM. In cases of severe glenoid bone loss where bone graft alone may be insufficient, a combination of bone graft and metallic augments should be considered.

Author Contributions: M.N.: data curation and writing—original draft preparation; L.N.: data curation, supervision, and writing—review and editing; H.B.: methodology, statistics, and writing—review and editing; S.W.L.H.: methodology and writing—review and editing; S.W.: data curation and visualization; X.L.C.: methodology and writing—review and editing; A.L.: conceptualization; methodology, supervision, resources, funding acquisition and writing—review and editing. All authors have read and agreed to the published version of the manuscript.

Funding: This research was funded by FORE (Foundation for Research and Teaching in Orthopaedics, Sports Medicine, Trauma and Imaging in the Musculoskeletal System); grant number FORE 2021-35.

Institutional Review Board Statement: The study received ethics committee approval from both centers (CCER 14-227 and COS-RGDS-2021-06-009-NEYTON-L).

Informed Consent Statement: Informed consent was obtained from all subjects involved in the study.

Data Availability Statement: All data relevant to the study are included in the article. Details regarding where data supporting reported results can be asked at the following e-mail address: hugo.bothorel@latour.ch.

Conflicts of Interest: Marko Nabergoj reports no conflict of interest. Lionel Neyton reports that he is a paid consultant for Arthrex and Tornier/Stryker and receives royalties from Tornier/Stryker. He is member of the Advisory Board of Sparta Biopharma and owns stock options. Hugo Bothorel reports no conflict of interest. Sean WL Ho reports no conflict of interest. Sidi Wang reports no conflict of interest. Xueling Chong reports no conflict of interest. Dr. Lädermann reports that he is a paid consultant for Arthrex, Inc., Stryker, and Medacta, and he receives royalties from Stryker. He is the founder of the FORE Foundation, Med4cast, and BeeMed. The funders had no role in the design of the study; in the collection, analyses, or interpretation of data; in the writing of the manuscript, or in the decision to publish the results.

References

1. Frankle, M.A.; Teramoto, A.; Luo, Z.P.; Levy, J.C.; Pupello, D. Glenoid morphology in reverse shoulder arthroplasty: Classification and surgical implications. *J. Shoulder Elb. Surg.* **2009**, *18*, 874–885. [CrossRef]
2. Klein, S.M.; Dunning, P.; Mulieri, P.; Pupello, D.; Downes, K.; Frankle, M.A. Effects of acquired glenoid bone defects on surgical technique and clinical outcomes in reverse shoulder arthroplasty. *J. Bone Jt. Surg. Am.* **2010**, *92*, 1144–1154. [CrossRef]
3. Blix, M. Die Länge und die Spannung des Muskels. 1 Skandinavisches. *Arch. Physiol.* **1892**, *3*, 295–318.
4. Lädermann, A.; Denard, P.J.; Boileau, P.; Farron, A.; Deransart, P.; Terrier, A.; Ston, J.; Walch, G. Effect of humeral stem design on humeral position and range of motion in reverse shoulder arthroplasty. *Int. Orthop.* **2015**, *39*, 2205–2213. [CrossRef]
5. Roche, C.P.; Diep, P.; Hamilton, M.; Crosby, L.A.; Flurin, P.H.; Wright, T.W.; Zuckerman, J.D.; Routman, H.D. Impact of inferior glenoid tilt, humeral retroversion, bone grafting, and design parameters on muscle length and deltoid wrapping in reverse shoulder arthroplasty. *Bull. Hosp. Jt. Dis.* **2013**, *71*, 284–293.

6. Boileau, P.; Watkinson, D.; Hatzidakis, A.M.; Hovorka, I. Neer Award 2005: The Grammont reverse shoulder prosthesis: Results in cuff tear arthritis, fracture sequelae, and revision arthroplasty. *J. Shoulder Elb. Surg.* **2006**, *15*, 527–540. [CrossRef]
7. Frankle, M.A.; Siegal, S.; Pupello, D.R.; Gutierrez, S.; Griewe, M.; Mighell, M.A. 11: Coronal plane tilt angle affects risk of catastrophic failure in patients treated with a reverse shoulder prosthesis. *J. Shoulder Elb. Surg.* **2007**, *16*, e46. [CrossRef]
8. Lädermann, A.; Tay, E.; Collin, P.; Piotton, S.; Chiu, C.H.; Michelet, A.; Charbonnier, C. Effect of critical shoulder angle, glenoid lateralization, and humeral inclination on range of movement in reverse shoulder arthroplasty. *Bone Jt. Res.* **2019**, *8*, 378–386. [CrossRef] [PubMed]
9. Lädermann, A.; Collin, P.; Denard, P.J. Range of motion after reverse shoulder arthroplasty: Which combinations of humeral stem and glenosphere work best? *Obere Extrem.* **2020**, *15*, 172–178. [CrossRef]
10. Endell, D.; Imiolczyk, J.-P.; Grob, A.; Moroder, P.; Scheibel, M. Full-wedge metallic reconstruction of glenoid bone deficiency in reverse shoulder arthroplasty. *Obere Extrem.* **2020**, *15*, 213–216. [CrossRef]
11. Constant, C.R.; Murley, A.H. A clinical method of functional assessment of the shoulder. *Clin. Orthop. Relat. Res.* **1987**, 160–164. [CrossRef]
12. Cunningham, G.; Lädermann, A.; Denard, P.J.; Kherad, O.; Burkhart, S.S. Correlation Between American Shoulder and Elbow Surgeons and Single Assessment Numerical Evaluation Score After Rotator Cuff or SLAP Repair. *Arthroscopy* **2015**, *31*, 1688–1692. [CrossRef]
13. Collin, P.; Matsukawa, T.; Denard, P.J.; Gain, S.; Lädermann, A. Pre-operative factors influence the recovery of range of motion following reverse shoulder arthroplasty. *Int. Orthop.* **2017**, *41*, 2135–2142. [CrossRef] [PubMed]
14. Bercik, M.J.; Kruse, K., II; Yalizis, M.; Gauci, M.O.; Chaoui, J.; Walch, G. A modification to the Walch classification of the glenoid in primary glenohumeral osteoarthritis using three-dimensional imaging. *J. Shoulder Elb. Surg.* **2016**, *25*, 1601–1606. [CrossRef] [PubMed]
15. Walch, G.; Badet, R.; Boulahia, A.; Khoury, A. Morphologic study of the glenoid in primary glenohumeral osteoarthritis. *J. Arthroplast.* **1999**, *14*, 756–760. [CrossRef]
16. Sirveaux, F.; Favard, L.; Oudet, D.; Huquet, D.; Walch, G.; Mole, D. Grammont inverted total shoulder arthroplasty in the treatment of glenohumeral osteoarthritis with massive rupture of the cuff. Results of a multicentre study of 80 shoulders. *J. Bone Jt. Surg. Br.* **2004**, *86*, 388–395. [CrossRef]
17. Melis, B.; DeFranco, M.; Lädermann, A.; Mole, D.; Favard, L.; Nerot, C.; Maynou, C.; Walch, G. An evaluation of the radiological changes around the Grammont reverse geometry shoulder arthroplasty after eight to 12 years. *J. Bone Jt. Surg. Br.* **2011**, *93*, 1240–1246. [CrossRef]
18. Simovitch, R.; Flurin, P.H.; Wright, T.; Zuckerman, J.D.; Roche, C.P. Quantifying success after total shoulder arthroplasty: The minimal clinically important difference. *J. Shoulder Elb. Surg.* **2018**, *27*, 298–305. [CrossRef] [PubMed]
19. Werner, B.C.; Chang, B.; Nguyen, J.T.; Dines, D.M.; Gulotta, L.V. What Change in American Shoulder and Elbow Surgeons Score Represents a Clinically Important Change After Shoulder Arthroplasty? *Clin. Orthop. Relat. Res.* **2016**, *474*, 2672–2681. [CrossRef] [PubMed]
20. Ascione, F.; Routman, H.D. Severe Glenoid Erosion (B2, B3, C, E2, E3) Treated with RSA. In *Complex and Revision Shoulder Arthroplasty: An Evidence-Based Approach to Evaluation and Management*, 1st ed.; Tashjian, R.Z., Ed.; Springer Nature Switzerland AG: Cham, Switzerland, 2019; pp. 59–73. [CrossRef]
21. Boileau, P.; Moineau, G.; Roussanne, Y.; O'Shea, K. Bony increased-offset reversed shoulder arthroplasty: Minimizing scapular impingement while maximizing glenoid fixation. *Clin. Orthop. Relat. Res.* **2011**, *469*, 2558–2567. [CrossRef]
22. Neyton, L.; Boileau, P.; Nove-Josserand, L.; Edwards, T.B.; Walch, G. Glenoid bone grafting with a reverse design prosthesis. *J. Shoulder Elb. Surg.* **2007**, *16*, S71–S78. [CrossRef]
23. Page, R.S.; Haines, J.F.; Trail, I. Impaction Bone Grafting of the Glenoid in Revision Shoulder Arthroplasty: Classification, Technical Description and Early Results. *Shoulder Elb.* **2017**, *1*, 81–88. [CrossRef]
24. Steinmann, S.P.; Cofield, R.H. Bone grafting for glenoid deficiency in total shoulder replacement. *J. Shoulder Elb. Surg.* **2000**, *9*, 361–367. [CrossRef] [PubMed]
25. Gupta, A.; Thussbas, C.; Koch, M.; Seebauer, L. Management of glenoid bone defects with reverse shoulder arthroplasty-surgical technique and clinical outcomes. *J. Shoulder Elb. Surg.* **2018**, *27*, 853–862. [CrossRef]
26. Neyton, L.; Walch, G.; Nove-Josserand, L.; Edwards, T.B. Glenoid corticocancellous bone grafting after glenoid component removal in the treatment of glenoid loosening. *J. Shoulder Elb. Surg.* **2006**, *15*, 173–179. [CrossRef] [PubMed]
27. Jones, R.B.; Wright, T.W.; Roche, C.P. Bone grafting the glenoid versus use of augmented glenoid baseplates with reverse shoulder arthroplasty. *Bull. Hosp. Jt. Dis.* **2015**, *73*, S129–S135.
28. Levigne, C.; Boileau, P.; Favard, L.; Garaud, P.; Mole, D.; Sirveaux, F.; Walch, G. Scapular notching in reverse shoulder arthroplasty. *J. Shoulder Elb. Surg.* **2008**, *17*, 925–935. [CrossRef]
29. Wong, M.T.; Langohr, G.D.G.; Athwal, G.S.; Johnson, J.A. Implant positioning in reverse shoulder arthroplasty has an impact on acromial stresses. *J. Shoulder Elb. Surg.* **2016**, *25*, 1889–1895. [CrossRef]
30. Gutierrez, S.; Greiwe, R.M.; Frankle, M.A.; Siegal, S.; Lee, W.E., 3rd. Biomechanical comparison of component position and hardware failure in the reverse shoulder prosthesis. *J. Shoulder Elb. Surg.* **2007**, *16*, S9–S12. [CrossRef] [PubMed]

31. Gutierrez, S.; Walker, M.; Willis, M.; Pupello, D.R.; Frankle, M.A. Effects of tilt and glenosphere eccentricity on baseplate/bone interface forces in a computational model, validated by a mechanical model, of reverse shoulder arthroplasty. *J. Shoulder Elb. Surg.* **2011**, *20*, 732–739. [CrossRef]
32. Ernstbrunner, L.; Werthel, J.D.; Wagner, E.; Hatta, T.; Sperling, J.W.; Cofield, R.H. Glenoid bone grafting in primary reverse total shoulder arthroplasty. *J. Shoulder Elb. Surg.* **2017**, *26*, 1441–1447. [CrossRef] [PubMed]
33. Hill, J.M.; Norris, T.R. Long-term results of total shoulder arthroplasty following bone-grafting of the glenoid. *J. Bone Jt. Surg. Am.* **2001**, *83*, 877–883. [CrossRef]
34. Malhas, A.; Rashid, A.; Copas, D.; Bale, S.; Trail, I. Glenoid bone loss in primary and revision shoulder arthroplasty. *Shoulder Elb.* **2016**, *8*, 229–240. [CrossRef] [PubMed]
35. Tashjian, R.Z.; Granger, E.; Chalmers, P.N. Structural glenoid grafting during primary reverse total shoulder arthroplasty using humeral head autograft. *J. Shoulder Elb. Surg.* **2018**, *27*, e1–e8. [CrossRef] [PubMed]
36. Wagner, E.; Houdek, M.T.; Griffith, T.; Elhassan, B.T.; Sanchez-Sotelo, J.; Sperling, J.W.; Cofield, R.H. Glenoid Bone-Grafting in Revision to a Reverse Total Shoulder Arthroplasty. *J. Bone Jt. Surg. Am.* **2015**, *97*, 1653–1660. [CrossRef]
37. Malahias, M.A.; Chytas, D.; Kostretzis, L.; Brilakis, E.; Fandridis, E.; Hantes, M.; Antonogiannakis, E. Bone grafting in primary and revision reverse total shoulder arthroplasty for the management of glenoid bone loss: A systematic review. *J. Orthop.* **2020**, *20*, 78–86. [CrossRef]
38. Singh, J.; Odak, S.; Neelakandan, K.; Walton, M.J.; Monga, P.; Bale, S.; Trail, I. Survivorship of autologous structural bone graft at a minimum of 2 years when used to address significant glenoid bone loss in primary and revision shoulder arthroplasty: A computed tomographic and clinical review. *J. Shoulder Elb. Surg.* **2021**, *30*, 668–678. [CrossRef] [PubMed]
39. Werner, B.S.; Bohm, D.; Abdelkawi, A.; Gohlke, F. Glenoid bone grafting in reverse shoulder arthroplasty for long-standing anterior shoulder dislocation. *J. Shoulder Elb. Surg.* **2014**, *23*, 1655–1661. [CrossRef] [PubMed]
40. Bonnevialle, N.; Geais, L.; Muller, J.H.; Shoulder Friends, I.; Berhouet, J. Effect of RSA glenoid baseplate central fixation on micromotion and bone stress. *JSES Int.* **2020**, *4*, 979–986. [CrossRef]

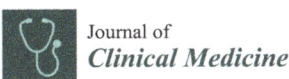

Article

Inverted-Bearing Reverse Shoulder Arthroplasty: Consequences on Scapular Notching and Clinical Results at Mid-Term Follow-Up

Alessandro Castagna [1,2], Mario Borroni [2], Luigi Dubini [1], Stefano Gumina [3,4], Giacomo Delle Rose [2] and Riccardo Ranieri [1,*]

[1] Department of Biomedical Sciences, Humanitas University, Via Rita Levi Montalcini 4, Rozzano (Mi), 20090 Milan, Italy
[2] IRCCS Humanitas Clinical and Research Center, Via Manzoni 56, Rozzano (Mi), 20089 Milan, Italy
[3] Department of Anatomy, Histology, Forensic Medicine and Orthopaedics, Sapienza University of Rome, Piazzale Aldo Moro 5, 00185 Roma, Italy
[4] Istituto Clinico Ortopedico Traumatologico (ICOT), Via Franco Faggiana 1668, 04100 Latina, Italy
* Correspondence: dr.riccardoranieri@gmail.com; Tel.: +39-33-8857-1926

Citation: Castagna, A.; Borroni, M.; Dubini, L.; Gumina, S.; Delle Rose, G.; Ranieri, R. Inverted-Bearing Reverse Shoulder Arthroplasty: Consequences on Scapular Notching and Clinical Results at Mid-Term Follow-Up. *J. Clin. Med.* **2022**, *11*, 5796. https://doi.org/10.3390/jcm11195796

Academic Editors: Markus Scheibel and Patrick Joel Denard

Received: 1 August 2022
Accepted: 25 September 2022
Published: 29 September 2022

Publisher's Note: MDPI stays neutral with regard to jurisdictional claims in published maps and institutional affiliations.

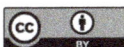

Copyright: © 2022 by the authors. Licensee MDPI, Basel, Switzerland. This article is an open access article distributed under the terms and conditions of the Creative Commons Attribution (CC BY) license (https://creativecommons.org/licenses/by/4.0/).

Abstract: Background: Scapular notching following reverse shoulder arthroplasty (RSA) is caused by both biological and mechanical mechanisms. Some authors postulated that osteolysis that extends over the inferior screw is caused mainly by biological notching. Inverted-bearing RSA (IB-RSA) is characterized by a polyethylene glenosphere and a metallic humeral liner, decreasing the poly debris formation and potentially reducing high grades of notching. This study aims to report the results of IB-RSA on a consecutive series of patients at mid-term follow-up, focusing on the incidence of Sirveaux grade 3 and 4 scapular notching. Methods: A retrospective study on 78 consecutive patients who underwent primary IB-RSA between 2015–2017 was performed. At a 4 years minimum follow-up, 49 patients were evaluated clinically with Constant score (CS), Subjective shoulder value (SSV), American Shoulder and Elbow score (ASES), pain and range of motion, and with an X-ray assessing baseplate position (high, low), implant loosening, and scapular notching. Results: At a mean follow-up of 5.0 ± 0.9, all the clinical parameters improved ($p < 0.05$). One patient was revised for an infection and was excluded from the evaluation, two patients had an acromial fracture, and one had an axillary neuropraxia. Scapular notching was present in 13 (27%) patients (six grade 1, seven grade 2) and no cases of grade 3 and 4 were observed. Scapular nothing was significantly associated with high glenoid position ($p < 0.001$) and with lower CS (70 ± 15 vs. 58 ± 20; $p = 0.046$), SSV (81 ± 14 vs. 68 ± 20; $p = 0.027$), ASES (86 ± 14 vs. 70 ± 22; $p = 0.031$), and anterior elevation (148 ± 23 vs. 115 ± 37; $p = 0.006$). A 44 mm- compared to 40 mm-glenosphere was associate with better CS (63 ± 17 vs. 78 ± 11; $p = 0.006$), external (23 ± 17 vs. 36 ± 17; $p = 0.036$), and internal rotation (4.8 ± 2.7 vs. 7.8 ± 2.2; $p = 0.011$). Conclusions: IB-RSA is a safe and effective procedure for mid-term follow-up. Inverting biomaterials leads to a distinct kind of notching with mainly mechanical features. Scapular notching is associated with a high baseplate position and has a negative influence on range of motion and clinical outcome.

Keywords: reverse shoulder arthroplasty; cuff tear arthropathy; polyethylene; scapular notching; range of motion; larger glenosphere

1. Introduction

Scapular notching is a common phenomenon associated with reverse shoulder arthroplasty (RSA) with a variable rate of 4.6–50.8% and up to 96% [1,2]. It can be considered a consequence of the inverted biomechanics of the shoulder, creating a semi-constrained joint. From a pathophysiological point of view, there are two different types of notching [3]: (1) mechanical notching, secondary to the contact of the humeral liner with the scapular pillar during movements in adduction, extension, and external rotation [4]; (2) biological notching, which is a chronic foreign-body reaction caused by polyethylene (PE) debris formation, leading to progressive osteolysis [5]. The radiological Sirveaux classification aims to quantify scapular notching, identifying four grades according to the amount of osteolysis [6] (Figure 1): some authors postulated that grades 1 and 2 are mainly due to mechanical notching, while grades 3 and 4, when it occurs above the inferior screw, are likely the results of the biological reaction [3].

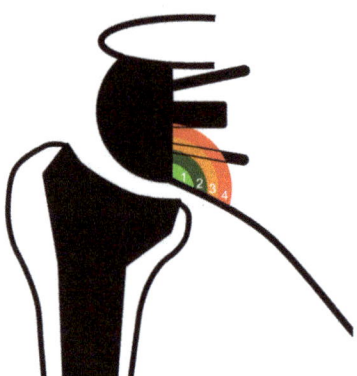

Figure 1. Notching classification according to Sirveaux et al. [6]: grade 1—defect confined to the pillar; grade 2—defect reaching the lower screw; grade 3—defect over the lower screw; grade 4—defect extended under the baseplate.

The clinical impact of scapular notching is controversial: some authors have found that notching has no influence on functional score [2,7,8], while other authors showed that it is associated with lower clinical results [6,9–11], and recently, Spiry et al. demonstrated a significant relationship between severe notching and late glenoid loosening [12].

For these reasons, since the introduction of the classic Grammont design, different solutions have been developed to avoid this complication and improve clinical results. Firstly, optimal glenoid positioning is a crucial factor to minimize this complication [5,8,11]. Secondly, lateralizing implants on both glenoid and humeral sides have shown to decrease the rate of notching [1,3,13–17].

While all these solutions act mainly on mechanical notching, an alternative solution is the inverted-bearing RSA (IB-RSA), where the prosthesis is characterized by a glenosphere made of PE and a metallic humeral liner [13,18,19]. This solution should theoretically minimize the wear of the PE, which is mainly due to the contact of the PE humeral liner with the scapula in the classic design [18], and decrease the biological component of scapular notching.

The primary endpoint of the study is to report the results of IB-RSA on a consecutive series of patients at mid-term follow-up, focusing on the incidence of grade 3 and 4 scapular notching. Secondary endpoints are other radiological and clinical outcomes. The hypothesis is that IB-RSA is a safe procedure and avoids scapular notching higher than Sirveaux grade 2.

2. Materials and Methods

This is a monocentric retrospective study on consecutive patients who underwent IB-RSA between 2015–2017 and evaluated at minimum 4 years follow-up. Patients treated for cuff tear arthropathy, primary osteoarthritis, inflammatory arthritis, and fracture sequelae who were available for clinical and radiological follow-up were included. We excluded patients who were operated on for acute fractures, patients treated for revision arthroplasty, and patients who received associated glenoid bone graft or metal glenosphere. A total of

78 patients who met the inclusion and exclusion criteria were operated on during the index period. Among these, 6 were dead, 17 were lost or impossible to contact, and 6 refused the control, leaving 49 patients reviewed clinically and radiologically at a mean follow-up of 5.0 ± 0.9 years. Thirty-three (67%) were female and 16 (33%) male. The mean age at surgery was 71 ± 7 years. The most common indication was rotator cuff arthropathy (49%), followed by primary osteoarthritis (31%), massive rotator cuff tear (12%), and fracture sequelae (8%).

2.1. Surgical Procedure

The SMR metal baseplate has a central peg and two screws, and the SMR long stem is an inlay design with a 150° neck-shaft angle. The SMR Reverse HP has a 40- or 44-mm diameter to improve ROM and it is characterized by an inversion of the materials with the aim to reduce polyethylene debris and, by a smart design (inferior sphere extension and superior narrowing), to facilitate the implantation and improving range of motion. It is made of a highly cross-linked PE (X-UHMWPE) and is coupled with CoCrMo liners. The glenoid implant provides intrinsic lateralization of the center of rotation of 5.2 mm. The glenosphere also presents a 4mm eccentricity option, but it is not utilized in primary cases at our institution. The humeral stem is implanted with 0° of retroversion using a forearm ancillary guide. A 40 mm glenosphere was used in 39 cases and a 44 mm glenopshere in 10 cases.

All the patients received both a general anesthetic and an interscalene block. The operation was performed in beach chair position, through a deltopectoral approach. The SMR RSA (LimaCorporate S.p.A, 33038 Villanova di San Daniele del Friuli, Udine, Italy) with the HP glenosphere was implanted in all the cases (Figure 2).

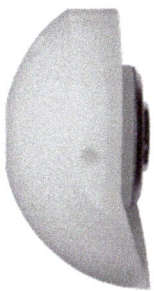 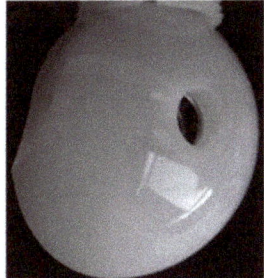

Figure 2. SMR reverse HP glenosphere (LimaCorporate S.p.A, 33038 Villanova di San Daniele del Friuli, Udine, Italy).

2.2. Clinical and Radiological Evaluation

Clinical evaluation performed pre- and post-operatively included the Constant–Murley score (CS) [20], the Subjective Shoulder Value (SSV) [21], the American Shoulder and Elbow Surgeon (ASES) score [22], the visual analogue scale (VAS) for pain and the range of motion (ROM) in term of active anterior elevation (AE), active external rotation (ER) in position 1, and active internal rotation (IR) (Constant-Murley subcategory). All complications and reoperation were recorded.

At last follow-up, radiographical evaluation was performed on the true anteroposterior projection on the glenohumeral joint line plane, with the humerus in neutral, external, and internal rotation. All the images were evaluated by two senior orthopedic residents trained in shoulder surgery. No attempt was made to determine the reliability of the observations, and when differences in assessments were noted, the observers reached a consensus. The positioning of the glenoid implant and the presence of radiolucent lines (RLL) were evaluated according to the classification system previously described for this baseplate in the anatomic prosthesis [23]. Loosening was considered to be present if the glenoid component had progressively migrated, as demonstrated by shift, tilt, or subsidence, or if complete radiolucency ≥ 2 mm was present in each zone [24]. On the humeral side, humeral RLL and loosening and partial or total greater tuberosity (GT) resorption were evaluated according to Melis et al. [24]. Inferior scapular notching was graded according to the classification system of Sirveaux et al. [6]. Pillar spurs and ossification, either individually or together, in the scapular-humeral space were recorded. According to the position of the inferior margin of the metallic baseplate in relation to the inferior border of the glenoid, the baseplate was evaluated to be high (inferior margin higher than inferior glenoid border) or low (inferior margin flush or lower than inferior glenoid border). Baseplate inclination was measured as the angle between the baseplate plane (line passing through the inferior e superior margin of the baseplate) and the supraspinatus fossa [16].

2.3. Statistical Analysis

The d'Agostino-Pearson test was used to analyze the distribution of the data collected, after which a paired t-test or the Mann-Whitney test was used to evaluate for statistical significance. Qualitative data were compared using the Chi2 and Fisher exact tests. Statistical analysis was performed with EasyMedStat software (Version 3.20; Amiens, France; www.easymedstat.com (accessed on 24 September 2022)).

3. Results

3.1. Clinical Results

Among the 49 patients, one patient was revised for infection and was excluded in the final evaluation, leaving 48 patients available for the study. Two patients had an acromial fracture and were treated conservatively. One patient suffered a postoperative infection which was revised in two stages. One patient had an axillary neuropraxia, which partially recovered. No loosening and no component disassembly was observed at the last follow-up.

All the clinical scores and range of motion improved at the last follow-up compared to the preoperative status (Table 1).

Table 1. Preoperative and postoperative clinical outcomes.

Outcome	Preop	Postop	p Value
CS	23 ± 13	67 ± 17	<0.001
ASES	37 ± 21	81 ± 18	<0.001
SSV	27 ± 24	77 ± 16	<0.001
Pain	7.3 ± 2.4	1.0 ± 1.8	<0.001
AE	66° ± 37°	140° ± 32°	<0.001
ER	15° ± 14°	26° ± 17°	0.042
IR	3.9 ± 2.1	5.4 ± 2.9	<0.001

CS, Constant Score; ASES, American Shoulder and Elbow Surgeon; SSV, Subjective shoulder value; AE; anterior elevation; ER, external rotation; IR, internal rotation.

Patients with 44 mm glenosphere showed a significantly higher CS and range of motion compared to patients with 40 mm glenosphere (Table 2).

Table 2. Clinical outcomes according to glenosphere size. No preoperative or demographical differences were found between the two groups.

Outcome	40 mm (38)	44 mm (10)	p Value
CS	63 ± 17	78 ± 11	0.006
ASES	79 ± 19	87 ± 15	0.206
SSV	75 ± 17	84 ± 12	0.141
AE	133 ± 33°	157 ± 19°	0.051
ER	23 ± 17°	36 ± 17°	0.036
IR	4.8 ± 2.7	7.8 ± 2.2	0.011

CS, Constant Score; ASES, American Shoulder and Elbow Surgeon; SSV, Subjective shoulder value; AE; anterior elevation; ER, external rotation; IR, internal rotation.

3.2. Radiological Results

At the radiological evaluation, an RLL < 2 mm around the glenoid was observed in five (10%) cases and ≥ 2 mm in a single zone in one case, which appeared to be progressive. In three cases we observed an initial subsidence of the base plate due to incomplete glenoid preparation, which stabilized within the first year without any progressive change at the last follow-up (Figure 3).

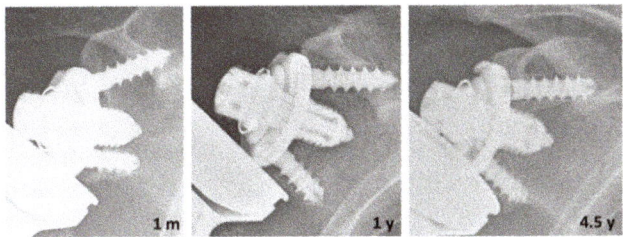

Figure 3. Subsidence of the glenoid due to incomplete glenoid preparation (baseplate not completely in contact with subchondral bone) which stabilizes at last follow-up in high glenoid position with the development of grade 2 scapular notching. m, months; y, year.

An RLL < 2 mm around the humerus was observed in 10 (21%) cases and was confined only to position 4 in 7 of the 10 cases. The distribution of RLL is shown in Figure 4.

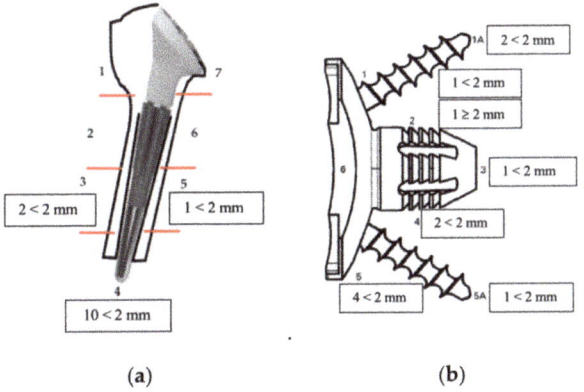

Figure 4. Image representing the frequency (number of cases) of RLL per zone of the humerus (**a**) and the glenoid (**b**).

GT was partially resorbed in 11 (23%) cases and totally in one (2%) case. Calcar was partially resorbed in 12 (25%) cases and totally in two (4%) cases. Cortical narrowing in zones 2 and 6 was present in 38 (79%) cases with 13 (27%) patients showing spot welds or condensation lines around the stem tip.

3.3. Scapular Notching

Scapular notching was present in 13 (27%) patients: 6 cases were grade 1 and 7 cases were grade 2. No cases of grades 3 and 4 were observed. All cases presented a bone spur formation at the scapular neck. Notching was significantly associated with high baseplate position (12/12 cases of notching in case of high baseplate vs. 1/36 in case of low position; $p < 0.001$). Patients with and without notching did not show a significant difference in baseplate inclination ($14° \pm 9°$ vs. $16° \pm 8°$, $p = 0.408$). Glenoid RLL were significantly more frequent in patients with scapular notching (31% vs. 6% $p = 0.038$). Notching was not associated with GT ($p = 0.611$) and calcar resorption ($p = 0.716$). Patients with scapular notching presented lower clinical results (Table 3).

Table 3. Clinical outcomes according to notching at the last follow-up. No preoperative or demographical differences were found between the two groups.

Outcome	No Notching (35)	Notching (13)	p Value
CS	70 ± 15	58 ± 20	0.046
ASES	86 ± 14	70 ± 22	0.031
SSV	81 ± 14	68 ± 20	0.027
Pain	0.9 ± 1.9	1.2 ± 1.6	0.058
AE	$148° \pm 23°$	$115° \pm 37°$	0.006
ER	$28° \pm 15°$	$20° \pm 21°$	0.142
IR	5.7 ± 2.5	5.1 ± 3.6	0.561

CS, Constant Score; ASES, American Shoulder and Elbow Surgeon; SSV, Subjective shoulder value; AE; anterior elevation; ER, external rotation; IR, internal rotation.

4. Discussion

This study showed that IB-RSA is a safe and effective procedure and does not present specific implant-associated complications at mid-term follow-up.

Scapular notching remain the most common complication associated with RSA [1,3]. In this series, notching occurred in 27% cases. Even though this rate still is not completely satisfying, it is lower compared to the notching rates (40–68%) of similar standard bearing RSA with a classic Grammont humeral stem with or without a lateralized glenoid [1,8,15,16,25]. Moreover, it must be underlined that the notching observed in this series has peculiar features. First, at this follow-up, no grade higher than 2 was observed (Figure 5).

As postulated by Friedman et al., grade 3 and 4 extending over the inferior screw are likely the results of a biologic response to polyethylene particles and osteolysis [3]. Secondly, in all cases with notching, a bone spur on the scapular neck was present. Third, the notching was almost only present in cases with a high position of the baseplate, a condition that is proven to be associated with mechanical contact of the prosthesis with the scapula [5,8,11,26]. All these features seem to be linked to a pure mechanical notching, proving that IB-RSA with a hard humeral liner leads to a distinct type of scapular notching and avoids PE wear-induced osteolysis at mid-term follow-up. Similar findings were shown by Kohut et al. using a different IB-RSA [27]. Based on our findings, optimal (as low as possible) and secure (optimal preparation of the subchondral bone) positioning of the glenoid is mandatory to avoid scapular notching (Figure 6).

Further studies are needed in order to analyze the notching evolution with IB-RSA at longer follow-up and verify if the notching remains mainly mechanical, or if the osteolysis will spread over the screw reaching the central peg, with a potential risk of loosening [12]. Moreover, histological studies on retrieved implants will be useful to clarify this phenomenon in vivo. In contrast with other authors [8,16], we did not find a statistical difference in baseplate inclination between patients with and without notching in our series. This finding may have different explanations. First, the limited number of patients included in this series compared to other series [8,16]. Second, the design of the glenosphere presenting an inferior extension may compensate for a slight superior inclination of the baseplate (Figure 2). Third, we believe that scapular notching is more linked to the inclination of the baseplate relative to the scapular neck [11] or to the intrinsic neck morphology [3] compared to the inclination relative to the supraspintus fossa.

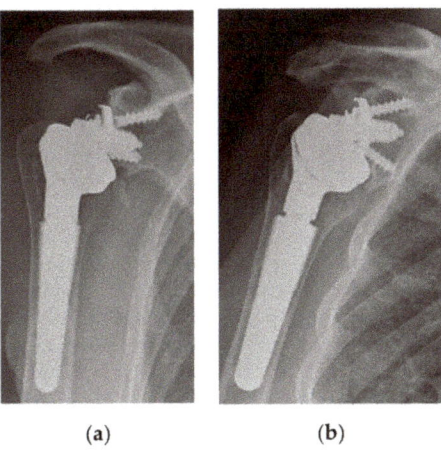

Figure 5. Two cases with a high glenoid position that developed a grade 1 (**a**) and grade 2 (**b**) of notching with the formation of a bone spur.

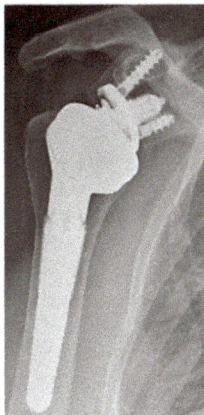

Figure 6. Correct position of the glenoid.

Another interesting observation was that in this series, GT and calcar resorption were not associated with scapular notching, which contrasts the finding of Mazaleyrat et al. [28] using a standard bearing RSA. This observation can be related to the fact that with IB-RSA PE, wear-induced osteolysis is minimized with a potential effect on proximal humerus resorption. The high rate of humeral stress shielding observed in this series is likely due to the methaphyseal fixation of the stem, which is associated with these radiographical changes [24,28]. Regarding the higher rate of glenoid RLL among patients with notching, we believe that this finding is due to the presence in this group of the three patients with early subsidence with the development of non-progressive RLL and notching. However, further studies at longer follow-ups are necessary to clarify the evolution of this observation.

The impact of scapular notching on clinical function is controversial. Some authors did not find an influence of notching on clinical function [2,7,8,12], while other authors clearly stated that scapular notching is associated with lower functional scores and decreased range of motion [6,9,10,29], especially in case of high grades. In this series, notching development has a significant negative influence on functional scores and anterior elevation at mid-term follow-up. We believe that this finding is due to the fact that the notching observed with this prosthesis is mainly mechanical and strictly linked to the incorrect high position of the glenoid. This leads to premature contact of the humeral component with the scapula and the acromion and consequent limitation of the motion [26].

Clinical scores and range of motion were overall improved at mid-term follow-up and were comparable with other series of IB-RSA [27,30] or standard RSA [6–10,16]. Interestingly, patients with a 44 mm diameter showed significantly better external and internal rotation, better CS, and a positive trend for better anterior elevation. Biomechanical studies showed that increasing the glenosphere diameter may have a favorable effect on range of motion [31–33]. Clinically, some authors found similar improvements when increasing the diameter to 42 or 44 mm [34,35]. The use of bigger glenospheres is advisable in order to improve the results. However, this finding should be taken with caution, since it is not possible to use a 44 mm glenosphere in all patients due to technical issues.

Regarding complications, only one patient was revised because of an infection and two patients had an acromial fracture. The reported rate of acromial fracture with classic reverse design is generally lower [1,36], but due to the low number of patients included in this series, it is impossible to evaluate whether increasing the glenosphere diameter could be associated with a higher risk of acromial fracture. However, Kohut et al. [27], in a larger series comparing 40/44 mm with 36 mm glenosphere, did not report an increased risk of acromial fracture. One important phenomenon that we observed in three cases is an initial glenoid migration, which stabilized within the first year and remains in a high and severe superiorly tilted baseplate (Figure 2). We noticed that in all these cases, the superior part of the glenoid was not perfectly in contact with the subchondral bone, probably due to an incorrect technique and uncompleted cartilage removal. Based on this observation, we recommended a good preparation of the subchondral bone in order to match the baseplate profile.

This study presents the following strengths: the series included all consecutive patients prospectively enrolled during the index period; the same prosthesis and the same technique was used in all the cases; radiographical and clinical evaluation was performed by two surgeons (R.R. and L.D.) not involved in the surgical procedure. However, this study presents some limitations. Firstly, its retrospective nature. Secondly, the lack of a control group. To definitively confirm our observation, comparative studies comparing IB-RSA and standard RSA will be needed in the future. Thirdly, because of the limited number of patients included it is impossible to draw definitive conclusions regarding complications and revisions rate. Fourth, other anatomical measures (i.e., scapular neck angle, neck-shaft angle, glenoid inclination) that may have a role in scapular notching were not measured.

5. Conclusions

IB-RSA is a safe and effective procedure without specific implant-associated complications at mid-term follow-up. Overall, using a 44-mm-diameter glenosphere compared to 40-mm-lead to an improved range of motion. Inverting biomaterials lead to a distinct kind of notching, which mainly showed mechanical features and no observed cases of grade 3 or 4. Scapular notching is associated with a high baseplate position and has a negative influence on range of motion and clinical outcome.

Author Contributions: Conceptualization, R.R. and A.C.; methodology, R.R.; software, R.R.; validation, A.C., M.B. and G.D.R.; formal analysis, R.R.; investigation, R.R. and L.D.; data curation, R.R. and L.D.; writing—original draft preparation, R.R.; writing—review and editing, A.C., S.G., M.B. and G.D.R.; supervision, A.C. and M.B. All authors have read and agreed to the published version of the manuscript.

Funding: This research received no external funding.

Institutional Review Board Statement: The study was conducted in accordance with the Declaration of Helsinki and approved by the Institutional Ethics Committee of IRCCS Humanitas Research Hospital (protocol code 41/22 and 19 July 2022).

Informed Consent Statement: Informed consent was obtained from all subjects involved in the study.

Data Availability Statement: Not applicable.

Conflicts of Interest: Alessandro Castagna declares conflict of interest: Lima consultant and royalties. The other authors declare no conflict of interest.

References

1. Alentorn-Geli, E.; Samitier, G.; Torrens, C.; Wright, T.W. Reverse Shoulder Arthroplasty. Part 2: Systematic Review of Reoperations, Revisions, Problems, and Complications. *Int. J. Shoulder Surg.* **2015**, *9*, 60–67. [CrossRef]
2. Werner, C.M.L.; Steinmann, P.A.; Gilbart, M.; Gerber, C. Treatment of Painful Pseudoparesis Due to Irreparable Rotator Cuff Dysfunction with the Delta III Reverse-Ball-and-Socket Total Shoulder Prosthesis. *J. Bone Jt. Surg. Am.* **2005**, *87*, 1476–1486. [CrossRef]
3. Friedman, R.J.; Barcel, D.A.; Eichinger, J.K. Scapular Notching in Reverse Total Shoulder Arthroplasty. *J. Am. Acad. Orthop. Surg.* **2019**, *27*, 200–209. [CrossRef]
4. Lädermann, A.; Gueorguiev, B.; Charbonnier, C.; Stimec, B.V.; Fasel, J.H.D.; Zderic, I.; Hagen, J.; Walch, G. Scapular Notching on Kinematic Simulated Range of Motion After Reverse Shoulder Arthroplasty Is Not the Result of Impingement in Adduction. *Medicine* **2015**, *94*, e1615. [CrossRef]
5. Nyffeler, R.W.; Werner, C.M.L.; Simmen, B.R.; Gerber, C. Analysis of a Retrieved Delta III Total Shoulder Prosthesis. *J. Bone Jt. Surg. Br.* **2004**, *86*, 1187–1191. [CrossRef] [PubMed]
6. Sirveaux, F.; Favard, L.; Oudet, D.; Huquet, D.; Walch, G.; Molé, D. Grammont Inverted Total Shoulder Arthroplasty in the Treatment of Glenohumeral Osteoarthritis with Massive Rupture of the Cuff. Results of a Multicentre Study of 80 Shoulders. *J. Bone Jt. Surg. Br.* **2004**, *86*, 388–395. [CrossRef] [PubMed]
7. Wall, B.; Nové-Josserand, L.; O'Connor, D.P.; Edwards, T.B.; Walch, G. Reverse Total Shoulder Arthroplasty: A Review of Results According to Etiology. *J. Bone Jt. Surg. Am.* **2007**, *89*, 1476–1485. [CrossRef]
8. Lévigne, C.; Boileau, P.; Favard, L.; Garaud, P.; Molé, D.; Sirveaux, F.; Walch, G. Scapular Notching in Reverse Shoulder Arthroplasty. *J. Shoulder Elb. Surg.* **2008**, *17*, 925–935. [CrossRef]
9. Simovitch, R.; Flurin, P.-H.; Wright, T.W.; Zuckerman, J.D.; Roche, C. Impact of Scapular Notching on Reverse Total Shoulder Arthroplasty Midterm Outcomes: 5-Year Minimum Follow-Up. *J. Shoulder Elb. Surg.* **2019**, *28*, 2301–2307. [CrossRef] [PubMed]
10. Mollon, B.; Mahure, S.A.; Roche, C.P.; Zuckerman, J.D. Impact of Scapular Notching on Clinical Outcomes after Reverse Total Shoulder Arthroplasty: An Analysis of 476 Shoulders. *J. Shoulder Elb. Surg.* **2017**, *26*, 1253–1261. [CrossRef]
11. Simovitch, R.W.; Zumstein, M.A.; Lohri, E.; Helmy, N.; Gerber, C. Predictors of Scapular Notching in Patients Managed with the Delta III Reverse Total Shoulder Replacement. *J. Bone Jt. Surg. Am.* **2007**, *89*, 588–600. [CrossRef] [PubMed]
12. Spiry, C.; Berhouet, J.; Agout, C.; Bacle, G.; Favard, L. Long-Term Impact of Scapular Notching after Reverse Shoulder Arthroplasty. *Int. Orthop.* **2021**, *45*, 1559–1566. [CrossRef]
13. Bloch, H.R.; Budassi, P.; Bischof, A.; Agneskirchner, J.; Domenghini, C.; Frattini, M.; Borroni, M.; Zoni, S.; Castagna, A. Influence of Glenosphere Design and Material on Clinical Outcomes of Reverse Total Shoulder Arthroplasty. *Shoulder Elb.* **2014**, *6*, 156–164. [CrossRef] [PubMed]
14. Franceschetti, E.; Ranieri, R.; Giovanetti de Sanctis, E.; Palumbo, A.; Franceschi, F. Clinical Results of Bony Increased-Offset Reverse Shoulder Arthroplasty (BIO-RSA) Associated with an Onlay 145° Curved Stem in Patients with Cuff Tear Arthropathy: A Comparative Study. *J. Shoulder Elb. Surg.* **2020**, *29*, 58–67. [CrossRef] [PubMed]
15. Athwal, G.S.; MacDermid, J.C.; Reddy, K.M.; Marsh, J.P.; Faber, K.J.; Drosdowech, D. Does Bony Increased-Offset Reverse Shoulder Arthroplasty Decrease Scapular Notching? *J. Shoulder Elb. Surg.* **2015**, *24*, 468–473. [CrossRef] [PubMed]
16. Boileau, P.; Morin-Salvo, N.; Bessière, C.; Chelli, M.; Gauci, M.-O.; Lemmex, D.B. Bony Increased-Offset-Reverse Shoulder Arthroplasty: 5 to 10 Years' Follow-Up. *J. Shoulder Elb. Surg.* **2020**, *29*, 2111–2122. [CrossRef]
17. Erickson, B.J.; Frank, R.M.; Harris, J.D.; Mall, N.; Romeo, A.A. The Influence of Humeral Head Inclination in Reverse Total Shoulder Arthroplasty: A Systematic Review. *J. Shoulder Elb. Surg.* **2015**, *24*, 988–993. [CrossRef] [PubMed]
18. Kohut, G.; Dallmann, F.; Irlenbusch, U. Wear-Induced Loss of Mass in Reversed Total Shoulder Arthroplasty with Conventional and Inverted Bearing Materials. *J. Biomech.* **2012**, *45*, 469–473. [CrossRef]
19. Irlenbusch, U.; Kääb, M.J.; Kohut, G.; Proust, J.; Reuther, F.; Joudet, T. Reversed Shoulder Arthroplasty with Inversed Bearing Materials: 2-Year Clinical and Radiographic Results in 101 Patients. *Arch. Orthop. Trauma Surg.* **2015**, *135*, 161–169. [CrossRef]
20. Constant, C.R.; Murley, A.H. A Clinical Method of Functional Assessment of the Shoulder. *Clin. Orthop. Relat. Res.* **1987**, *214*, 160–164. [CrossRef]
21. Gilbart, M.K.; Gerber, C. Comparison of the Subjective Shoulder Value and the Constant Score. *J. Shoulder Elb. Surg.* **2007**, *16*, 717–721. [CrossRef]

22. Richards, R.R.; An, K.N.; Bigliani, L.U.; Friedman, R.J.; Gartsman, G.M.; Gristina, A.G.; Iannotti, J.P.; Mow, V.C.; Sidles, J.A.; Zuckerman, J.D. A Standardized Method for the Assessment of Shoulder Function. *J. Shoulder Elb. Surg.* **1994**, *3*, 347–352. [CrossRef]
23. Castagna, A.; Randelli, M.; Garofalo, R.; Maradei, L.; Giardella, A.; Borroni, M. Mid-Term Results of a Metal-Backed Glenoid Component in Total Shoulder Replacement. *J. Bone Jt. Surg. Br.* **2010**, *92*, 1410–1415. [CrossRef]
24. Melis, B.; DeFranco, M.; Lädermann, A.; Molé, D.; Favard, L.; Nérot, C.; Maynou, C.; Walch, G. An Evaluation of the Radiological Changes around the Grammont Reverse Geometry Shoulder Arthroplasty after Eight to 12 Years. *J. Bone Jt. Surg. Br.* **2011**, *93*, 1240–1246. [CrossRef]
25. Boileau, P.; Watkinson, D.; Hatzidakis, A.M.; Hovorka, I. Neer Award 2005: The Grammont Reverse Shoulder Prosthesis: Results in Cuff Tear Arthritis, Fracture Sequelae, and Revision Arthroplasty. *J. Shoulder Elb. Surg.* **2006**, *15*, 527–540. [CrossRef]
26. Nyffeler, R.W.; Werner, C.M.L.; Gerber, C. Biomechanical Relevance of Glenoid Component Positioning in the Reverse Delta III Total Shoulder Prosthesis. *J. Shoulder Elb. Surg.* **2005**, *14*, 524–528. [CrossRef] [PubMed]
27. Kohut, G.; Reuther, F.; Joudet, T.; Kääb, M.J.; Irlenbusch, U. Inverted-Bearing Reverse Total Shoulder Arthroplasty: Scapular Notching Does Not Affect Clinical Outcomes and Complications at up to 7 Years of Follow-Up. *J. Shoulder Elb. Surg.* **2022**, *31*, 868–874. [CrossRef]
28. Mazaleyrat, M.; Favard, L.; Boileau, P.; Berhouet, J. Humeral Osteolysis after Reverse Shoulder Arthroplasty Using Cemented or Cementless Stems Comparative Retrospective Study with a Mean Follow-up of 9 Years. *Orthop. Traumatol. Surg. Res.* **2021**, *107*, 102916. [CrossRef] [PubMed]
29. Ernstbrunner, L.; Suter, A.; Catanzaro, S.; Rahm, S.; Gerber, C. Reverse Total Shoulder Arthroplasty for Massive, Irreparable Rotator Cuff Tears Before the Age of 60 Years: Long-Term Results. *JBJS* **2017**, *99*, 1721–1729. [CrossRef] [PubMed]
30. Jones, C.W.; Barrett, M.; Erickson, J.; Chatindiara, I.; Poon, P. Larger Polyethylene Glenospheres in Reverse Shoulder Arthroplasty: Are They Safe? *JSES Int.* **2020**, *4*, 944–951. [CrossRef]
31. Chou, J.; Malak, S.F.; Anderson, I.A.; Astley, T.; Poon, P.C. Biomechanical Evaluation of Different Designs of Glenospheres in the SMR Reverse Total Shoulder Prosthesis: Range of Motion and Risk of Scapular Notching. *J. Shoulder Elb. Surg.* **2009**, *18*, 354–359. [CrossRef]
32. Langohr, G.D.G.; Willing, R.; Medley, J.B.; Athwal, G.S.; Johnson, J.A. Contact Mechanics of Reverse Total Shoulder Arthroplasty during Abduction: The Effect of Neck-Shaft Angle, Humeral Cup Depth, and Glenosphere Diameter. *J. Shoulder Elb. Surg.* **2016**, *25*, 589–597. [CrossRef] [PubMed]
33. Roche, C.; Flurin, P.-H.; Wright, T.; Crosby, L.A.; Mauldin, M.; Zuckerman, J.D. An Evaluation of the Relationships between Reverse Shoulder Design Parameters and Range of Motion, Impingement, and Stability. *J. Shoulder Elb. Surg.* **2009**, *18*, 734–741. [CrossRef] [PubMed]
34. Mollon, B.; Mahure, S.A.; Roche, C.P.; Zuckerman, J.D. Impact of Glenosphere Size on Clinical Outcomes after Reverse Total Shoulder Arthroplasty: An Analysis of 297 Shoulders. *J. Shoulder Elb. Surg.* **2016**, *25*, 763–771. [CrossRef] [PubMed]
35. Müller, A.M.; Born, M.; Jung, C.; Flury, M.; Kolling, C.; Schwyzer, H.-K.; Audigé, L. Glenosphere Size in Reverse Shoulder Arthroplasty: Is Larger Better for External Rotation and Abduction Strength? *J. Shoulder Elb. Surg.* **2018**, *27*, 44–52. [CrossRef]
36. Neyton, L.; Erickson, J.; Ascione, F.; Bugelli, G.; Lunini, E.; Walch, G. Grammont Award 2018: Scapular Fractures in Reverse Shoulder Arthroplasty (Grammont Style): Prevalence, Functional, and Radiographic Results with Minimum 5-Year Follow-Up. *J. Shoulder Elb. Surg.* **2019**, *28*, 260–267. [CrossRef]

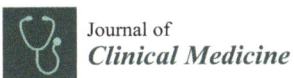

Journal of Clinical Medicine

Article

Conversion of Hemiarthroplasty to Reverse Shoulder Arthroplasty with Humeral Stem Retention

Falk Reuther [1,*], Ulrich Irlenbusch [2], Max J. Kääb [3] and Georges Kohut [4]

1. Department of Trauma Surgery and Orthopaedics, DRK Kliniken Berlin Koepenick, Salvador-Allende-Str. 2-8, 12559 Berlin, Germany
2. Clinic for Orthopaedics and Trauma Surgery, Erfurt Sports Clinic, Am Urbicher Kreuz 7, 99099 Erfurt, Germany; prof.irlenbusch@sportklinik-erfurt.de
3. Clinic for Sports Medicine and Orthopaedics, Sporthopaedicum Straubing, Bahnhofplatz 27, 94315 Straubing, Germany; max.kaeaeb@gmx.de
4. Clinic for Orthopaedics and Trauma Surgery, Clinique Générale Fribourg, Rue Hans Geiler 6, 1700 Fribourg, Switzerland; gkohut@cliniquegenerale.ch
* Correspondence: f.reuther@drk-kliniken-berlin.de; Tel.: +49-(30)-30353313

Abstract: The purpose of this study is to evaluate the mid-term clinical results of an ongoing case series on conversion reverse shoulder arthroplasty (RSA) with a modular prosthesis system. We included 17 elderly patients revised for failed hemiarthroplasty after proximal humeral fracture, of which 13 were converted using a modular reverse shoulder prosthesis. Four could not be converted due to overstuffing. For the conversion RSA, we determined the Constant score, American Shoulder and Elbow Surgeons Shoulder Score, visual analogue scale for pain and satisfaction, and range of motion preoperatively, at one year, and at the last follow-up. All measured clinical outcomes improved significantly at both follow-up time points ($p < 0.05$). The mean duration of surgery was 118.4 min (range: 80.0 to 140.0 min). We observed complications in three patients; these included one late infection and two aseptic stem loosenings. Modular shoulder arthroplasty is a suitable procedure for conversion RSA in elderly patients. All measured postoperative clinical outcomes improved significantly, the complication rate was acceptable, and no prosthesis-related complications occurred. Conversion RSA, although not feasible in every case, is a viable treatment option in the elderly, which can provide successful mid-term results.

Keywords: reverse shoulder arthroplasty; conversion; failed hemiarthroplasty; shoulder hemiprosthesis; modular reverse prosthesis

1. Introduction

Proximal humeral fractures in elderly patients are a common indication for shoulder arthroplasty. Treatment options mainly involve hemiarthroplasty (HA) and reverse shoulder arthroplasty (RSA). Choosing the appropriate treatment option is influenced by many factors, such as the fracture pattern, tuberosity involvement, bone quality, surgeon preference, and the age and activity level of the patient [1].

HA is a well-known procedure for managing proximal humeral fractures. However, with the advent of RSA, the use of HA has become debatable owing to its unpredictable and non-homogeneous outcomes, its technical difficulties, and the fact that it is rarely indicated [2]. Moreover, HA is associated with a high rate of tuberosity complications (up to 50%) [2].

Failure of HA has been attributed to several causes including pain, deep infection, impaired shoulder function, rotator cuff degeneration, cartilage wear of the glenoid, aseptic loosening of the humeral component, and implant instability or dislocation [3,4]. Failed HA may be revised in several ways. Typical treatment options include revision to conventional total shoulder arthroplasty, revision to RSA, and resection arthroplasty [5–9]. Revision to

RSA may be carried out by exchanging the complete hemiprosthesis (traditional revision RSA) or by retaining the existing humeral stem (conversion RSA). Indicated primarily for concomitant rotator cuff dysfunction, revision to RSA improves shoulder function and relieves pain; however, it is associated with a high complication rate [6,7,9–11].

The removal of the humeral stem is associated with a relatively high risk of humeral shaft fracture, which may jeopardize the anchoring of the new stem and result in implant failure [11–13]. Furthermore, removal of a well-fixed stem can be technically difficult, especially in cases where there is poor bone quality, and may require osteotomy of the humeral shaft [10,11,14]. Levy et al. observed that the high rate (32%) of prosthesis-related complications in their study of traditional revision RSA with stem exchange for failed HA was mainly associated with bone loss in the proximal humerus, glenoid, or both [7]. Therefore, to prevent bone loss and reduce the risk of intra- and postoperative complications, it would be best to retain the hemiprosthesis stem [10,14,15].

With the advent of modular convertible shoulder prosthesis systems, retaining the humeral stem during revision of HA to RSA has become a viable option. Indeed, the authors of some studies have shown encouraging results accompanied by reduced rates of complications and implant failures [13–18]. Moreover, clinical data have suggested that minimal changes in height and offset [14], shorter operating times [11,13,15], fewer intraoperative complications [11,13,15], and fewer subsequent revision surgeries [10,11,15] are associated with conversion RSA with modular prostheses compared to traditional revision RSA with stem exchange. However, these data are limited to a few short- and mid-term studies, primarily because revision of HA to RSA is a rare indication.

Our aim with this study is to provide further insight into the outcomes of this rare procedure by reporting the mid-term clinical results of an ongoing case series on conversion RSA with a modular prosthesis system in patients revised for failed HA after a proximal humeral fracture.

2. Materials and Methods

2.1. Study Design and Patient Selection

This study was a subgroup analysis of an ongoing, multicenter, prospective cohort study of 519 patients with various indications and operated with an Affinis Inverse or Affinis Facture Inverse system (Mathys Ltd., Bettlach, Switzerland) between 6 May 2008 and 1 June 2015. Of these, 17 patients met the following inclusion criteria: revision required for failed HA after proximal humeral fracture, Affinis Fracture or Articula system (Mathys Ltd., Bettlach, Switzerland) implanted as primary prosthesis, and stem removal not required during revision. Reasons for revision included secondary tuberosity dislocation or malunion after primary arthroplasty, luxation or instability after primary arthroplasty, rotator cuff disorder after primary arthroplasty, and glenoid erosion after HA, all resulting in pain and/or loss of function.

Conversion RSA was considered in patients who showed no stem loosening or infection and had adequate soft tissue tension for humeral stem retention, as assessed intraoperatively. Thirteen patients, enrolled from four centers in Germany and Switzerland, were considered suitable for conversion RSA (Figure 1). Of these patients, two were lost due to early revision, two to dementia or old age, and one to dislocation, leaving eight patients at the final follow-up. In the remaining four patients, conversion was not possible due to overstuffing; these patients were treated with traditional revision RSA with stem exchange.

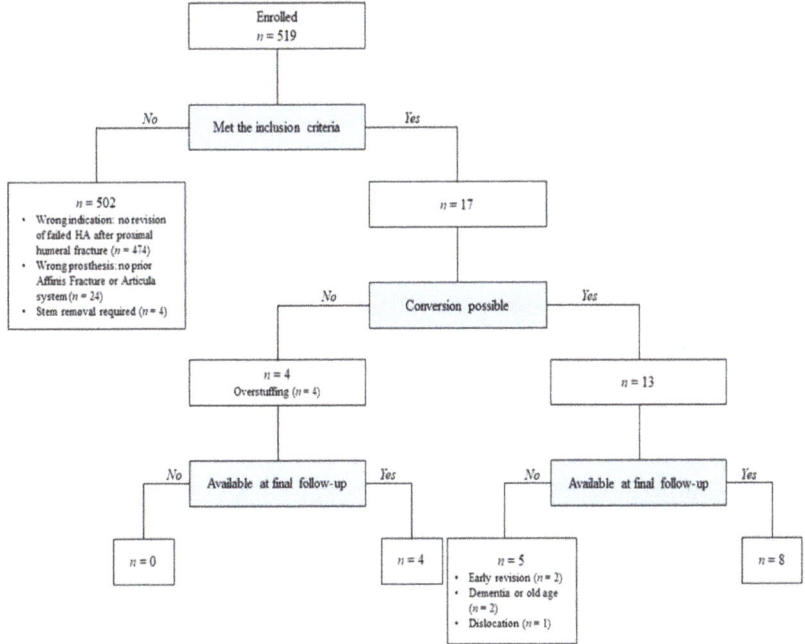

Figure 1. Flow diagram of the patient selection.

Patients underwent a clinical examination preoperatively, after one year, and at the final follow-up. The mean final follow-up period was 55.1 months (range: 12.0 to 91.1 months).

2.2. Implant Characterstics

HA was performed using a fracture prosthesis (Affinis Fracture or Articula system), which is part of a modular implant system that allows conversion to RSA using the same humeral stem as in HA. For conversion RSA, the head component and the metaphyseal element were replaced with a reverse metaphyseal element (Affinis Fracture Inverse system) (Figure 2). This element can be fixed to the humeral stem with 10 mm of possible height adjustment and free torsion. On the glenoid side, either a 39 or 42 mm glenosphere can be chosen. The reverse metaphyseal element exists in a 0 or 3 mm offset version. If both metaphyseal parts are at the same level, converting HA to RSA would lengthen the humerus by 23 mm and medialize the center of rotation by at least 19 mm (from 4 to 23 or 25 mm lateral offset, Figure 3). This equates to the minimal lengthening in a worst-case scenario, where the central part was placed completely distally during the implantation of the fracture HA and revised with a 39 mm glenosphere and a 0 mm offset reverse metaphyseal element. When placing the reverse metaphyseal element completely proximally during the revision surgery with the largest glenosphere and the highest offset, a maximum lengthening of 38 mm and medialization of the center of rotation of 21 mm can be achieved.

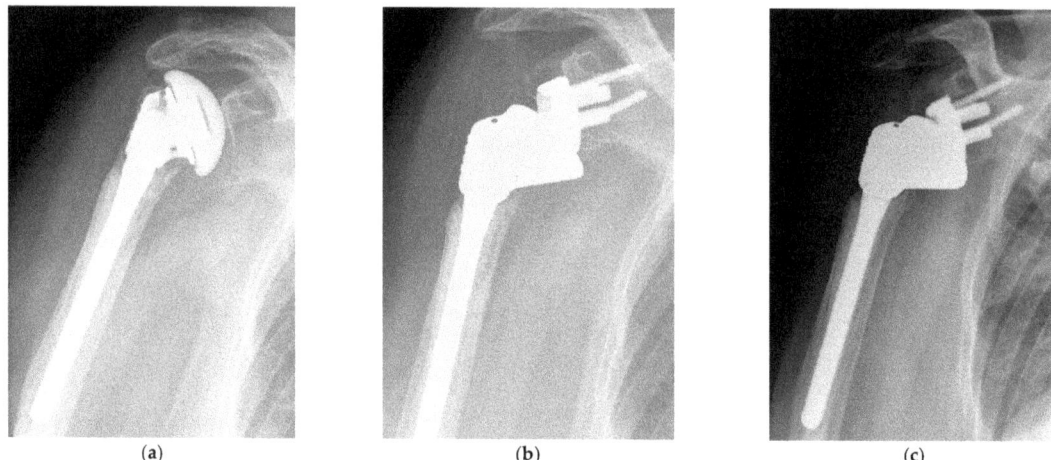

Figure 2. Failure of hemiarthroplasty and conversion to reverse shoulder arthroplasty. (**a**) Preoperative anteroposterior radiograph of a hemiarthroplasty with a firmly cemented stem showing insufficiency of the supraspinatus tendon and superior migration of the humeral head; (**b**) Postoperative anteroposterior radiograph of a conversion reverse shoulder arthroplasty with humeral stem retention; (**c**) Four-year postoperative anteroposterior radiograph showing prosthesis in situ.

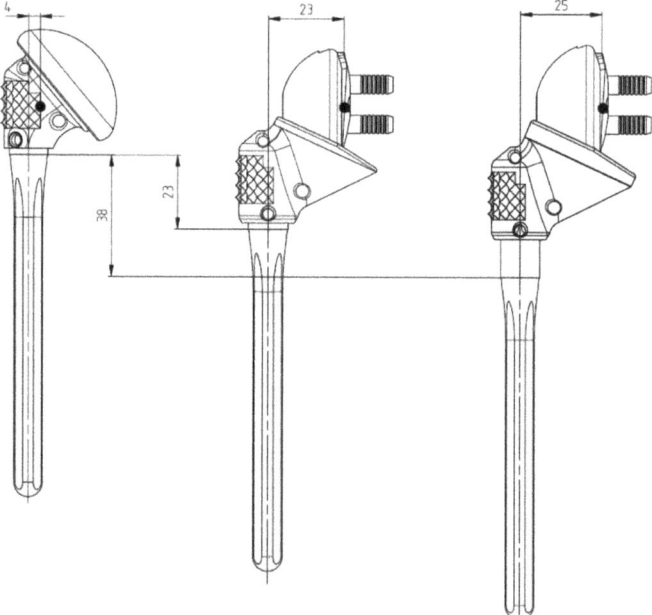

Figure 3. Modular reverse shoulder prosthesis. If both metaphyseal parts are at the same level, conversion leads to 23 mm of distalization and medializes the center of rotation by 19 mm (left). This corresponds to the worst-case scenario if the reverse metaphyseal element was placed most distally during the primary implantation of hemiarthroplasty (middle). The maximum lengthening of the conversion is 38 mm by choosing a 42 mm glenosphere and an offset of 3 mm (right). The length of the anatomic and the reverse prosthesis can be adjusted by 10 mm to reduce distalization. The center of rotation is medialized between 19 mm and 21 mm.

2.3. Operating Technique

Surgeons used a standard deltopectoral approach in all cases. The recording of the operating time began at the moment of the first incision and ended at postoperative skin closure.

Initially, the humeral head was mobilized, and the metaphyseal part of the prosthesis was freed from the tuberosities if present. Next, the prosthetic head and the metaphyseal part were removed. On the humeral side, we removed the cement and bone from the proximal end of the stem enough to allow the insertion of the trial prosthetic epiphysis at the deepest position possible with the prosthetic system.

On the opposite side of the joint, we exposed the glenoid, then reamed and drilled it so that the metaglene could be inserted using a standard technique. Trial glenospheres and epiphyses were used to confirm the optimal configuration of the prosthesis before the definitive prosthetic components were implanted. Bony parts of the greater and lesser tuberosities, if present, were then reattached to the prosthetic epiphysis with heavy, non-absorbable sutures.

2.4. Clinical Evaluation

We measured the Constant score, American Shoulder and Elbow Surgeons (ASES) Shoulder Score, visual analogue scale (VAS) for pain and satisfaction, and range of motion preoperatively, after one year, and at the final follow-up. All complications were carefully monitored and recorded throughout the study.

2.5. Statistical Analysis

We compared the pre- and postoperative clinical parameters using a two-sided exact Wilcoxon rank sum test. In all cases, p values < 0.05 were considered significant. We presented the data as the mean (range) unless otherwise indicated. In cases of loss to follow-up (including death), we used the last observation for calculation.

3. Results

The patient demographics and characteristics are detailed in Table 1. The mean age of patients at the time of surgery was 73.6 years (range: 64.9 to 89.6 years), the mean final follow-up period was 55.1 months (range: 12.0 to 91.1 months), and the mean duration of surgery was 118.4 (range: 80.0 to 140.0) minutes.

Table 1. Patient demographics and characteristics.

Variable	Value
Sex (female/male)	9/4
Operated side (right/left)	6/7
Age at surgery (years)	73.6 (64.9–89.6)
Time since implantation of hemiprosthesis (months)	16.7 (3.9–61.7)
Follow-up period (months)	55.1 (12.0–91.1)

The values of the age at surgery, time since implantation of hemiprosthesis, and follow-up period are reported as means (ranges). Total number of patients: 13.

3.1. Clinical Outcomes

The clinical outcomes, such as the Constant score, ASES Shoulder Score, VAS for pain and satisfaction, and ROM, improved significantly, both at one year postoperatively ($p < 0.05$) and at the last follow-up visit ($p < 0.05$) (Table 2).

Table 2. Clinical outcomes.

Clinical Outcome	Preoperative (n = 13)	At 12 Months (n = 11)	p Value *	At Last Follow-up (n = 8)	p Value **
Constant score	21.7 (4.0–52.0)	50.1 (37.0–71.0)	0.0001	57.9 (42.0–96.0)	0.0001
ASES Shoulder Score	24.3 (6.7–46.8)	63.8 (46.7–86.7)	<0.001	66.9 (46.7–98.3)	<0.001
VAS for pain	7.3 (5.0–9.0)	2.3 (0.0–5.0)	<0.001	2.3 (0.0–5.0)	<0.001
VAS for satisfaction	2.0 (0.0–6.2)	7.9 (5.0–10.0)	<0.001	8.0 (7.0–10.0)	<0.001
Active ROM in abduction (°)	38.8 (10.0–100.0)	103.2 (50.0–180.0)	<0.001	111.9 (50.0–160.0)	0.006
Active ROM in forward flexion (°)	46.2 (10.0–130.0)	111.8 (60.0–160.0)	0.0001	122.5 (60.0–180.0)	0.001

Values reported as means (ranges). p values from two-sided exact Wilcoxon rank sum test between preoperative and 12-month follow-up (*) and between preoperative and last follow-up (**). ASES: American Shoulder and Elbow Surgeons; n: number of patients; ROM: range of motion; VAS: visual analogue scale.

3.2. Complications

Three patients presented with complications. One patient had a late infection at 5.2 months postoperatively and was treated by debridement and exchange of the bearing components; the patient had no clinical signs of ongoing infection at the last follow-up. Two patients had aseptic stem loosening. One occurred 49.2 months postoperatively and was treated by stem exchange. The other occurred 7.5 months postoperatively, and the humeral component was revised. However, the implant was later removed, and the patient was treated with antibiotics due to a late infection occurring 26.0 months after stem revision.

4. Discussion

In this study, we evaluated the conversion of failed HA to RSA using a modular prosthetic system and assessed the clinical outcomes at different time intervals postoperatively. We reported significant postoperative improvements in the Constant score, ASES Shoulder Score, VAS for pain and satisfaction, and ROM.

During the revision of failed HA, the correct balancing of soft tissue tension is important. Insufficient tension can result in instability of the prosthesis, whereas excessive tension can result in acromial fracture, poor deltoid function, and/or neurological lesions [19]. Moreover, restoring adequate tension can be complicated by scarring and altered muscle function. However, most current modular prostheses allow the height of the humeral head to be adjusted enough to modify the compressive forces across the glenohumeral joint, and thereby achieve adequate soft tissue tension.

Postoperative arm lengthening is a typical occurrence after RSA. Lädermann et al. reported a mean postoperative lengthening of 23 ± 12 mm in primary and revision RSA using a different prosthesis than we did [19], while Teschner et al. measured a mean increase in implant height of 24 ± 2.6 mm in the conversion of failed HA to RSA using the same prosthesis as we did [14]. Both of these values are similar to the lengthening that can be achieved with the reverse modular prosthesis used in our series (23 mm) (Figure 3). Moreover, we did not observe any complications related to the under- or over-tensioning of the deltoid tissue. We therefore believe that the modular prosthesis used in our series allowed for the optimal soft tissue balance required for retaining a firmly implanted humeral stem.

Although several modular convertible shoulder prostheses are available today for the successful conversion of HA to RSA [14], stem retention may not always be possible, especially when the humeral stem is poorly positioned or not well fixed [10,11]. In these cases, stem revision is needed [10,11]. Similarly, conversion RSA is not feasible in cases with infection or where the stem cannot be distalized enough, as seen in the present study. Finally, the use of stemless anatomical implants in primary procedures does not allow conversion RSA. We also found that not every patient in the present study could benefit from conversion RSA. Of the 17 cases where conversion RSA was considered, four cases (23%) could not be converted due to overstuffing. A similar rate was found in a recent study where 22% of the patients could not be converted despite the presence of a modular prosthesis [10], indicating a limitation of today's convertible modular prosthetic systems. Other limitations include the need for highly skilled surgeons and a meticulous surgical technique for implanting a convertible modular prosthetic system during the primary procedure [16]. These limitations necessitate the continued use of modular non-convertible shoulder prostheses.

Revision surgery of failed HA remains technically challenging and may be associated with less predictable clinical outcomes and various complications [18]. Nevertheless, in the current study, we found a significant improvement in the mean Constant score (from 21.7 preoperatively to 57.9 at the last follow-up; $p = 0.0001$). Other studies on the revision of failed HA to RSA also found similar increases in the mean Constant scores: from 12.67 to 45.08 [6] and from 8.9 to 41.0 [18].

Besides the functional scores, intraoperative parameters such as the operating time are also important contributors to successful conversion RSA. In recent studies comparing conversions and revisions, conversion procedures resulted in shorter operating times [10,11,13,15]. We found similar results in our study: the mean operating time for conversion RSA was shorter than that for traditional revision RSA [118.4 min (range: 80.0 to 140.0) versus 150.0 min (range: 100.0 to 230.0), our unpublished results].

Despite successful clinical outcomes, complication rates remain high after conversion RSA, ranging from 22% to 43% [11]. We found complications in three (23%) patients who underwent conversion RSA. Revision with stem exchange was needed in two (15%) patients due to aseptic loosening. Although we observed an overall complication rate similar to that reported in other studies of RSA after failed shoulder arthroplasty [6,20,21], more clinical evidence is needed to draw definite conclusions in this regard. Previous studies also showed that modular prosthesis designs minimized the risk of periprosthetic humeral shaft fractures [18]. We confirmed this finding; no periprosthetic fractures or other implant-related complications were observed in our study.

Our study had a number of limitations; these included the absence of standardized radiographs for the accurate measuring of arm length and the small sample size owing to the nature of the indication, which limited the interpretation of our findings. This is why—although challenging—studies with larger patient cohorts are needed to investigate the full potential of modular systems in the conversion of failed HA to RSA. Finally, the results from the type of modular convertible shoulder prosthesis used in our study are not sufficient to make generalized conclusions on the outcomes of conversion RSA. For this, a clinical comparison with different implant types will be needed.

5. Conclusions

Modular shoulder arthroplasty is a suitable procedure for the conversion of failed HA to RSA in elderly patients, allowing a successful conversion in the majority of cases. In our study, all measured postoperative clinical outcomes improved significantly. Moreover, retaining the prosthetic stem was associated with a short operating time. Finally, the observed complication rate was acceptable, and no prosthesis-related complications occurred. Although not feasible in every case, conversion RSA is a viable treatment option in the elderly, which can provide successful mid-term results with an acceptable complication rate. Nevertheless, studies with larger sample sizes should be carried out to provide greater insight into conversion RSA outcomes in this rare indication.

Author Contributions: Conceptualization, F.R., U.I., M.J.K. and G.K.; methodology, F.R., U.I., M.J.K. and G.K.; investigation, F.R., U.I., M.J.K. and G.K.; writing—original draft preparation, G.K.; writing—review and editing, F.R., U.I., M.J.K. and G.K. All authors have read and agreed to the published version of the manuscript.

Funding: This research was partially funded by Mathys Ltd. Bettlach. Funds helped cover a medical advisor contract and travel expenses for Georges Kohut, Ulrich Irlenbusch, Max Josef Kääb, and Falk Reuther. Mathys Ltd. Bettlach also supported the independent statistical analysis. Related to a certain study (study ID 0701).

Institutional Review Board Statement: The study was conducted according to the guidelines of the Declaration of Helsinki and approved by the Ethics Committee of the Comité intercantonal d'éthique (Switzerland) on 24 September 2008 (number 01/2008).

Informed Consent Statement: Informed consent was obtained from all subjects involved in the study.

Data Availability Statement: The data presented in this study are available on request from the corresponding author. The data are not publicly available due to ethical restrictions.

Acknowledgments: Medical Minds GmbH provided medical writing and editorial support.

Conflicts of Interest: Falk Reuther, Ulrich Irlenbusch, Max J. Kääb, and Georges Kohut declare that they have received benefits for professional use from Mathys Ltd. Bettlach directly related to the subject of this manuscript (see Funding). Besides this, Mathys Ltd. Bettlach had no role in the collection or interpretation of data, in the writing of the manuscript, or in the decision to publish the results.

References

1. Shukla, D.R.; McAnany, S.; Kim, J.; Overley, S.; Parsons, B.O. Hemiarthroplasty versus reverse shoulder arthroplasty for treatment of proximal humeral fractures: A meta-analysis. *J. Shoulder Elb. Surg.* **2016**, *25*, 330–340. [CrossRef] [PubMed]
2. Boileau, P.; Winter, M.; Cikes, A.; Han, Y.; Carles, M.; Walch, G.; Schwartz, D. Can surgeons predict what makes a good hemiarthroplasty for fracture? *J. Shoulder Elb. Surg.* **2013**, *22*, 1495–1506. [CrossRef] [PubMed]
3. Fevang, B.T.L.; Lie, S.A.; Havelin, L.I.; Skredderstuen, A.; Furnes, O. Risk factors for revision after shoulder arthroplasty: 1825 shoulder arthroplasties from the Norwegian Arthroplasty register. *Acta Orthop.* **2009**, *80*, 83–91. [CrossRef] [PubMed]
4. Wiater, B.P.; Moravek, J.E.; Wiater, J.M. The evaluation of the failed shoulder arthroplasty. *J. Shoulder Elb. Surg.* **2014**, *23*, 745–758. [CrossRef]
5. De Wilde, L.M.M.; Van Petegem, P.; Verdonk, R. Revision of shoulder replacement with a reversed shoulder prosthesis (Delta III): Report of five cases. *Acta Orthop. Belg.* **2001**, *67*, 348–353.
6. Gohlke, F.; Rolf, O. Revision of failed fracture hemiarthroplasties to reverse total shoulder prosthesis through the transhumeral approach: Method incorporating a pectoralis-major-pedicled bone window. *Oper. Orthop. Und Traumatol.* **2007**, *19*, 185–208. [CrossRef]
7. Levy, J.C.; Virani, N.; Pupello, D.; Frankle, M. Use of the reverse shoulder prosthesis for the treatment of failed hemiarthroplasty in patients with glenohumeral arthritis and rotator cuff deficiency. *J. Bone Jt. Surgery. Br. Vol.* **2007**, *89*, 189–195. [CrossRef]
8. Levy, J.; Frankle, M.; Mighell, M.; Pupello, D. The use of the reverse shoulder prosthesis for the treatment of failed hemiarthroplasty for proximal humeral fracture. *J. Bone Jt. Surg. Am. Vol.* **2007**, *89*, 292–300. [CrossRef]
9. Saltzman, B.M.; Chalmers, P.N.; Gupta, A.K.; Romeo, A.; Nicholson, G.P. Complication rates comparing primary with revision reverse total shoulder arthroplasty. *J. Shoulder Elb. Surg.* **2014**, *23*, 1647–1654. [CrossRef]
10. Crosby, L.A.; Wright, T.W.; Yu, S.; Zuckerman, J.D. Conversion to reverse total shoulder arthroplasty with and without humeral stem retention: The role of a convertible-platform stem. *J. Bone Jt. Surg. Am. Vol.* **2017**, *99*, 736–742. [CrossRef]
11. Kirsch, J.M.; Khan, M.; Thornley, P.; Gichuru, M.; Freehill, M.T.; Neviaser, A.; Moravek, J.; Miller, B.S.; Bedi, A. Platform shoulder arthroplasty: A systematic review. *J. Shoulder Elb. Surg.* **2018**, *27*, 756–763. [CrossRef]
12. Chacon, A.; Virani, N.; Shannon, R.; Levy, J.C.; Pupello, D.; Frankle, M. Revision Arthroplasty with Use of a Reverse Shoulder Prosthesis-Allograft Composite. *J. Bone Jt. Surg. Am. Vol.* **2009**, *91*, 119–127. [CrossRef]
13. Dilisio, M.F.; Miller, L.R.; Siegel, E.J.; Higgins, L.D. Conversion to Reverse Shoulder Arthroplasty: Humeral Stem Retention Versus Revision. *Orthopedics* **2015**, *38*, e773–e779. [CrossRef]
14. Teschner, H.; Vaske, B.; Albrecht, U.-V.; Meller, R.; Liodakis, E.; Wiebking, U.; Krettek, C.; Jagodzinski, M. Conversion of hemi into reverse shoulder arthroplasty: Implant design limitations. *Arch. Orthop. Trauma Surg.* **2014**, *134*, 1683–1689. [CrossRef]
15. Wieser, K.; Borbas, P.; Ek, E.T.; Meyer, D.C.; Gerber, C. Conversion of stemmed hemi- or total to reverse total shoulder arthroplasty: Advantages of a modular stem design. *Clin. Orthop. Relat. Res.* **2015**, *473*, 651–660. [CrossRef]
16. Werner, B.C.; Dines, J.S.; Dines, D.M. Platform systems in shoulder arthroplasty. *Curr. Rev. Musculoskelet. Med.* **2016**, *9*, 49–53. [CrossRef]

17. Castagna, A.; Delcogliano, M.; De Caro, F.; Ziveri, G.; Borroni, M.; Gumina, S.; Postacchini, F.; De Biase, C.F. Conversion of shoulder arthroplasty to reverse implants: Clinical and radiological results using a modular system. *Int. Orthop.* **2013**, *37*, 1297–1305. [CrossRef]
18. Werner, B.S.; Boehm, D.; Gohlke, F. Revision to reverse shoulder arthroplasty with retention of the humeral component. *Acta Orthop.* **2013**, *84*, 473–478. [CrossRef]
19. Lädermann, A.; Williams, M.D.; Melis, B.; Hoffmeyer, P.; Walch, G. Objective evaluation of lengthening in reverse shoulder arthroplasty. *J. Shoulder Elb. Surg.* **2009**, *18*, 588–595. [CrossRef]
20. Melis, B.; Bonnevialle, N.; Neyton, L.; Lévigne, C.; Favard, L.; Walch, G.; Boileau, P. Glenoid loosening and failure in anatomical total shoulder arthroplasty: Is revision with a reverse shoulder arthroplasty a reliable option? *J. Shoulder Elb. Surg.* **2012**, *21*, 342–349. [CrossRef]
21. Walker, M.; Willis, M.P.; Brooks, J.P.; Pupello, D.; Mulieri, P.J.; Frankle, M.A. The use of the reverse shoulder arthroplasty for treatment of failed total shoulder arthroplasty. *J. Shoulder Elb. Surg.* **2012**, *21*, 514–522. [CrossRef]

Article

Two-Stage Exchange Arthroplasty for Periprosthetic Shoulder Infection Is Associated with High Rate of Failure to Reimplant and Mortality

Doruk Akgün *,†,‡, Mats Wiethölter †,‡, Nina Maziak ‡, Alp Paksoy ‡, Daniel Karczewski ‡, Markus Scheibel ‡ and Philipp Moroder ‡

Center for Musculoskeletal Surgery, Charité-Universitätsmedizin Berlind, Charitéplatz 1, 10117 Berlin, Germany; mats-jonas.wiethoelter@charite.de (M.W.); nina.maziak@charite.de (N.M.); paksoyalp97@gmail.com (A.P.); daniel.karczewski@charite.de (D.K.); markus.scheibel@charite.de (M.S.); philipp.moroder@charite.de (P.M.)
* Correspondence: doruk.akguen@charite.de; Tel.: +49-30-450-652-319; Fax: +49-30-450-515-905
† Equally Contributed.
‡ Corporate Member of Freie Universität Berlin, Humboldt-Universität zu Berlin, and Berlin Institute of Health.

Abstract: Background: Patients with a periprosthetic joint infection (PJI) of the shoulder, who fail to undergo reimplantation in an attempted two-stage exchange seem to be neglected in the current literature. The aim of this study was to assess the clinical course of patients after the first stage in the process of an attempted two-stage exchange for shoulder PJI. Methods: After a retrospective review of our institutional database between 2008 and 2018, 49 patients, who were treated with an intended two-stage exchange for shoulder PJI, were identified. Patients' demographics, laboratory and health status parameters, along with records of clinical outcome were collected. The primary outcome measurements analyzed were infection eradication, successful reimplantation, and patient survival. Results: Reimplantation was completed in only 35 (71%) of 49 cases and eradication of infection was achieved in 85.7% of patients with successful reimplantation after a mean follow-up duration of 5.1 years (1.1 to 10.2 years). Reasons for failure to reimplant were premature death in 36%, high general morbidity in 29%, satisfaction with the current status in 21%, or severe infection with poor bone and soft tissues in 14% of the patients. Of the 14 cases without reimplantation, eradication rate of infection was 57% after a mean follow-up of 5 years (2.6 to 11 years). The overall mortality rate of the entire cohort was 25% at the latest follow-up and 10% within ninety days after implant removal. Patients who deceased or did not undergo reimplantation during the follow-up were significantly older and had a significantly higher Charlson comorbidity index (CCI). Conclusions: While the two-stage exchange arthroplasty can lead to high rates of infection eradication, a considerable subset of patients never undergoes the second stage for a variety of reasons. Shoulder PJI and its treatment are associated with a high risk of mortality, especially in patients with older age and higher CCI.

Keywords: periprosthetic shoulder infection; two-stage exchange; mortality; reimplantation

1. Introduction

Periprosthetic joint infection (PJI) of the shoulder represents a devastating complication and is the main cause of revision within the first few years after shoulder arthroplasty [1–3]. Its treatment continues to pose a challenge for the orthopedic community [3,4]. Although the preferred surgical treatment of chronic shoulder PJI is still unknown and pooled data demonstrate single-stage exchange may be superior to two-stage exchange in selected cases, two-stage exchange arthroplasty with implant removal, insertion of an antibiotic spacer, followed by reimplantation of an arthroplasty, continues to be the most common treatment strategy for shoulder PJI [5,6]. The reported infection eradication rate of two-stage exchange arthroplasty varies in literature between 63% and 100% [4,6]. However, the majority of these studies focus on the clinical outcomes after successful reimplantation and overlook a substantial number of patients who undergo resection arthroplasty alone and do not complete the second stage of an attempted two-stage exchange arthroplasty [7,8]. Thus, these studies may not accurately reflect the overall success rate of two-stage exchange arthroplasty for shoulder PJI. Furthermore, most studies are limited to small case series and most importantly, there is a lack of data and high variability of how these studies define diagnosis and treatment success of shoulder PJI, which could result in an overestimation of the outcome parameters. An improved understanding of the interstage period and application of a standardized, multidimensional definition of shoulder PJI diagnosis and also treatment success is crucial to accurately depict the clinical outcome of two-stage exchange arthroplasty.

The purpose of the current study was to assess the clinical course of patients after implant removal in the process of an attempted two-stage exchange arthroplasty for shoulder PJI including infection eradication, successful reimplantation, and patient survival as main outcome parameters.

2. Materials and Methods

2.1. Study Design and Cohort

We conducted a retrospective analysis of all patients who were scheduled for a two-stage exchange arthroplasty in our institution between 2008 and 2018 due to a shoulder PJI. A total of 49 patients were identified from our prospectively collected institutional database and were included in the study. The study protocol was reviewed and approved by the institutional ethics committee (EA4/040/14).

The mean age of the patients at the time of the first stage of the two-stage exchange arthroplasty was 70 ± 11 years (range: 37–88 years) and 30 patients (61%) were female. The main reasons for primary shoulder arthroplasty were cuff arthropathy (10 patients), primary osteoarthritis (17 patients), fracture (19 patients), or posttraumatic osteoarthritis (3 patients). A total of 10 patients (20.4%) had undergone at least one previous septic revision in another hospital, 10 (20.4%) had undergone at least one aseptic revision, and 29 (59%) had developed a shoulder PJI after the initial arthroplasty. The type of arthroplasty at the time of the first stage revision surgery was hemiarthroplasty in 17 (35%), anatomic total shoulder arthroplasty in 9 (18%), and reverse shoulder arthroplasty in 23 patients (47%). The mean interval between the primary arthroplasty and implant removal surgery at our institution was 4.1 ± 3.7 years.

2.2. Data Collection

Comorbidities, history of the infected shoulder arthroplasty, the score of the Charlson comorbidity index (CCI) [9], laboratory values including serum C-reactive protein (CRP), and serum leucocyte count were recorded on admission. In addition, the following data were extracted for all patients: leucocyte count, microbiological and histopathological results of aspiration, number of revision surgeries between stages, length of interval between explantation and reimplantation, and microbiological and histopathological results of all surgeries. Furthermore, component loosening was evaluated radiologically and intraoperatively and documented in our database for every patient, as well as intraoperative findings such as cloudy fluid or gross intra-articular purulence. Patients were seen in our outpatient clinic postoperatively after 3, 6, and 12 months and after that period, annually. Clinical and radiological evaluations were performed by an orthopedic surgeon and infectious disease specialist. A standardized questionnaire evaluating the general health, joint and skin status, any additional surgical interventions, and antibiotic use was performed. Further follow-up was performed, contacting the patients by phone or during the visit in our outpatient clinic. The primary outcome measurements analyzed were treatment success in terms of infection eradication, successful reimplantation, and patient survival.

2.3. Definitions

Periprosthetic shoulder infection was diagnosed according to the last proposed definition criteria of the ICM [10]. According to these criteria, patients were classified into 4 infection subgroups: (1) definitive infection; (2) probable infection; (3) possible infection; (4) infection unlikely. Meeting one of the following criteria was diagnostic of definitive periprosthetic shoulder infection: (1) a sinus tract communicating with the prosthesis; (2) gross intra-articular pus; (3) two positive cultures with phenotypically identical virulent organisms. In the lack of these defining signs, weighted minor criteria (Table 1) are summed and used to distinguish between probable, possible, and unlikely infection.

The three categories in these less distinct scenarios are defined as follows:
- Six or greater with identified organism: probable infection.
- Six or greater without identified organism; possible infection.
- Fewer than six.
  - single positive culture virulent organism: possible infection.
  - two positive cultures low-virulence organism: possible infection.
  - negative cultures or only single positive culture for low virulent organism: infection unlikely.

Table 1. Demographic data, clinical, and laboratory findings of the study cohort and groups with and without subsequent reimplantation.

Variable	All Patients, n = 49	Reimplantation Group, n = 35	No Reimplantation Group, n = 14	p-Value [1]
Mean age, y *	69.7 ± 11	67.1 ± 10.6	76 ± 9.7	0.009
Gender ♦				
Male	19 (39)	15 (43)	4 (29)	0.5
Female	30 (61)	20 (57)	10 (71)	
CRP at admission (mg/L) *	21.1 ± 32.4	19 ± 36.2	26.8 ± 20	0.46
CCI *	4.1 ± 2.8	3.3 ± 2.1	6.2 ± 3.4	<0.001
Mortality after first stage ♦				
Ninety days	5 (10)	0 (0)	5 (36)	0.001
Last follow-up	12 (25)	4 (11)	8 (57)	0.002
Polymicrobial shoulder PJI ♦	14 (29)	8 (23)	6 (43)	0.18
Culture-negative shoulder PJI ♦	8 (16)	7 (20)	1 (7)	0.4
Infection eradication ♦	38 (78)	30 (86)	8 (57)	0.06

[1] Statistical analysis was only undertaken between reimplantation and no reimplantation groups. * The values are given as the mean and the standard deviation. ♦ The values are given as the number with the percentage of the group in parentheses. CCI—Charlson comorbidity index.

Of the 49 infected patients, 16 met the criteria for definitive infection, 25 for probable infection, and 8 for possible infection. Cutibacterium acnes was the most common infecting microorganism at the time of resection arthroplasty in 18/49 patients (37%), followed by coagulase-negative staphylococci (18/49, 37%), Staphylococcus aureus (8/49, 16%), and other microorganisms (9/49, 18%). In 14 of 49 cases (29%), a polymicrobial infection was evident and eight patients (16%) had no growth in the microbiology. Three of these eight patients with negative microbiology had a definitive infection due to presence of gross intraarticular pus and antibiotic treatment was started before taking samples, as patients were in sepsis. In the remaining five patients, the infection was classified as possible due to presence of minor criteria.

The definition for successfully treated shoulder PJI, in terms of infection eradication, was based on the Dephi-based international multidisciplinary consensus [11] and was further modified [12,13]. Infection was considered as eradicated if all of the following criteria were fulfilled at the latest follow-up: infection eradication, characterized by a healed wound without fistula and drainage; no recurrence of the infection; no occurrence of periprosthetic joint infection-related mortality; no subsequent surgical intervention for infection after reimplantation surgery; no long-term (>6 months) antimicrobial suppression therapy. Given that the Delphi criteria do not consider patients who do not undergo the reimplantation stage of the two-stage exchange arthroplasty, in this study successful infection eradication also included no subsequent surgical intervention for infection after explantation and no mortality related to infection in patients who did not undergo the reimplantation stage [8].

2.4. Two-Stage Exchange Arthroplasty Approach

All patients were treated according to a standardized two-stage exchange protocol. The first stage consisted of removal of all implants, as well as infected tissue, cement, and all other foreign material followed by irrigation and debridement. In most cases an antibiotic-impregnated cement spacer was inserted. Tissue cultures were incubated for 14 days. Antibiotic treatment was started intravenously (IV) after surgery or preoperatively in the case of patients presenting with sepsis after synovial aspiration. A standardized antimicrobial treatment was applied in every case based on a previously published concept under the surveillance of our infectious disease specialists [14]. A revision with irrigation, debridement, and concomitant spacer exchange was performed in case of a persistent infection (discharging wound and/or local sings of infection and/or increasing CRP without any other focus). A reimplantation was performed when the operation site was healed, with soft tissues in a good condition and ready for surgery, and the general health status of the patient was suitable for surgery. The reimplantation was used as another chance to execute another debridement of the surrounding soft tissues and bone before reimplantation of the definitive components. Intravenous antibiotic treatment was given for 2 weeks after reimplantation surgery and changed to oral regime mostly for another 4 weeks to complete a total treatment duration of 6 weeks after reimplantation.

2.5. Statistical Analysis

Chi-squared and Fisher's exact tests were used to find significant differences between categorical variables. The Kolmogorov–Smirnov test was used to test for normal distribution. The 2-sample t test (for parametric distributions) or Mann–Whitney U test (for nonparametric distributions) was used to compare continuous variables between groups. The results were given as the mean and standard deviation or as the number and percentage. For statistical analyses, IBM SPSS Statistics software (version 25.0; IBM, Armonk, NY, USA) was used. $p < 0.05$ was considered statistically significant.

3. Results

Reimplantation was completed in only 35 (71%) of 49 cases and eradication of infection was achieved in 85.7% of patients with successful reimplantation after a mean follow-up duration of 5.1 years (range: 1.1 to 10.2 years). Nine of thirty-five (26%) patients underwent one revision surgery between the resection arthroplasty and reimplantation and one of 35 patients (3%) underwent two revision surgeries, which included additional spacer exchange due to wound-related complications and bone grafting procedures because of poor glenoid bone stock. The mean interval between resection arthroplasty and reimplantation was 2.4 months (range: 0.4 to 8 months). In one case, a hemiarthroplasty; in three cases, a total shoulder arthroplasty; and in the remaining 31 cases, a reverse shoulder arthroplasty was performed at the time of reimplantation.

Of the 14 cases that did not undergo reimplantation, infection eradication was achieved in 57% of the cases (8 of 14 cases) after a mean follow-up of 5 years (range: 2.6 to 11 years). Reasons for failure to reimplant were premature death in 5 patients (36%), high general morbidity in 4 patients (29%), satisfaction with the current status in 3 patients (21%), or severe infection with poor bone and soft tissues in 2 patients (14%). Patients who did not undergo subsequent reimplantation were significantly older (76 vs. 67 years, $p = 0.009$), had a significantly higher Charlson comorbidity index (6.2 vs. 3.3, $p < 0.001$), and mortality rate (8/14 vs. 4/35, $p = 0.002$) compared to patients who achieved a successful reimplantation (Table 1). Furthermore, more polymicrobial infections were identified in patients who did not undergo reimplantation. However, this difference was statistically not significant (43% vs. 23%, p = 0.18).

A successful infection eradication was achieved in 38 patients of the entire cohort (78%) at the last follow-up. Patients with persistent infection had a significantly higher C-reactive protein on admission (49.4 vs. 14.3 mg/L, p = 0.003) and mortality (6/11 vs. 6/38, p = 0.02), compared to patients with successful eradication of infection (Table 2).

Table 2. Demographic data, clinical, and laboratory findings of the groups with infection eradication and infection persistence.

Variable	Infection Eradication n = 38	Infection Persistence n = 11	p-Value
Mean age, y *	69.1 ± 10.7	71 ± 12.4	0.5
CRP at admission (mg/L) *	14.3 ± 17	49.4 ± 60	0.003
CCI *	4 ± 2.8	4.8 ± 3	0.37
Mortality after first stage ♦			
Ninety days	0 (0)	5 (46)	<0.001
Last follow-up	6 (16)	6 (54)	0.02
Infection subgroups			
Definitive	11 (29)	5 (46)	0.47
Probable	22 (58)	3 (27)	0.1
Possible	5 (13)	3 (27)	0.4
Polymicrobial shoulder PJI ♦	11 (29)	3 (27)	1.0
Culture-negative shoulder PJI ♦	5 (13)	3 (27)	0.4

* The values are given as the mean and the standard deviation. ♦ The values are given as the number with the percentage of the group in parentheses. CCI: Charlson comorbidity index.

The overall mortality rate of the entire cohort was 25% (12 of 49 cases) at the latest follow-up, 10% (five cases) within ninety days after resection arthroplasty. Patients who deceased during the follow-up were significantly older (77 vs. 67.3 years, p = 0.005) and had a significantly higher Charlson comorbidity index (7.3 vs. 3.1, p < 0.001) (Table 3).

Table 3. Demographic data, clinical, and laboratory findings of the alive and deceased patients.

Variable	Patients Alive n = 37	Patients Deceased, n = 12	p-Value
Mean age, yr *	67.3 ± 10.6	77 ± 9	0.005
CRP at admission (mg/L) *	17 ± 20.2	34.2 ± 55.6	0.12
CCI *	3.1 ± 1.9	7.3 ± 2.8	<0.001
Polymicrobial shoulder PJI ♦	12 (29)	2 (27)	0.5
Culture-negative shoulder PJI ♦	6 (13)	2 (27)	1.0

* The values are given as the mean and the standard deviation. ♦ The values are given as the number with the percentage of the group in parentheses. CCI: Charlson comorbidity index.

4. Discussion

Despite the abundance of available literature focusing on two-stage exchange arthroplasty in patients with shoulder PJI, there is a widespread heterogeneity among most studies. The most important fact is the different definition criteria of the shoulder PJI diagnosis, as well as of its treatment success, leading to a lack of comparability. With the expected increase of performed shoulder arthroplasties over the next years, a consensus diagnostic definition and a consensus definition of treatment success for shoulder PJI are getting increasingly relevant and important not only to create a more comparable scientific reporting, but also to diagnose, counsel, and treat patients in a standardized matter.

There is considerable variation in reimplantation rates among studies in literature, ranging from 37% to 97% [7,15–21]. Only a few studies have dealt with these patients and tried to report on their clinical outcomes and causes for their attrition [7,18,22]. The current study aimed at evaluating all patients who underwent an attempted two-stage exchange arthroplasty for shoulder PJI, irrespective of the subsequent clinical course, and demonstrated that almost one-third of all patients who underwent the first stage of the procedure, did not complete a subsequent reimplantation. Despite having an acceptable infection eradication rate in patients with a permanent spacer, the clinical outcome scores are poor and progressive bone loss can occur with the extended retention of the spacer [18,22]. The current accepted goal of a two-stage exchange arthroplasty protocol is still the reimplantation of a new prosthesis to ensure best functional outcome for patients and every effort should be made to improve shoulder function by providing the opportunity for reimplantation.

A variety of reasons can lead to failure to reimplant, including mortality, medical comorbidities, uncontrollable infection leading to amputation of the limb or lifetime antibiotic suppression, and unwillingness of patients to undergo a second surgery, as well as patient's satisfaction with the current status. Similar to the hip and knee literature [23,24], premature mortality and high general morbidity were the most common causes for not being able to proceed with the intended reimplantation in this study. CCI and older age seemed to be risk factors for failure to reimplant, as the patients in the group without reimplantation had significantly higher CCI and were significantly older compared to patients with reimplantation. Patients with a higher CCI mostly have poorer health as well as a compromised immune status, which can be due to scar tissue and vascular damage. This local and systemic immune failure can massively decrease the minimal infecting dose of bacteria, predisposing to problems with infection eradication [25].

Furthermore, several studies in hip and knee literature were able to show an association of the microorganism type and likelihood of inability to achieve a reimplantation. To our knowledge, there are no existing studies investigating this association in patients with shoulder PJI. Barton et al. found that patients with a polymicrobial infection had a nearly 8-fold greater likelihood of inability to undergo reimplantation compared to patients with monomicrobial or culture-negative infections [23]. Although it did not achieve statistical significance, we were able to identify more polymicrobial infections in patients who did not undergo reimplantation, compared to patients with a successful reimplantation.

The treatment success rate in terms of infection eradication was as high as 86% among patients with reimplantation. This is comparable to the almost 90% infection control rate reported in a recent systematic review and meta-analysis of 30 studies reporting on two-stage exchange arthroplasty in patients with shoulder PJI [6]. However, when taking the patients without reimplantation into consideration, the overall infection eradication rate dropped to 78%, which is lower than most of the studies in the literature dealing with two-stage exchange arthroplasty. The majority of these studies do not encompass patients who do not complete the second stage of an attempted two-stage exchange arthroplasty and exclude them from their treatment success analysis, thereby leading to a possibly overestimated success of this surgical procedure. In addition, the considerably high inflammatory response in many patients of the study cohort may be a further factor affecting our infection eradication rate, as patients with persistent infection had a significantly higher C-reactive protein on admission compared to patients with successful eradication of infection. High virulent microorganisms mostly induce an acute response and much inflammation with the release of cytokines and elevation of CRP, leading to a potentially worse postoperative clinical course [26,27].

Although mortality and morbidity associated with two-stage exchange arthroplasty for hip and knee periprosthetic joint infection has been one of the main research topics [8,23,24], there is a lack of knowledge in shoulder PJI literature. Cancienne et al. recently showed a mortality rate of 2.2% within the first postoperative year in patients undergoing removal of an infected shoulder prosthesis [7]. This is significantly less than the mortality rate reported in the current study, which was 10% within ninety days after resection arthroplasty and 25% at the latest follow-up, which is similar to what has been reported previously in hip and knee literature [23,24,28]. The mortality in five patients, who deceased in the first 90 days after resection arthroplasty, was related to the infection, whereas the other patients died due to other health issues. This indicated that shoulder PJI and its treatment is associated with a high risk of mortality, especially in patients with older age and higher CCI, as shown in our study. In these patients, it may be reasonable to have a detailed discussion with the patient about their likelihood of treatment success, as well as postoperative mortality and consider alternative treatment options, such as long-term antibiotic suppression. Thus, an optimal treatment algorithm should be based on patient-specific general health status, risk factors, and patient expectations.

Only looking from the perspective of infection eradication would lead to overlook a great subset of patients who are too fragile to endure further surgery for reimplantation, decease prematurely, or refuse further surgery because of low functional demand after implant removal. We therefore suggest that the success of two-stage exchange arthroplasty should be accounted from the point of the first stage, rather than following reimplantation, to consider the failures occurring between the stages and better represent the clinical course of two-stage exchange arthroplasty in patients with shoulder PJI [8].

This study has some limitations. Although the patients' data were longitudinally collected in our database, the retrospective nature of the study may lead to bias. Despite being the largest cohort in literature dealing with this topic, the study may be underpowered, preventing the significant differences between analyzed groups. Furthermore, we did not include any assessment of functional outcomes, which may be seen as a potential weakness. However, the most compelling outcome measures of the current study were the infection eradication, reimplantation, and mortality rates. In addition, there is already an abundance of available literature focusing on the functional outcome of patients after two-stage exchange arthroplasty or antibiotic cement spacer retention. The complexity of our study cohort, due to multiple previous revision surgeries, can furthermore alter our results, making our results to be generalized and difficult to compre with other studies. Finally, infection-related mortality was difficult to confirm in patients who died outside of the hospital and the precise cause of death in these cases could not be determined, which can alter our treatment success rate.

5. Conclusions

While the two-stage exchange arthroplasty can lead to high rates of infection eradication, a third of patients never undergo the second stage of the procedure due to a variety of reasons, including premature mortality, high general morbidity, and low functional demand. Furthermore, shoulder PJI and its treatment is associated with a high risk of mortality, especially in patients with older age and higher CCI. This information needs to be accounted for when counseling frail and elderly patients on the chances and risks before undergoing two-stage exchange arthroplasty for shoulder PJI.

Author Contributions: Conceptualization, D.A. and M.W.; methodology, D.A. and N.M.; formal analysis, A.P. and D.K.; data curation, D.A.; writing—original draft preparation, D.A. and M.W.; writing—review and editing, A.P., M.S. and P.M.; supervision, P.M. and M.S. All authors have read and agreed to the published version of the manuscript.

Funding: This research received no external funding.

Institutional Review Board Statement: The study was conducted according to the guidelines of the Declaration of Helsinki and approved by the Institutional Review Board (or Ethics Committee) of Charite Universitätsmedizin ((EA4/040/14, 12 September 2018).

Informed Consent Statement: Informed consent was obtained from all subjects involved in the study.

Data Availability Statement: Data available on request due to restrictions, e.g., privacy or ethical.

Conflicts of Interest: The authors declare no conflict of interest.

References

1. Cooper:, M.E.; Trivedi, N.N.; Sivasundaram, L.; Karns, M.R.; Voos, J.E.; Gillespie, R.J. Diagnosis and Management of Periprosthetic Joint Infection After Shoulder Arthroplasty. *JBJS Rev.* **2019**, *7*, e3. [CrossRef] [PubMed]
2. Dodson, C.C.; Craig, E.V.; Cordasco, F.A.; Dines, D.M.; Dines, J.S.; DiCarlo, E.; Brause, B.D.; Warren, R.F. Propionibacterium acnes infection after shoulder arthroplasty: A diagnostic challenge. *J. Shoulder Elb. Surg.* **2010**, *19*, 303–307. [CrossRef] [PubMed]
3. Akgun, D.; Maziak, N.; Plachel, F.; Siegert, P.; Minkus, M.; Thiele, K.; Moroder, P. The role of implant sonication in the diagnosis of periprosthetic shoulder infection. *J. Shoulder Elb. Surg.* **2020**, *29*, e222–e228. [CrossRef] [PubMed]
4. Garrigues, G.E.; Zmistowski, B.; Cooper, A.M.; Green, A.; Group, I.C.M.S. Proceedings from the 2018 International Consensus Meeting on Orthopedic Infections: Management of periprosthetic shoulder infection. *J. Shoulder Elb. Surg.* **2019**, *28*, S67–S99. [CrossRef] [PubMed]
5. George, D.A.; Volpin, A.; Scarponi, S.; Haddad, F.S.; Romano, C.L. Does exchange arthroplasty of an infected shoulder prosthesis provide better eradication rate and better functional outcome, compared to a permanent spacer or resection arthroplasty? A systematic review. *BMC Musculoskelet. Disord.* **2016**, *17*, 52. [CrossRef]
6. Belay, E.S.; Danilkowicz, R.; Bullock, G.; Wall, K.; Garrigues, G.E. Single-stage versus two-stage revision for shoulder periprosthetic joint infection: A systematic review and meta-analysis. *J. Shoulder Elb. Surg.* **2020**, *29*, 2476–2486. [CrossRef] [PubMed]
7. Cancienne, J.M.; Brockmeier, S.F.; Carr, J.C., 2nd; Werner, B.C. Implant Removal and Spacer Placement for Infected Shoulder Arthroplasty: Risk Factors for Repeat Procedures, Spacer Retention, and Mortality. *HSS J.* **2018**, *14*, 228–232. [CrossRef]
8. Gomez, M.M.; Tan, T.L.; Manrique, J.; Deirmengian, G.K.; Parvizi, J. The Fate of Spacers in the Treatment of Periprosthetic Joint Infection. *J. Bone Joint Surg. Am.* **2015**, *97*, 1495–1502. [CrossRef]
9. Charlson, M.E.; Pompei, P.; Ales, K.L.; MacKenzie, C.R. A new method of classifying prognostic comorbidity in longitudinal studies: Development and validation. *J. Chronic Dis.* **1987**, *40*, 373–383. [CrossRef]
10. Garrigues, G.E.; Zmistowski, B.; Cooper, A.M.; Green, A.; Group, I.C.M.S. Proceedings from the 2018 International Consensus Meeting on Orthopedic Infections: The definition of periprosthetic shoulder infection. *J. Shoulder Elb. Surg.* **2019**, *28*, S8–S12. [CrossRef] [PubMed]
11. Diaz-Ledezma, C.; Higuera, C.A.; Parvizi, J. Success after treatment of periprosthetic joint infection: A Delphi-based international multidisciplinary consensus. *Clin. Orthop. Relat. Res.* **2013**, *471*, 2374–2382. [CrossRef] [PubMed]
12. Akgun, D.; Perka, C.; Trampuz, A.; Renz, N. Outcome of hip and knee periprosthetic joint infections caused by pathogens resistant to biofilm-active antibiotics: Results from a prospective cohort study. *Arch. Orthop. Trauma Surg.* **2018**, *138*, 635–642. [CrossRef]
13. Akgun, D.; Muller, M.; Perka, C.; Winkler, T. High cure rate of periprosthetic hip joint infection with multidisciplinary team approach using standardized two-stage exchange. *J. Orthop. Surg. Res.* **2019**, *14*, 78. [CrossRef] [PubMed]
14. Zimmerli, W.; Trampuz, A.; Ochsner, P.E. Prosthetic-joint infections. *N. Engl. J. Med.* **2004**, *351*, 1645–1654. [CrossRef] [PubMed]
15. Grubhofer, F.; Imam, M.A.; Wieser, K.; Achermann, Y.; Meyer, D.C.; Gerber, C. Staged Revision With Antibiotic Spacers for Shoulder Prosthetic Joint Infections Yields High Infection Control. *Clin. Orthop. Relat. Res.* **2018**, *476*, 146–152. [CrossRef]
16. Assenmacher, A.T.; Alentorn-Geli, E.; Dennison, T.; Baghdadi, Y.M.K.; Cofield, R.H.; Sanchez-Sotelo, J.; Sperling, J.W. Two-stage reimplantation for the treatment of deep infection after shoulder arthroplasty. *J. Shoulder Elb. Surg.* **2017**, *26*, 1978–1983. [CrossRef] [PubMed]
17. Buchalter, D.B.; Mahure, S.A.; Mollon, B.; Yu, S.; Kwon, Y.W.; Zuckerman, J.D. Two-stage revision for infected shoulder arthroplasty. *J. Shoulder Elb. Surg.* **2017**, *26*, 939–947. [CrossRef]
18. Pellegrini, A.; Legnani, C.; Macchi, V.; Meani, E. Two-stage revision shoulder prosthesis vs. permanent articulating antibiotic spacer in the treatment of periprosthetic shoulder infections. *Orthop. Traumatol. Surg. Res.* **2019**, *105*, 237–240. [CrossRef] [PubMed]
19. Brown, M.; Eseonu, K.; Rudge, W.; Warren, S.; Majed, A.; Bayley, I.; Higgs, D.; Falworth, M. The management of infected shoulder arthroplasty by two-stage revision. *Shoulder Elb.* **2020**, *12*, 70–80. [CrossRef]
20. Patrick, M.; Vincent, H.K.; Farmer, K.W.; King, J.J.; Struk, A.M.; Wright, T.W. Management of infected shoulder arthroplasty: A comparison of treatment strategies. *J. Shoulder Elb. Surg.* **2019**, *28*, 1658–1665. [CrossRef]
21. Klingebiel, S.; Theil, C.; Gosheger, G.; Schneider, K.N.; Ackmann, T.; Timme, M.; Schorn, D.; Liem, D.; Rickert, C. Clinical Outcome of Two-Stage Revision after Periprosthetic Shoulder Infection. *J. Clin. Med.* **2021**, *10*, 218. [CrossRef] [PubMed]
22. Cronin, K.J.; Hayes, C.B.; Sajadi, K.R. Antibiotic cement spacer retention for chronic shoulder infection after minimum 2-year follow-up. *J. Shoulder Elb. Surg.* **2020**, *29*, e325–e329. [CrossRef] [PubMed]
23. Barton, C.B.; Wang, D.L.; An, Q.; Brown, T.S.; Callaghan, J.J.; Otero, J.E. Two-Stage Exchange Arthroplasty for Periprosthetic Joint Infection Following Total Hip or Knee Arthroplasty Is Associated With High Attrition Rate and Mortality. *J. Arthroplasty* **2019**, *35*, 1384–1389. [CrossRef]
24. Wang, Q.; Goswami, K.; Kuo, F.C.; Xu, C.; Tan, T.L.; Parvizi, J. Two-Stage Exchange Arthroplasty for Periprosthetic Joint Infection: The Rate and Reason for the Attrition After the First Stage. *J. Arthroplasty* **2019**, *34*, 2749–2756. [CrossRef]
25. Akgun, D.; Muller, M.; Perka, C.; Winkler, T. A positive bacterial culture during re-implantation is associated with a poor outcome in two-stage exchange arthroplasty for deep infection. *Bone Joint J.* **2017**, *99*, 1490–1495. [CrossRef] [PubMed]
26. Akgun, D.; Wietholter, M.; Siegert, P.; Danzinger, V.; Minkus, M.; Braun, K.F.; Moroder, P. The role of serum C-reactive protein in the diagnosis of periprosthetic shoulder infection. *Arch. Orthop. Trauma Surg.* **2021**, *141*, 1–7. [CrossRef]

27. Hoiby, N.; Ciofu, O.; Johansen, H.K.; Song, Z.J.; Moser, C.; Jensen, P.O.; Molin, S.; Givskov, M.; Tolker-Nielsen, T.; Bjarnsholt, T. The clinical impact of bacterial biofilms. *Int. J. Oral Sci.* **2011**, *3*, 55–65. [CrossRef] [PubMed]
28. Petis, S.M.; Perry, K.I.; Mabry, T.M.; Hanssen, A.D.; Berry, D.J.; Abdel, M.P. Two-Stage Exchange Protocol for Periprosthetic Joint Infection Following Total Knee Arthroplasty in 245 Knees without Prior Treatment for Infection. *J. Bone Joint Surg. Am.* **2019**, *101*, 239–249. [CrossRef]

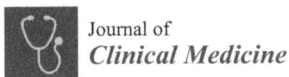

Article

Measuring Patient Value after Total Shoulder Arthroplasty

Alexandre Lädermann [1,2,3], Rodolphe Eurin [4], Axelle Alibert [4], Mehdi Bensouda [4] and Hugo Bothorel [5,*]

1. Division of Orthopaedics and Trauma Surgery, La Tour Hospital, 1217 Meyrin, Switzerland; alexandre.laedermann@gmail.com
2. Faculty of Medicine, University of Geneva, 1211 Geneva, Switzerland
3. Division of Orthopaedics and Trauma Surgery, Department of Surgery, Geneva University Hospitals, 1205 Geneva, Switzerland
4. General Management Department, La Tour Hospital, 1217 Meyrin, Switzerland; rodolphe.eurin@latour.ch (R.E.); axelle.alibert@latour.ch (A.A.); mehdi.bensouda@latour.ch (M.B.)
5. Research Department, La Tour Hospital, 1217 Meyrin, Switzerland
* Correspondence: hugo.bothorel@latour.ch; Tel.: +41-22-719-78-33

Abstract: Evaluating the value of health care is of paramount importance to keep improving patients' quality of life and optimizing associated costs. Our objective was to present a calculation method based on Michael Porter's formula and standard references to estimate patient value delivered by total shoulder arthroplasty (TSA). We retrospectively reviewed the records of 116 consecutive TSAs performed between June 2015 and June 2019. Patient value was defined as quality of care divided by direct costs of surgery. Quality metrics included intra- and postoperative complications as well as weighted improvements in three different patient-reported outcome measures at a minimum of one-year follow-up. Direct costs of surgery were retrieved from the management accounting analyses. Substantial clinical benefit (SCB) thresholds and the standard reimbursement system were used as references for quality and cost dimensions. A multivariable linear regression was performed to identify factors associated with patient delivered value. Compared to a reference of 1.0, the quality of care delivered to patients was 1.3 ± 0.3 (range, 0.6–2.0) and the associated direct cost was 1.0 ± 0.2 (range, 0.7–1.6). Ninety patients (78%) had a quality of care ≥ 1.0 and 61 patients (53%) had direct costs related to surgery ≤ 1.0. The average value delivered to patients was 1.3 ± 0.4 (range, 0.5–2.5) with 91 patients (78%) ≥ 1.0, was higher for non-smokers (beta, 0.12; $p = 0.044$), anatomic TSA (beta, 0.53; $p < 0.001$), increased with higher pre-operative pain (beta, 0.08; $p < 0.001$) and lower pre-operative Constant score (beta, -0.06; $p = 0.001$). Our results revealed that almost 80% of TSAs provided substantial patient value. Patient pre-operative pain/function, tobacco use, and procedure type are important factors associated with delivered patient value.

Keywords: total shoulder arthroplasty; patient reported outcome measures; PROMs; VBHC; value-based health care; patient value; quality; costs

Citation: Lädermann, A.; Eurin, R.; Alibert, A.; Bensouda, M.; Bothorel, H. Measuring Patient Value after Total Shoulder Arthroplasty. *J. Clin. Med.* **2021**, *10*, 5700. https://doi.org/10.3390/jcm10235700

Academic Editor: Johannes C. Reichert

Received: 18 October 2021
Accepted: 1 December 2021
Published: 4 December 2021

Publisher's Note: MDPI stays neutral with regard to jurisdictional claims in published maps and institutional affiliations.

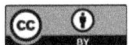

Copyright: © 2021 by the authors. Licensee MDPI, Basel, Switzerland. This article is an open access article distributed under the terms and conditions of the Creative Commons Attribution (CC BY) license (https://creativecommons.org/licenses/by/4.0/).

1. Introduction

In the past decades, healthcare challenges have considerably increased due to the global aging of the population and higher treatment costs following advances in medical technologies and medicinal products. In such a context, healthcare actors first focused their interests on reducing costs while giving fewer priorities to patient care quality and efficiency. Therefore, a new disruptive concept emerged to move the current system toward a sustainable and patient-centered model that optimizes both health outcomes and associated costs: the value-based health care (VBHC).

In their work published in 2006, Michael Porter and Elizabeth Teisberg defined value as health outcomes achieved per dollar spent [1]. While this value equation is becoming increasingly prominent, it remains nonetheless difficult to implement in every day clinical practice in absence of a validated method to quantify value and a standard scale for interpretation and benchmarking purposes. In their published article, Reilly et al. [2]

proposed an innovative method that allows a surgeon to evaluate the value delivered to his patients after total knee or hip arthroplasties according to the average department results. While we applaud them for this work, the applied methodology relies on the presence of several surgeons for establishing the reference. Moreover, the condition mentioned above can be misleading since it can lead to "false positive" or "false negative" results for a particular surgeon if the entire orthopedic department has low or high outcomes.

With the increasing use of patient-reported outcome measures (PROMs), different thresholds have been published to help understand the amount of PROMs improvement that is clinically relevant to patients [3]. Moreover, the standard direct cost for a specific surgical procedure can be estimated from the national hospital reimbursement system based on diagnosis-related groups (DRG). Therefore, the purpose of the present study was to propose a new calculation method to evaluate the delivered patient value using standard references, thereby shifting the value-based competition from a local orthopedic department to a broader level.

2. Materials and Methods

2.1. Study Design

The authors retrospectively reviewed the records of consecutive prospectively collected primary TSAs performed at La Tour hospital (Meyrin, Switzerland). The study was conducted according to the Declaration of Helsinki principles, was approved prior to beginning by the Commission cantonale d'éthique de la recherche (CCER) de Genève (Shoulder Outcomes Clinical Study, n° 2014-277), and all patients provided written informed consent for the use of their data for research purposes.

2.2. Patient Selection, Demographic and Operative Data

Between June 2015 and June 2019, 284 patients had a primary shoulder arthroplasty performed by the senior author (A.L.). Patients were included in the study if they were operated on at La Tour hospital and underwent a TSA ($n = 139$). Patients were excluded if they did not have a complete pre-operative evaluation due to the need for emergency care ($n = 13$), if they deceased due to other reasons than surgery before the 1-year follow-up visit ($n = 5$), and if they were lost to follow-up (LTFU, $n = 6$). This left a study cohort of 116 patients aged 77.8 ± 7.6 years (median, 78.0; range, 57–94) at index surgery, comprising 86 women (74%) and 30 men (26%), available for analyses (Table 1, Figure 1). The principal diagnoses were rotator cuff tear arthropathy ($n = 62$, 53%), primary glenohumeral osteoarthrosis ($n = 39$, 34%), secondary glenohumeral osteoarthrosis ($n = 7$, 6%), acute trauma ($n = 4$, 3%), osteonecrosis ($n = 1$, 1%), and others in 3 cases (3%). The type of procedure was anatomic TSA for 24 patients (aTSA, 21%) and reverse TSA for the other 92 patients (rTSA, 79%). The operations were performed by a single senior surgeon (A.L.). A majority of the patients were operated on the dominant arm ($n = 77$, 66%) through a deltopectoral approach ($n = 62$, 53%) or subscapularis and deltoid sparing approach ($n = 47$, 41%) [4,5]. A patient specific guide was used in 13 cases (11%) to help the prothesis implantation and cementation was required in 23 cases on the glenoid side (20%, for aTSA only) and in 7 cases on the humeral side (6%). The patient management time in the operating room (OR) was 121 ± 26 min (median, 125; range, 60–210 min) and patient length of stay was 3.6 ± 2.0 days (median, 3.0; range, 1.2–12.9 days).

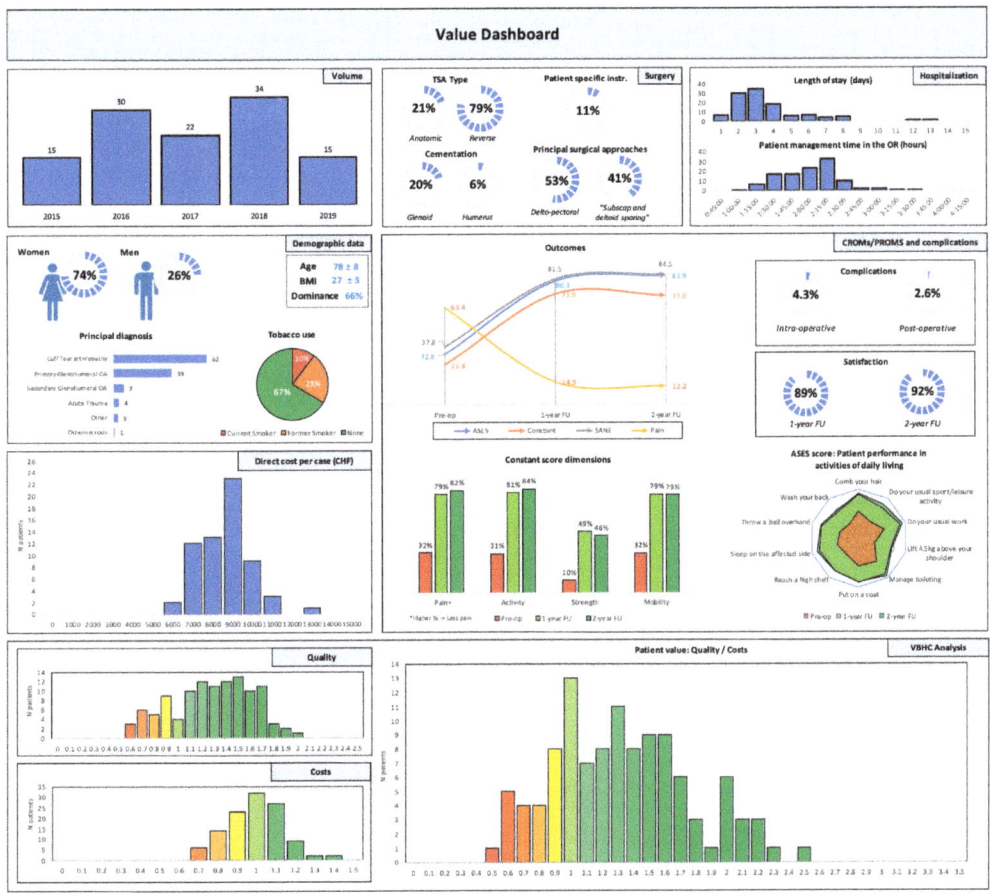

Figure 1. Value dashboard.

Table 1. Pre- and intra-operative data.

	Final Cohort (*n* = 116 Patients)			
	n	(%)		
	Mean	±SD	Median	(Range)
Preoperative data				
Age	77.8	±7.6	78.0	(57.0–94.0)
Body mass index	27.4	±4.8	26.7	(17.6–42.8)
Male gender	30	(25.9%)		
Principal diagnosis				
Rotator cuff tear arthropathy	62	(53.4%)		
Primary glenohumeral osteoarthrosis	39	(33.6%)		
Secondary glenohumeral osteoarthrosis	7	(6.0%)		
Acute trauma	4	(3.4%)		

Table 1. Cont.

	Final Cohort (n = 116 Patients)			
	n	(%)		
	Mean	±SD	Median	(Range)
Osteonecrosis	1	(0.9%)		
Others	3	(2.6%)		
Dominant arm affected	77	(66.4%)		
Intraoperative data				
Surgical procedure				
Anatomic Total Shoulder Arthroplasty (aTSA)	24	(20.7%)		
Reverse Total Shoulder Arthroplasty (rTSA)	92	(79.3%)		
Surgical approach				
Deltopectoral	62	(53.4%)		
Subscapularis and deltoid sparing	47	(40.5%)		
Anterior Deltoid Detachment with Lateral Split	3	(2.6%)		
Subscapularis sparing	3	(2.6%)		
Transdeltoid	1	(0.9%)		
Use of patient specific instrumentation				
Software (planification)	116	(100.0%)		
Hardware (guide)	13	(11.2%)		
Cementation				
Humeral side	7	(6.0%)		
Glenoid side	23	(19.8%)		

2.3. Study Variables

The outcome of interest was the delivered patient value. The data analyzed in this study comprised the characteristics of the patient (age, gender, BMI, arm dominance, principal diagnosis), surgery (anatomic/reverse TSA, approach, cementation, patient management time in the operating room, intraoperative complications), hospitalization (length of stay, direct cost), complications, patient satisfaction, and PROMs.

2.4. Clinical Evaluation

Patients were evaluated at a minimum follow-up of one year (59 at 1 year and 57 at 2 years). The clinical outcomes included periprosthetic joint infection (PJI), implant revision, and other intra- or postoperative complications. The PROMs included the American Shoulder and Elbow Surgeons (ASES) score [6], the Constant score [7], the Single Assessment Numeric Evaluation (SANE) score [8,9], and the pain on a visual analogue scale (VAS). The ASES score (from 0 worst to 100 best) comprises one pain item and 10 questions relative to patient function/disability. The Constant score (from 0 worst to 100 best) has four different dimensions, including pain, activity, strength, and mobility. The SANE score (from 0 worst to 100 best) was assessed with a single question: "How would you rate your affected shoulder today as a percentage of normal (0% to 100% scale with 100% being normal)" and the pain on VAS (from 0 best to 10 worst) was rescaled to a range of 0–100 points. The reference used for each PROM improvement was the substantial clinical benefit calculated by Simovitch et al. in a combined cohort of 1856 reverse and anatomic TSA (31.5 points for the ASES score, 19.1 points for the Constant score, 32 points for pain on VAS) [3]. Although being a useful metric, we did not include the SANE score improvement in the quality evaluation since its SCB has not been robustly validated in the scientific literature yet [10]. Furthermore, the SANE score has been reported to be moderately/strongly correlated with the ASES score [11]. The authors also used the minimal clinically important differences (MCID) for the aforementioned scores for descriptive analyses (13.6 points for the ASES score, 5.7 points for the Constant score, 16 points for pain on VAS) [3].

2.5. Equation for Patient Value

The equation used for the calculation of patient value was based on the one previously published by Reilly et al. [2]:

$$\text{Patient value} = \frac{\text{Quality}}{\text{Cost}} = \frac{(\text{Weighted clinical outcomes} + \text{Weighted PROMs improvement})}{\text{Direct cost}}$$

The value equation can therefore be written as follows:

$$Value = \frac{W_1\left(\frac{\Delta P_{ASES}}{SCB_{ASES}}\right) + W_2\left(\frac{\Delta P_{Constant}}{SCB_{Constant}}\right) + W_3\left(\frac{\Delta P_{VAS\ Pain}}{SCB_{VAS\ Pain}}\right) + W_4\left(P_{Intra-op\ Comp}\right) + W_5\left(P_{Post-op\ Comp}\right) + W_6\left(P_{P\ JI}\right) + W_7\left(P_{revision}\right)}{\left(\frac{P_{direct\ cost}}{DRG_{direct\ cost}}\right)}$$

As detailed in the article of Reilly et al. [2], all negative pre- to postoperative improvements were forced to 0, and clinical outcomes were coded as binary depending on the event occurrence. The absence of event resulted in a patient score equaling 0 for that outcome, while the presence of it resulted in a patient score equaling the total weight. The weighting for the clinical outcomes and PROMs was performed by the senior surgeon (AL) according to his strong clinical experience and scientific knowledge. For clarity, a quality of 1.0 indicated an improvement in PROMs which was equal to the defined SCBs and an absence of any complication, PJI or revision. A cost of 1.0 indicated a TSA that cost the exact direct cost reference (see below). The result of the equation (quality/cost) was rounded at the first decimal place and indicated a substantial delivered value if ≥ 1.0 or an unsubstantial delivered value if < 1.0.

2.6. Costs

The cost was defined as the direct cost related to the surgical procedure (material and medicine costs only). This data was exported from the management accounting REKOLE® analyses that are performed annually at our institution. The standard reimbursement for a TSA was calculated by multiplying the hospital base rate (9550 CHF) by the DRG standard cost-weight, which varied between 1.929 and 2.096 from 2015 to 2019. The standard TSA reimbursement for a patient with basic insurance only was therefore 19,081 CHF in 2015, 20,017 CHF in 2016, 18,651 in 2017, 18,422 CHF in 2018, and 18,479 CHF in 2019. In our consecutive series of patients with basic insurance only ($n = 47$, 38%), the direct cost per case represented 44% of the total cost (44% ± 7%; median, 44%; range, 32–60%). Thus, we considered that 44% of the standard TSA reimbursement should be used as the direct cost reference, which gives: 8396 CHF in 2015, 8807 CHF in 2016, 8206 in 2017, 8106 CHF in 2018, and 8131 CHF in 2019.

2.7. Statistical Analyses

For baseline characteristics, variables were reported as mean ± standard deviation or proportions. Shapiro–Wilk tests were used to assess the normality of distributions. Differences between preoperative and postoperative continuous values were evaluated using either the paired Student's t-test (if Gaussian distribution) or the Wilcoxon signed-rank test (if non-Gaussian distribution). The correlation between the quality and cost was analyzed using the Pearson's coefficient. A multivariable linear regression model was performed to identify which pre-operative factors (Constant and ASES scores, VAS pain, primary diagnosis), patient characteristics (age, gender, BMI, arm dominance, and tobacco use), and intra-operative factors (patient management time in the operating room, surgical procedure, surgical approach, cementation and use of patient specific instrumentation) were independently associated with patient delivered value.

The variables included in the multivariable regression model were identified using the backward selection method with a threshold of significance set at a p value < 0.05 (pre-operative Constant score, pre-operative VAS pain, tobacco use, and surgical procedure). Statistical analyses were performed using R version 3.6.2 (R Foundation for Statistical Computing, Vienna, Austria), and p-values < 0.05 were considered statistically significant.

3. Results

3.1. Clinical Outcomes

The weighting for the clinical outcomes were as follows: 0.1 for the ASES and Constant scores, 0.2 for the VAS pain, 0.1 for an intra- or postoperative complication, and 0.2 for a PJI or an implant revision.

From the final cohort of 116 patients, 5 (4.3%) had an intra-operative complication and 17 (15%) experienced a postoperative complication (Table 2). Three patients (3.4%) underwent an implant revision within the 2 postoperative years due to a component dislocation (revised at 2 months), an implant dissociation (revised at 2 months), and a humeral implant loosening ($n = 1$ revised at 6 months). It is worth noting that none of our patients had a PJI, and that patient satisfaction was 89% at 1-year follow-up and 92% at 2-year follow-up.

Table 2. Intra and post-operative complications.

	Final Cohort (n = 116 Patients)	
	n	(%)
Intraoperative complications	5	(4.3%)
Unplanned humeral fractures	5	(4.3%)
Postoperative complications	17	(14.7%)
Acromial fracture	7	(6.0%)
Component loosening	2	(1.7%)
Deltoid Muscle Dysfunction	2	(1.7%)
Instability-Dislocation	2	(1.7%)
Component dissociation	1	(0.9%)
Instability-Subluxation	1	(0.9%)
Rotator Cuff Tear	1	(0.9%)
Nerve Palsy (other than axillary)	1	(0.9%)
Implant revisions	3	(2.6%)

At their last follow-up (1.5 ± 0.5 years), our patients significantly improved their VAS pain (49 ± 29 points) as well as SANE (45.1 ± 25.6 points), Constant (45.2 ± 20.2 points), and ASES scores (48.2 ± 23.8) (Table 3). The MCID threshold for the Constant score, ASES score, and VAS pain was achieved by 97%, 89%, and 83% of the patients, while the SCB threshold for similar scores was, respectively, reached by 88%, 77%, and 68% of the cases.

Table 3. Pre- and post-operative outcomes.

	Preoperative Status				Postoperative Status (Last Follow-Up)				Absolute Improvement			
	Mean	±SD	Median	(Range)	Mean	±SD	Median	(Range)	Mean	±SD	Median	(Range)
SANE score	37.6	±22.2	30.0	(0.0–90.0)	82.4	±16.9	90.0	(20.0–100.0)	45.1	±25.6	45.0	(0.0–100.0)
Constant score	25.7	±15.0	24.0	(0.0–62.4)	70.8	±16.4	74.2	(24.0–99.2)	45.2	±20.2	47.1	(0.0–83.0)
Strength	2.4	±4.3	0.0	(0.0–17.6)	11.5	±6.2	11.0	(0.0–25.0)	9.7	±6.4	9.9	(0.0–25.0)
Mobility	12.8	±10.7	10.0	(0.0–40.0)	31.5	±7.3	32.0	(8.0–40.0)	18.6	±11.6	19.5	(0.0–40.0)
Pain	4.8	±3.2	4.0	(0.0–15.0)	12.0	±3.8	14.0	(0.0–15.0)	7.3	±4.3	7.0	(0.0–15.0)
Activity	6.2	±3.5	6.0	(0.0–15.0)	16.1	±4.3	18.0	(0.0–20.0)	10.0	±5.3	10.0	(0.0–20.0)
ASES score	32.6	±16.2	32.5	(0.0–82.0)	81.1	±19.8	87.0	(13.0–100.0)	48.2	±23.8	50.0	(0.0–100.0)
Pain	18.5	±11.4	15.0	(0.0–50.0)	42.6	±10.1	45.0	(10.0–50.0)	24.5	±14.4	25.0	(0.0–50.0)
Activity	14.1	±8.6	13.0	(0.0–42.0)	38.4	±11.9	43.0	(3.0–50.0)	24.4	±12.8	26.5	(0.0–50.0)
VAS Pain *	64	±22	70	(0–100)	15	±20	10	(0–80)	49	±29	50	(0–100)

SANE, Single Assessment Numeric Evaluation; ASES, American Shoulder and Elbow Surgeons; VAS, Visual Analogue Scale; * A decrease in VAS Pain indicates a good result. A positive improvement is noted if the VAS Pain decreases. All pre- versus post-operative scores were statistically significant ($p < 0.001$).

3.2. Costs

The total cost per case was 17,954 ± 3383 CHF (median, 17,433; range, 12,757–27,517 CHF) with an average direct cost of 8311 ± 1243 CHF (median, 8442; range, 5347–12,849 CHF).

3.3. Patient Value

According to the patient value equation presented in the methods section, the quality of care delivered to patients was 1.3 ± 0.3 (median, 1.3; range, 0.6–2.0), and the associated cost was 1.0 ± 0.2 (median, 1.0; range, 0.7–1.6). Ninety patients (78%) had a quality of care ≥1.0 and 61 patients (53%) had a direct cost related to surgery ≤1.0 (Figure 2). No significant correlation was found between cost and quality ($r = -0.17$, CI = -0.34–0.02; $p = 0.076$). Considering these two dimensions, the average value delivered to patients was 1.3 ± 0.4 (median, 1.3; range, 0.5–2.5), with 91 patients (78%) equaling or exceeding 1.0 (Figure 1). Among the 55 patients with a cost >1.0, 36 (65%) had still a substantial delivered value owing to a high quality of care. Likewise, among the 26 patients with a quality of care <1.0, 5 (19%) had a substantial delivered value thanks to a lower cost than expected. The multivariable linear regression revealed that patient delivered value was significantly higher for non-smokers (beta, 0.12; 95%CI, 0.00–0.23; $p = 0.044$), patients operated with anatomic TSA (beta, 0.53; 95%CI, 0.39–0.66; $p < 0.001$), increased with higher (worse) pre-operative VAS pain (beta for 10 points of VAS pain, 0.08; 95%CI, 0.06–0.11; $p < 0.001$) but reduced with higher pre-operative Constant score (beta for 10 points of Constant score, -0.06; 95%CI, -0.03–-0.10; $p = 0.001$).

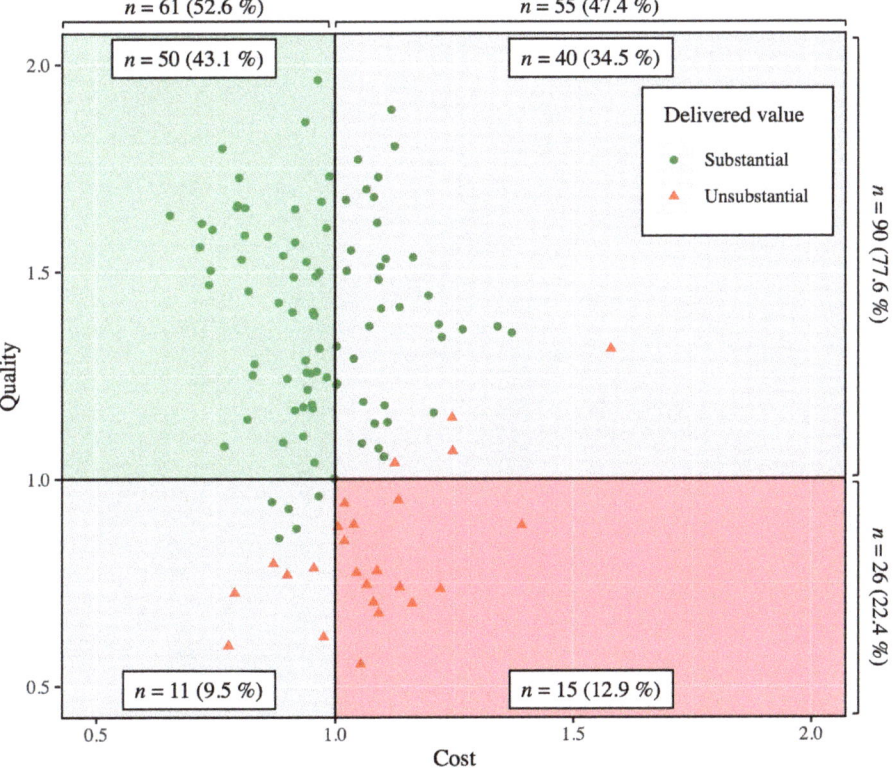

Figure 2. Scatter plot illustrating cost versus quality measures with patient delivered value.

4. Discussion

Evaluating the value of health care is of paramount importance to keep improving patients' quality of life and optimizing associated costs. Hospitals' digitalization is still ongoing and offers a great potential for patients' evaluation along their entire care path. Beyond this, the real challenge that often arises in VBHC discussions is the absence of external benchmarks which compels us to compare our results within our institution or at different time intervals. The authors of the present study therefore created a new value-based dashboard for TSA, which allows an objective comparison with standard references.

According to our results, 78% of the TSAs performed at our institution offered a substantial value to patients. It is worth noting that 41 patients (35%) had a substantial delivered value although they had either a quality of care below the expectations or an excessive direct cost (Figure 2). This emphasizes the importance of evaluating both indicators together rather than interpreting them independently from each other.

Different authors recently evaluated the value delivered by TSA at short term using different methods [12–14]. Menendez et al. [14] defined the delivered value as the postoperative ASES score divided by the hospitalization time-driven activity-based costs. More comparable to our value calculation method, Berglund et al. [13] divided the ratio of PROM improvement (in units of MCID) by the total hospitalization cost. Both aforementioned studies found that reverse TSA was associated with a decreased delivered value compared to anatomic TSA, which corroborates our findings. Although it was expected given that reverse TSA has a higher cost associated with the management of rotator cuff deficiencies, it is important to note that such an association can be reversed at some point since different studies already revealed mid- or long-term concerns on anatomic TSA (glenoid loosening, difficult revision procedures, and disappointing outcomes) [15–17]. Furthermore, the indications for these two procedures can be different and further analyses with matched cohorts are needed [18].

In our study, the delivered value was higher for shoulders with a lower preoperative function or higher pre-operative pain since greatest clinical improvements are usually observed for patients with worse preoperative health [19]. Our analyses also revealed that current or former smokers had a lower delivered value compared to non-smokers. The negative impact of tobacco use on outcomes after TSA is well reported [20–23] and emphasizes smoking cessation programs [24]. In the next decades, machine learning algorithms might be able to accurately predict postoperative patient outcomes based on their preoperative characteristics [25]. Such prognostic tools would help manage patient expectations [26] and avoid surgery for patients who would not benefit from it, thereby reducing associated risks for the patients while lowering costs for the health care system.

Different authors already worked on the creation of VBHC dashboards/scorecards [2,27]. Riley et al. published an innovative method to illustrate patient value following total hip and knee arthroplasties [2]. This method consisted of comparing the results of different surgeons within the same institution, which motivates them to outperform for the sake of their patients. However, the use of internal references such as orthopedic department averages for direct costs or PROMs can be misleading. For instance, implementing this method in small institutions where only one surgeon works in a specific medical field would be unwarranted. Furthermore, this method could reveal outstanding results for a surgeon even though the entire department has bad outcomes. In our study, we proposed to use SCB thresholds for the interpretation of PROMs improvements and to estimate the direct cost reference by using the DRG-based standard reimbursement system. The proposed dashboard can guide toward patient value improvement before a new methodology and strong external benchmarks using data from several hospitals are created.

Continuous improvements based on measuring the own performance in order to provide the best possible value to customers has been a key success factor for successful companies across all industries. VBHC is bringing this principle into health care, to the great benefit of patients and the system. The mentality of the different health care players is changing, and the competition slowly shifts from micro-costing only to patient outcome and cost optimization. It is setting the stage for a new way of thinking, collaborating, and competing, thereby opening new opportunities to reinforce excellence in care. The combination of medical expertise with an open mindset for change and self-evaluation is essential. In this sense, VBHC is redefining the basis of what leadership is for healthcare professionals. An essential development will be the emergence of new reimbursement models rewarding better outcomes. This will again require a fundamental change in people's mindset, while providing a great opportunity for early adopters to accelerate change.

Our study has several limitations. First, our analyses only illustrate the delivered patient value at short follow-up. Furthermore, patients for whom complications were noted might have been double-penalized since such clinical outcomes might also affect PROMs. To reduce the aforementioned bias, an artificial floor was used for patients who had a negative change in PROMs. Second, the weighting of clinical outcomes was solely based on the senior surgeon's experience. The logic was to attribute an equal weight (0.2) to the five principal outcomes that are crucial for shoulder arthroplasty success: global function (ASES and Constant scores), pain, complication (intra- or post-operatively), PJI, and revision. If a principal outcome comprised different sub-outcomes (e.g., Global function), the weight was then split proportionally to have a similar weighting between sub-outcomes (e.g., 0.1 for the ASES score and 0.1 for the Constant score). A Delphi method engaging the patients, insurance providers, and other key important players would have been more appropriate. Third, our outcome and cost indicators were not risk-adjusted, which can represent a bias if comparisons are made between two surgeons with differences in case mix and patient populations. Fourth, the direct cost reference was estimated to be 44% of the standard TSA reimbursement based on our patients with basic insurance only. A thorough analysis of the DRG-based standard reimbursement system should be performed and published so that each institution knows the theoretical amount supposed to cover direct costs. Fifth, the MCID and SCB values might change across different patient populations. Lastly, a broader analysis focusing on a specific pathology (e.g., glenohumeral arthritis) rather than on a particular treatment (e.g., TSA) would be more in line the VBHC concept.

5. Conclusions

The proposed calculation method provides an estimation of delivered patient value using standard references. Such a dashboard could be used to implement VBHC in everyday clinical practice. Our results revealed that TSAs performed at our institution provided substantial patient value in almost 80% of our cases. Patient pre-operative pain/function, tobacco use, and type of procedure (anatomic or reverse) are important factors associated with patient value after TSA. A VBHC community gathering all the different key players is definitely needed to establish solid guidelines and improve our practice according to experiences of each.

Author Contributions: Conceptualization, A.L. and H.B.; methodology, A.L. and H.B.; investigation, A.L. and H.B.; data curation, A.L. and H.B.; writing—original draft preparation, A.L. and H.B.; writing—review and editing, A.L., R.E., A.A., M.B. and H.B.; supervision, A.L. and H.B. All authors have read and agreed to the published version of the manuscript.

Funding: This research was founded by a grant from FORE (Foundation for Research and Teaching in Orthopaedics, Sports Medicine, Trauma and Imaging in the Musculoskeletal System): grant number 2021-56.

Institutional Review Board Statement: The study was conducted according to the guidelines of the Declaration of Helsinki and approved by the Ethics Committee (Commission cantonale d'éthique de la recherche (CCER) de Genève: Shoulder Outcomes Clinical Study, n° 2014-277).

Informed Consent Statement: Informed consent was obtained from all subjects involved in the study.

Data Availability Statement: Details regarding where data supporting reported results can be requested at the following e-mail address: hugo.bothorel@latour.ch.

Acknowledgments: The authors are grateful towards Yonas Abraham for the management accounting analyses, and towards Florian Rossiaud-Fischer and Ezra Bottequin for their help in manuscript editing.

Conflicts of Interest: Lädermann reports that he is a paid consultant for Arthrex, Inc., Stryker and Medacta and receives royalties from Stryker. He is the founder of FORE foundation, Med4cast, and of BeeMed. Eurin, Alibert, Bensouda, and Bothorel declare no conflict of interest that could influence the representation or interpretation of reported research results.

References

1. Porter, M.E.; Teisberg, E.O. *Redefining Health Care: Creating Value-Based Competition on Results*; Press, H.B.R., Ed.; Harvard Business Publishing: Brighton, MA, USA, 2006.
2. Reilly, C.A.; Doughty, H.P.; Werth, P.M.; Rockwell, C.W.; Sparks, M.B.; Jevsevar, D.S. Creating a Value Dashboard for Orthopaedic Surgical Procedures. *J. Bone Joint Surg. Am.* **2020**, *102*, 1849–1856. [CrossRef]
3. Simovitch, R.; Flurin, P.H.; Wright, T.; Zuckerman, J.D.; Roche, C.P. Quantifying success after total shoulder arthroplasty: The substantial clinical benefit. *J. Shoulder Elbow Surg.* **2018**, *27*, 903–911. [CrossRef] [PubMed]
4. Ladermann, A.; Denard, P.J.; Tirefort, J.; Collin, P.; Nowak, A.; Schwitzguebel, A.J. Subscapularis- and deltoid-sparing vs traditional deltopectoral approach in reverse shoulder arthroplasty: A prospective case-control study. *J. Orthop. Surg. Res.* **2017**, *12*, 112. [CrossRef] [PubMed]
5. Ladermann, A.; Lo, E.Y.; Schwitzguebel, A.J.; Yates, E. Subscapularis and deltoid preserving anterior approach for reverse shoulder arthroplasty. *Orthop. Traumatol. Surg. Res.* **2016**, *102*, 905–908. [CrossRef] [PubMed]
6. Richards, R.R.; An, K.N.; Bigliani, L.U.; Friedman, R.J.; Gartsman, G.M.; Gristina, A.G.; Iannotti, J.P.; Mow, V.C.; Sidles, J.A.; Zuckerman, J.D. A standardized method for the assessment of shoulder function. *J. Shoulder Elbow Surg.* **1994**, *3*, 347–352. [CrossRef]
7. Constant, C.R.; Murley, A.H. A clinical method of functional assessment of the shoulder. *Clin. Orthop. Relat. Res.* **1987**, *214*, 160–164. [CrossRef]
8. Gowd, A.K.; Charles, M.D.; Liu, J.N.; Lalehzarian, S.P.; Cabarcas, B.C.; Manderle, B.J.; Nicholson, G.P.; Romeo, A.A.; Verma, N.N. Single Assessment Numeric Evaluation (SANE) is a reliable metric to measure clinically significant improvements following shoulder arthroplasty. *J. Shoulder Elbow Surg.* **2019**, *28*, 2238–2246. [CrossRef] [PubMed]
9. Williams, G.N.; Gangel, T.J.; Arciero, R.A.; Uhorchak, J.M.; Taylor, D.C. Comparison of the Single Assessment Numeric Evaluation method and two shoulder rating scales. Outcomes measures after shoulder surgery. *Am. J. Sports Med.* **1999**, *27*, 214–221. [CrossRef] [PubMed]
10. Cohn, M.R.; Kunze, K.N.; Polce, E.M.; Nemsick, M.; Garrigues, G.E.; Forsythe, B.; Nicholson, G.P.; Cole, B.J.; Verma, N.N. Establishing clinically significant outcome thresholds for the Single Assessment Numeric Evaluation 2 years following total shoulder arthroplasty. *J. Shoulder Elbow Surg.* **2021**, *30*, e137–e146. [CrossRef]
11. Retzky, J.S.; Baker, M.; Hannan, C.V.; Srikumaran, U. Single Assessment Numeric Evaluation scores correlate positively with American Shoulder and Elbow Surgeons scores postoperatively in patients undergoing rotator cuff repair. *J. Shoulder Elbow Surg.* **2020**, *29*, 146–149. [CrossRef]
12. Berglund, D.D.; Law, T.Y.; Rosas, S.; Kurowicki, J.; Giveans, M.R.; Mijic, D.; Levy, J.C. The procedure value index: A new method for quantifying value in shoulder arthroplasty. *J. Shoulder Elbow Surg.* **2019**, *28*, 335–340. [CrossRef]
13. Berglund, D.D.; Mijic, D.; Law, T.Y.; Kurowicki, J.; Rosas, S.; Levy, J.C. Value comparison of humeral component press-fit and cemented techniques in reverse shoulder arthroplasty. *J. Shoulder Elbow Surg.* **2019**, *28*, 496–502. [CrossRef] [PubMed]
14. Menendez, M.E.; Mahendraraj, K.A.; Grubhofer, F.; Muniz, A.R.; Warner, J.J.P.; Jawa, A. Variation in the value of total shoulder arthroplasty. *J. Shoulder Elbow Surg.* **2021**, *30*, 1924–1930. [CrossRef] [PubMed]
15. Aibinder, W.R.; Bartels, D.W.; Sperling, J.W.; Sanchez-Sotelo, J. Mid-term radiological results of a cementless short humeral component in anatomical and reverse shoulder arthroplasty. *Bone Joint J.* **2019**, *101-B*, 610–614. [CrossRef] [PubMed]
16. Cheung, E.V.; Sperling, J.W.; Cofield, R.H. Revision shoulder arthroplasty for glenoid component loosening. *J. Shoulder Elbow Surg.* **2008**, *17*, 371–375. [CrossRef]
17. Izquierdo, R.; Voloshin, I.; Edwards, S.; Freehill, M.Q.; Stanwood, W.; Wiater, J.M.; Watters, W.C., 3rd; Goldberg, M.J.; Keith, M.; Turkelson, C.M.; et al. Treatment of glenohumeral osteoarthritis. *J. Am. Acad. Orthop. Surg.* **2010**, *18*, 375–382. [CrossRef]
18. Polisetty, T.S.; Colley, R.; Levy, J.C. Value Analysis of Anatomic and Reverse Shoulder Arthroplasty for Glenohumeral Osteoarthritis with an Intact Rotator Cuff. *J. Bone Joint Surg. Am.* **2021**, *103*, 913–920. [CrossRef]
19. Fehringer, E.V.; Kopjar, B.; Boorman, R.S.; Churchill, R.S.; Smith, K.L.; Matsen, F.A., 3rd. Characterizing the functional improvement after total shoulder arthroplasty for osteoarthritis. *J. Bone Joint Surg. Am.* **2002**, *84*, 1349–1353. [CrossRef]
20. Friedman, R.J.; Eichinger, J.; Schoch, B.; Wright, T.; Zuckerman, J.; Flurin, P.H.; Bolch, C.; Roche, C. Preoperative parameters that predict postoperative patient-reported outcome measures and range of motion with anatomic and reverse total shoulder arthroplasty. *JSES Open Access* **2019**, *3*, 266–272. [CrossRef]

21. Hatta, T.; Werthel, J.D.; Wagner, E.R.; Itoi, E.; Steinmann, S.P.; Cofield, R.H.; Sperling, J.W. Effect of smoking on complications following primary shoulder arthroplasty. *J. Shoulder Elbow Surg.* **2017**, *26*, 1–6. [CrossRef]
22. Schwartz, A.M.; Farley, K.X.; Boden, S.H.; Wilson, J.M.; Daly, C.A.; Gottschalk, M.B.; Wagner, E.R. The use of tobacco is a modifiable risk factor for poor outcomes and readmissions after shoulder arthroplasty. *Bone Joint J.* **2020**, *102-B*, 1549–1554. [CrossRef] [PubMed]
23. Tramer, J.S.; Khalil, L.S.; Fidai, M.S.; Meldau, J.; Sheena, G.J.; Muh, S.J.; Moutzouros, V.; Makhni, E.C. Mental health and tobacco use are correlated with PROMIS upper extremity and pain interference scores in patients with shoulder pathology. *Musculoskelet. Surg.* **2020**, 1–6. [CrossRef] [PubMed]
24. Walters, J.D.; George, L.W., 2nd; Walsh, R.N.; Wan, J.Y.; Brolin, T.J.; Azar, F.M.; Throckmorton, T.W. The effect of current and former tobacco use on outcomes after primary reverse total shoulder arthroplasty. *J. Shoulder Elbow Surg.* **2020**, *29*, 244–251. [CrossRef] [PubMed]
25. Kumar, V.; Roche, C.; Overman, S.; Simovitch, R.; Flurin, P.H.; Wright, T.; Zuckerman, J.; Routman, H.; Teredesai, A. Using machine learning to predict clinical outcomes after shoulder arthroplasty with a minimal feature set. *J. Shoulder Elbow Surg.* **2021**, *30*, e225–e236. [CrossRef]
26. Swarup, I.; Henn, C.M.; Nguyen, J.T.; Dines, D.M.; Craig, E.V.; Warren, R.F.; Gulotta, L.V.; Henn, R.F., III. Effect of pre-operative expectations on the outcomes following total shoulder arthroplasty. *Bone Joint J.* **2017**, *99-B*, 1190–1196. [CrossRef]
27. Winegar, A.L.; Jackson, L.W.; Sambare, T.D.; Liu, T.C.; Banks, S.R.; Erlinger, T.P.; Schultz, W.R.; Bozic, K.J. A Surgeon Scorecard Is Associated with Improved Value in Elective Primary Hip and Knee Arthroplasty. *J. Bone Joint Surg. Am.* **2019**, *101*, 152–159. [CrossRef]

MDPI
St. Alban-Anlage 66
4052 Basel
Switzerland
Tel. +41 61 683 77 34
Fax +41 61 302 89 18
www.mdpi.com

Journal of Clinical Medicine Editorial Office
E-mail: jcm@mdpi.com
www.mdpi.com/journal/jcm

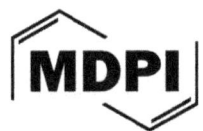

www.ingramcontent.com/pod-product-compliance
Lightning Source LLC
LaVergne TN
LVHW070432100526
838202LV00014B/1581